MASTER
MEDICINE

Obstetrics and Gynaecology

D1350320

Commissioning Editor: Ellen Green
Project Development Manager: Barbara Simmons
Project Manager: Frances Affleck
Designers: Judith Wright, George Ajayi

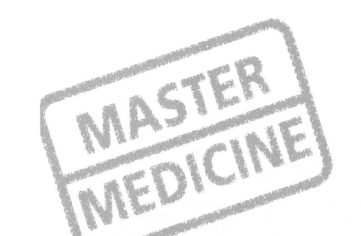

MASTER MEDICINE

Obstetrics and Gynaecology

A core text with self-assessment

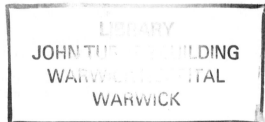
ANDREW McCARTHY

MD MRCOG MRCPI
Consultant Obstetrician
Hammersmith and Queen Charlotte's Hospital
London, UK

BILL HUNTER

FRCS FRCOG
Consultant Obstetrician and Gynaecologist
York District Hospital
York, UK

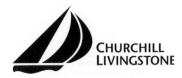

CHURCHILL LIVINGSTONE

EDINBURGH   LONDON   NEW YORK   OXFORD   PHILADELPHIA   ST LOUIS   SYDNEY   TORONTO   2003

CHURCHILL LIVINGSTONE
An imprint of Elsevier Limited

First edition 1998
Second edition 2003
    Reprinted 2003

ISBN 0443 070970

British Library Cataloguing in Publication Data
A catalogue record for this book is available from the British Library

Library of Congress Cataloging in Publication Data
A catalog record for this book is available from the Library of Congress

Notice
Medical knowledge is constantly changing. Standard safety precautions must be followed, but as new research and clinical experience
broaden our knowledge, changes in treatment and drug therapy may
become necessary or appropriate. Readers are advised to check the
most current product information provided by the manufacturer of
each drug to be administered to verify the recommended dose, the
method and duration of administration, and contraindications. It is the
responsibility of the practitioner, relying on experience and knowledge
of the patient, to determine dosages and the best treatment for each
individual patient. Neither the Publisher nor the author assume any lia-
bility for any injury and/or damage to persons or property arising from
this publication.

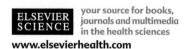

ELSEVIER
SCIENCE

your source for books,
journals and multimedia
in the health sciences

www.elsevierhealth.com

The
publisher's
policy is to use
**paper manufactured
from sustainable forests**

Printed in Spain

Contents

Using this book

Philosophy of the book

Most students need a textbook which will provide all the basic facts within a discipline and also facilitates understanding of the subject. This textbook achieves these objectives and also provides test questions for the student to explore their level of knowledge. It is also important for students to achieve a 'feel for the subject' and learn communication skills. No textbook can fulfil all these needs and it is assumed that the student using this text will also be pursuing an attachment to an obstetrical and gynaecological department.

This textbook is designed to provide basic information necessary to pass an undergraduate examination in obstetrics and gynaecology. It also expands on the core curriculum to allow the motivated student an opportunity to pursue the subject in greater detail. The information is presented in such a way as to aid recall for exam purposes but also to facilitate understanding of the subject. Key facts are highlighted, and principles of diagnosis and management emphasised. It is hoped that the book will also be a satisfactory basis for postgraduate practice and studies.

The practice of obstetrics and gynaecology brings the student into contact with a young and fit part of the population where expectations of outcome are high and where much counselling is required. This book attempts to put the practice of obstetrics and gynaecology into perspective within society, emphasising recent changes in management reflecting safety but also aspirations of women to avoid intervention. Just as it is impossible to provide every fact which a student might wish to memorise, it must be emphasised that this is not a replacement for time spent on the labour ward, talking with patients, participating in surgery and discussion with senior colleagues.

Layout and contents

The main part of the text describes important topics in major subject areas. Within each chapter, essential information is presented in a set order with explanations and logical 'links' between topics. Where relevant, key facts about basic sciences/anatomy are outlined. The aetiology, pathological features, clinical features, differential diagnosis and an approach to investigation are then described. Finally, the principles of management and the prognosis are presented.

You need to be sure that you are reaching the required standards, so the final section of each chapter is there to help you to check out your knowledge and understanding. The self-assessment is in the form of multiple choice questions (MCQs), patient management problems – case histories, data interpretation, picture quizzes short notes, and objective structured clinical examination (OSCEs). All of these are centred around common clinical problems that are important in judging your performance as a doctor. Detailed answers are given. These answers will also contain some information and explanations that you will not find elsewhere, so you have to do the assessment to get the most out of this book.

How to use this book

I expect you are using this book as part of your exam preparations. Your first task is to map out on a sheet of paper a series of three lists dividing the major subjects (corresponding to the chapter headings) into an assessment of your strong, reasonable and weak areas. This gives you a rough outline of your revision schedule, which you must then fit in with the time available. Clearly, if your exams are looming large you will have to be ruthless in the time allocated to your strong areas. The major subject should be further classified into individual topics. Encouragement to store information and to test your ongoing improvement is by the use of the self-assessment sections – you must not just read passively. It is important to keep checking your current level of knowledge, both strengths and weaknesses. This should be assessed objectively – self-rating in the absence of testing can be misleading. You may consider yourself strong in a particular area whereas it is more a reflection on how much you enjoy and are stimulated by the subject. Conversely, you may be stronger in a subject than you would expect simply because the topic does not appeal to you.

It is a good idea to discuss topics and problems with colleagues/friends; the areas which you understand least well will soon become apparent when you try to explain them to someone else.

Approaching the examinations

The discipline of learning is closely linked to preparation for examinations. Many of us opt for a process of superficial learning that is directed towards retention of facts and recall under exam conditions because full understanding is often not required. It is much better if you try to acquire a deeper knowledge and understanding, combining the necessity of passing exams with longer term needs.

First, you need to know how you will be examined. Does the examination involve clinical assessment such as history taking and clinical examination? If you are sitting a written examination what are the length and types of questions? How many must you answer and how much choice will you have?

Now you have to choose what sources you are going to use for your learning and revision. Textbooks come in different forms. At one extreme, there is the large reference book. This type of book should be avoided at this stage of revision and only used (if at all) for reference, when answers to questions cannot be found in smaller books. At the other end of the spectrum is the condensed 'lecture note' format, which often relies heavily on lists. Facts of this nature on their own are difficult to remember if they are not supported by understanding. In the middle of the range are the medium-sized textbooks. These are often of the most use whether you are approaching final university examinations or the first part of professional examinations. My advice is to choose one of the several medium-sized books on offer on the basis of which you find most readable. The best approach is to combine your lecture notes, textbooks (appropriate to the level of study) and past examination papers as a framework for your preparation.

Armed with information about the format of the exams, a rough syllabus, your own lecture notes and some books that you feel comfortable in using, your next step is to map out the time available for preparation. You must be realistic, allow time for breaks and work steadily, not cramming. If you do attempt to cram, you have to realise that only a certain amount of information can be retained in your short-term memory, so as the classification of ovarian tumours moves in, the treatment of pre-term labour moves out! Cramming simply retains facts. If the examination requires understanding you will be in trouble.

It is often a good idea to begin by outlining the topics to be covered and then attempting to summarise your knowledge about each in note form. In this way your existing knowledge will be activated and any gaps will become apparent. Self-assessment also helps determine the time to be allocated to each subject for exam preparation. If you are consistently scoring excellent marks in a particular subject it is not cost effective to spend a lot of time trying to achieve the 'perfect' mark.

In an essay, it is many times easier to obtain the first mark (try writing your name) than the last. You should also try to decide on the amount of time assigned to each

subject based on the likelihood of it appearing in the exam! Commonest things are usually commonest!

The main types of examination

Multiple choice questions

Unless very sophisticated, multiple choice questions test your recall of information. The aim is to gain the maximum marks from the knowledge that you can remember. The stem statement must be read with great care, highlighting the 'little' words such as *only, rarely, usually, never* and *always*. Overlooking negatives, such as *not, unusual* and *unsuccessful*, often causes marks to be lost. *May occur* has an entirely different connotation to *characteristic*. The latter may mean a feature which should be there and the absence of which would make you question the correctness of the diagnosis.

Remember to check the marking method before starting. Most multiple choice papers employ a negative system in which marks are lost for incorrect answers. The temptation is to adopt a cautious approach, answering a relatively small number of questions. However, this can lead to problems, as we all make simple mistakes or even disagree vehemently with the answer in the computer! Caution may lead you to answer too few questions to obtain a pass after the marks have been deducted for incorrect answers.

Short notes

Short notes are not negatively marked. Predetermined marks are given for each important key fact. Nothing is gained for style or superfluous information. The aim is to set out your knowledge in an ordered *concise* manner. Do not devote too much time to a single question thereby neglecting the rest, and remember to limit your answer to the question that has been set.

Objective structured clinical examination questions (OSCEs)

The objective structured clinical examination (OSCE) is now extensively used to examine clinical competencies. The questions may relate to a patient, a simulated patient, a mannikin or to a clinical photograph, radiograph, pathology specimen or laboratory report. Good questions test clinical skills, practical procedures and clinical reasoning rather than factual recall.

Data interpretation

Data interpretation involves the application of knowledge to solve a problem. In your revision you should aim for an understanding of principles; it is impossible to memorise all the different data combinations. In an exam, a helpful approach is to translate numbers into a description; for example, a serum potassium of 2.8 mmol/L is *low* and the ECG tracing of a heart rate of 120/min shows a *tachycardia*. This type of question is usually not negatively marked so put down an answer even if you are far from sure that it is right.

Slide/picture questions

Recognition is the first step in a picture question. This should be coupled with a systematic approach looking for, and listing, abnormalities. For example, breast shadows, bony skeleton, soft tissues, retrocardiac space, etc., can be examined in a chest X-ray. Describe in your mind what you see and try to match it with common problems. Again, even if you are in doubt, put an answer down. Any accompanying statement or data should be used alongside the visual image as it may give a clue as to the answer required; it may also be essential in distinguishing between two conditions that are of the same appearance.

Patient management problems

A more sophisticated form of exam question is an evolving case history, with information being presented sequentially and you being asked to give a response at each stage. They are constructed so that a wrong response in the first part of the question does not mean that no more marks can be obtained from the subsequent parts. Each part should stand on its own. Patient management problems are designed to test the recall and application of knowledge through an understanding of the principles involved.

Conclusions

You should amend the framework for using this book according to your own needs and the examinations you are facing. Whatever approach you adopt your aim should be for an understanding of the principles involved rather than rote learning of a large number of poorly connected facts.

SECTION 1
Obstetrics

1 Physiology of obstetrics

Overview

The greatest adaptation to pregnancy is the increase in intravascular volume of the mother to cater for the increased blood flow to organs such as the womb and to provide the necessary substrate for increased metabolic demands of pregnancy. Plasma volume increases by 40% and is accompanied by an increase in red cell mass of 20% resulting in haemodilution. There is also an associated fall in peripheral vascular resistance. There is a massive increase in blood flow to the uterus, but there are also significant increases in blood flow to other organs such as the kidney. An increase in procoagulant activity helps reduce blood loss at delivery, though it is also associated with an increased risk of clinical thrombosis. Progesterone may play an important role in keeping the uterus relaxed until the onset of labour when uterine contractions become coordinated and more frequent.

Introduction

During the course of a woman's life, the years between the teens and the menopause are not expected to represent a major threat to health or well-being. While serious diseases do affect people in this age distribution they are relatively rare; the incidence of ischaemic heart disease does become more common after the age of 35–40 years. Nonetheless most women will have to cope with pregnancy over these years. This represents a major challenge to physiological systems, and is also associated with specific disease processes which can result in maternal mortality and morbidity. The specialty of obstetrics is devoted to ensuring that specialists who care for women are aware of the altered physiological state of pregnancy and have specialist knowledge of associated diseases. Much of the physiological change and the problems that arise are best described with reference to the stage of pregnancy at which they occur.

A woman will normally conceive with ovulation 2 weeks following the first day of her last menstrual period provided she has a regular 28-day menstrual cycle. If her menstrual cycle is longer, this needs to be considered in assessing the expected date of delivery. The expected date of delivery is calculated by Naegele's rule, by which one adds 7 days and 9 calendar months to the first day of the last menstrual period, i.e. if the last menstrual period fell on January 6th, then the expected date of delivery will be October 13th. Thus human pregnancy lasts 9 months approximately, or 266 days (38 weeks) exactly from conception, or 40 weeks approximately from the last menstrual period.

The date of conception is only occasionally known to the patient, and therefore the clinician will be guided by the patient's last menstrual period (LMP) to calculate the expected date of delivery as above. Thus the pregnancy will continue for 40 weeks from the LMP. Pregnancy is divided into trimesters for convenience (see Table 1).

Table 1 Pregnancy: trimesters and stages of development

Weeks from LMP	Weeks	Stage of development
1–13, or first trimester	2–4	Fertilisation (pre-embryonic)
	4–10	Embryonic development
14–27, or second trimester		Fetal development
	23 onwards	Viability
28–40, or third trimester		Maturation
37–42, or term		Delivery of the mature fetus
Delivery–6 weeks, the puerperium		Involution of physiological changes

For the pregnancy to proceed successfully, it is necessary for the mother to adapt to the needs of the fetus, to prepare for its safe delivery, and for the fetus to develop in such a way as to be able to survive when delivered at term. There is a progressive adaptation to the pregnant state by the mother throughout the trimesters, which is then reversed in the puerperium. Many of the adaptive responses to pregnancy are exaggerated in multiple pregnancies. Adaptation by the mother occurs in parallel with development of the fetoplacental unit, which in turn is dependent on physiological change in the uterus.

1.1 Maternal physiology

Learning objectives

You should understand:

- the principles of vascular adaptation

- the advantage to the mother of the adaptive changes that occur

- how some of these changes result in commonly experienced symptoms of pregnancy

A variety of maternal physiological changes occur during pregnancy. These changes occur to facilitate fetal development and the process of labour. The major changes occur in the cardiovascular and coagulation systems.

Haematological changes

- Plasma volume increases by 40% (approximately 1.25 litres) in pregnancy, with a progressive rise until 32 weeks followed by a plateau. This increase allows a rise in blood flow to specific vascular beds such as the renal and uterine circulations.
- The total number of circulating red cells (approximately 1.4 litres, the red cell mass) increases by approximately 20% by term. This increase is greater (30%) if iron supplements are taken. Both the increase in plasma volume and the increase in red cell mass are related to fetal weight. The increase in red cell mass helps to accommodate the 15% increase in oxygen requirement during pregnancy.
- The haemoglobin concentration falls in normal pregnancy because of the larger increase in plasma volume relative to the increase in red cell mass, i.e. there is a haemodilutional effect. Total haemoglobin rises, however, and therefore there is an increased iron requirement which is met by increased iron absorption.

- There is a low-grade increase in coagulant activity. This is thought to prepare the mother for delivery of the placenta, a time when there is risk of substantial haemorrhage. Platelet counts fall slightly in pregnancy. This is accompanied by a two-fold rise in the fibrinogen level, and also by increases in Factors VII, VIII and X. Fibrinolytic activity is decreased but returns to normal 1 hour following delivery. This suggests the placenta is the source of inhibition of fibrinolysis. Whilst the increase in clotting factors in pregnancy is beneficial in preventing excessive blood loss at the time of delivery, this is at the expense of an increased risk of thromboembolism.

The increase in red cell mass also helps prepare the mother for delivery when up to approximately 500 ml of blood is lost and this is increased with delivery of twins or at caesarean section to approximately 1 litre. Most of this blood loss occurs within 1 hour of delivery. The main mechanism preventing blood loss is contraction of the uterus compressing the vasculature.

Cardiovascular and respiratory changes

- Pregnancy is accompanied by a 40% rise in cardiac output from the first trimester, from 3.5 L/min to 6 L/min. This is due to an increase in both heart rate and stroke volume. In the later stages of pregnancy cardiac output may be reduced by up to 20% if the woman lies in the supine position. This is as a result of the gravid uterus compressing the vena cava, reducing venous return to the heart. This is known as the 'supine hypotensive syndrome' and may result in maternal symptoms and fetal distress.
- Blood pressure falls in the first half of pregnancy due to a marked reduction in peripheral vascular resistance. The underlying cause of the reduced resistance is unknown. Blood pressure tends to rise to pre-pregnant levels in the latter part of pregnancy. These changes in cardiovascular status can cause significant compromise in patients with underlying heart disease, as will be discussed later. Successful adaptation to increased intravascular volume appears to be related to perinatal outcome and risk of development of hypertension. There is an increased tendency towards varicosities in pregnancy affecting the vulval and anal regions as well as the lower limbs.
- Oxygen consumption increases by approximately 15% in pregnancy, most of the increased consumption meeting maternal needs, and approximately one third meeting the needs of the fetoplacental unit. There is an increase of 40% in ventilation in pregnancy (probably due to progesterone) mediated by an increase in tidal volume, with no change in

respiratory rate. There is little change in PO_2 and pH in pregnancy, and a slight fall in PCO_2.

In contrast to cardiovascular adaptation, respiratory changes are of a lesser degree and seldom critical. However, in patients with marked respiratory compromise prior to pregnancy (such as with cystic fibrosis) or in those who develop respiratory compromise during pregnancy, these changes can be very important.

Renal changes

- There is dilatation of the renal pelvis and ureters in normal pregnancy, often giving the impression of an obstructive uropathy. This occurs because of the pressure effect of the pregnant uterus and the relaxing effect of progesterone on ureteric smooth muscle tone. This change predisposes to acute pyelonephritis.
- Glomerular filtration rate and renal plasma flow increase by approximately 50% from the first half of pregnancy. This results in some reduction in plasma levels of urea and creatinine. Plasma osmolality is reduced by 8–10 mosmol/L.
- Urinary protein loss increases in pregnancy. Levels in excess of 500 mg in 24 hours should be considered abnormal.

Endocrine changes

- Insulin secretion doubles in normal pregnancy. This is associated with increased resistance to insulin due to the antagonistic effects of placental hormones. Blood glucose remains unchanged. Glycosuria may occur in normal pregnancy as a result of altered renal handling of glucose. As a result of this only blood glucose levels should be used in assessing glucose tolerance.
- Thyroid binding globulin concentration doubles in pregnancy whereas free T_4 and free T_3 fall slightly. There is an increased incidence of goitre in pregnancy in areas of iodine deficiency.
- The anterior pituitary increases to twice the normal size in pregnancy. This increases the risk of ischaemic damage in watershed areas of the pituitary in the presence of postpartum haemorrhage (Sheehan's syndrome), though in practice the incidence is very low. Total and free serum cortisol are both increased in pregnancy, as is urinary free cortisol with maintenance of diurnal variation.

Musculoskeletal changes

There are extensive changes to the musculoskeletal system in pregnancy. These are to prepare the skeleton for delivery, and mainly involve softening and relaxation of the joints in the lower back and pelvis.

Skin changes in pregnancy

Various other changes occur in connective tissue, contributing to increased water content of the skin with a predisposition to skin rashes, nose bleeds and gum bleeding. Hyperpigmentation also occurs, spider naevi and palmar erythema become more frequent, and sebaceous glands become more active.

Calcium and phosphate in pregnancy

- Calcium requirements increase during pregnancy, especially during the third trimester when fetal requirements are maximal. Calcium is transported actively across the placenta.
- Gut absorption of calcium increases substantially to meet this demand, due to an increased level of 1,25 dihydroxy vitamin D.
- Serum levels of total calcium and phosphate fall, in parallel with a fall in protein level. Ionised calcium levels, however, remain stable.
- Lactation also results in increased demand for calcium, which must be met by adequate dietary intake in the puerperium. Increased gut absorption of calcium is maintained during lactation.

Liver changes

- Unlike renal and uterine blood flow, hepatic blood flow does not increase in pregnancy.
- Alkaline phosphatase levels are commonly increased to 50% above the normal values.
- Albumin levels fall by 10 g/L, resulting in a fall in total protein.

1.2 Uterine physiology

Learning objectives

You should:

- understand how the uterus increases in size
- appreciate how uterine blood flow must increase
- understand the function of the cervix

The major physiological changes described above are necessary to ensure the mother can meet the demands of the pregnancy. It is clear, however, that it is the uterus which must adapt in the most remarkable fashion.

The uterus is capable of accommodating the fetus, placenta and amniotic fluid and then reverting to its pre-pregnancy size within weeks of delivery. Adaptation also involves the ability to transport oxygen and nutrients through the uterus to its contents via a hugely increased blood supply. Furthermore, the uterus must be capable of retaining its contents until fetal maturity is reached, and then releasing them in such a way as to ensure fetal well-being and to minimise maternal blood loss.

Morphology

The uterus at term holds approximately 5 litres of contents, a 500-fold increase above its non-pregnant capacity, accompanied by at least a 10-fold increase in weight. This is predominantly due to hypertrophy of the muscle cells, though there is also a marked increase in the number of blood vessels.

Uterine blood supply

Uterine blood flow must serve the intervillous space of the placenta, and allow sufficient increase in blood flow to the body of the uterus to meet its increased needs. The blood supply is via both the uterine and ovarian arteries. Uteroplacental blood flow is estimated at 500 ml/min in late pregnancy.

Cervix

The cervix provides structural support for the pregnant uterus. During pregnancy a mucous plug occupies the canal of the cervix and prevents passage of vaginal products or bacteria into the uterus. Prior to labour, as the cervix begins to soften and dilate, the mucous plug is shed, resulting in a 'show'. The cervix is predominantly composed of connective tissue with a high collagen and elastin content and there is also smooth muscle present (approximately 15%). The process of cervical softening occurs in the weeks prior to labour and involves realignment of the collagen fibres and degradation by proteolytic enzymes. The cervix dilates in labour due to the transmission of uterine activity. This results in progressive dilatation, with elastin contributing to a ratchet-like mechanism.

1.3 Placental and fetal physiology

Learning objectives

You should:

- know how the placenta implants into the uterus
- have a clear understanding of the components of the feto-placental unit

The placenta provides a critical link between the pregnant mother and her fetus. Successful function depends on an adequate blood supply both on the maternal and fetal sides.

Placentation

Implantation involves attachment of the blastocyst to maternal endometrium followed by invasion by trophoblast. Early development of the fertilised ovum is followed by controlled proliferation of trophoblast cells. The blastocyst forms at the 32-cell stage, and at this stage the trophectoderm is recognisable (Fig. 1). The inner cell mass is apparent at this stage and is the precursor of the embryo. The trophectoderm overlying the embryonic pole interacts with the uterine lining, facilitates implantation and is the source of the placental trophoblast. Embryonic mesodermal cells migrate into the placenta within weeks of implantation and give rise to the different components of the fetoplacental vasculature. Even though paternal genes are expressed on trophoblast, maternal immunity does not lead to rejection of the fetus.

The feto-placental unit is composed of the fetus and other tissue of blastocyst origin, the placenta and membranes (Box 1). All such tissue is genetically of blastocyst origin, and therefore genetically identical. Sometimes chromosomal changes occur in the placenta during its

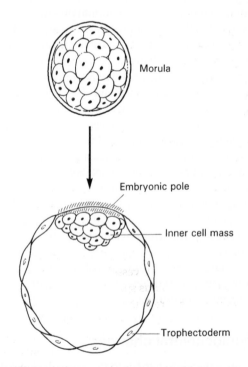

Fig. 1 The morula develops into the blastocyst at the 32-cell stage. This figure demonstrates the relationship between the inner cell mass (precursor of the embryo) and the embryonic pole (source of trophoblast, i.e. placenta).

development that are not present in the fetus. This is termed 'confined placental mosaicism' and can cause problems in prenatal diagnosis where reliance is placed on placental biopsy. The placenta is intimately related to the fetal membranes, and is formed as a specialised area of the chorion, the chorion frondosum.

The fetus develops within the amniotic cavity and is attached to the placenta through the umbilical cord. The amniotic cavity is fluid-filled and cushions the fetus within the uterus. The amnion is the layer of membrane which lines this cavity and it is capable of expanding with the course of the pregnancy. The second layer of membrane is the chorion, which is seen to be in apposition to the amnion at delivery. The membranes receive their nutrients from blood vessels in the maternal decidua. The placenta represents a specific area of differentiation of the chorion.

Trophoblast represents a major component of the placenta, and it is the trophoblast which forms the interface with maternal tissue and which adheres to the uterine epithelium. This trophoblast may be present as cytotrophoblast (individual cells), or syncytiotrophoblast where a syncytium is formed by the fusion of cytotrophoblast. The trophoblast is distributed over the chorionic villi, and also in specialised forms within the decidual layer, as depicted in Figure 2. The placenta is anchored at specialised junctions to the maternal decidua. The intervillous space is supplied with maternal blood through the spiral arteries. These arteries are altered to allow much-increased blood flow during the course of the pregnancy. The most important physiological change (referred to as maternal trophoblastic invasion) involves migration of specialised trophoblast cells into the lumen of these arteries, resulting in loss of the smooth muscle layer of the arteries. This creates low-resistance flaccid blood vessels and therefore optimal supply to the intervillous space.

As shown in Figure 3, the maternal and fetal blood is separated by the trophoblast layer, the villous stroma and the fetal capillary endothelium. The syncytiotrophoblast forms from cell fusion and represents a structural and immunological barrier between mother and fetus. It is also involved in respiratory and nutrient exchange, and as an endocrine organ through synthesis of steroid and peptide hormones.

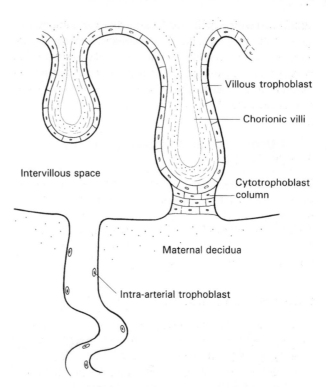

Fig. 2 Chorionic villi projecting into the intervillous space, and the adjacent maternal decidua with a maternal spiral artery supplying the intervillous space. Intra-arterial trophoblast is demonstrated, which causes trophoblastic invasion, and cytotrophoblast is seen anchoring the chorionic villi to the maternal decidua.

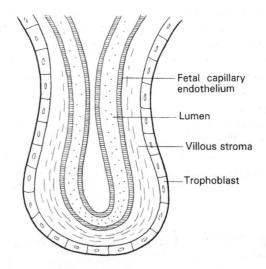

Fig. 3 A chorionic villus showing the layers which are present between maternal and fetal blood, the fetal capillary endothelium, the villous stroma and the trophoblast layer. The chorionic villi project into the intervillous space.

Fetoplacental blood supply

The umbilical cord links the fetus with the placenta. It is composed of the umbilical vessels surrounded by

Wharton's jelly which cushions the cord from compression. There are normally two arteries which carry relatively deoxygenated blood from the fetus to the placenta, and a single umbilical vein which returns oxygenated blood from the placenta to the fetus. The umbilical cord is not innervated.

First trimester and organogenesis

The developmental stages are generally described in the study of embryology, but there are some important points of relevance to clinical care in obstetrics.

- Implantation occurs 7–14 days after conception.
- Organogenesis occurs at between 2 and 8 weeks after conception. The neural plate begins to develop during the third week after conception. This emphasises that periconceptual treatment to prevent neural tube defects with folic acid must realistically begin prior to conception.
- Cardiac development also begins at an early stage. The fetal heart begins to beat about 3 weeks following conception. This also emphasises how optimal control of blood sugar in a diabetic population (at risk of an increased incidence of congenital heart and other defects) must be ensured throughout the periconceptual period.

Fetal development

Once organogenesis has taken place, the major changes which occur are of growth of the different organs. The most important developmental changes occur in the fetal heart and lungs. The lungs undergo sequential maturational changes such that survival of the pre-term fetus is dependent on the stage of pulmonary maturation.

1.4 Physiology of the onset of labour

Learning objectives

You should:

- understand how the uterus and cervix change progressively prior to labour
- be familiar with the mechanisms which may be important in the initiation of labour

As described above, the mother adapts physiologically to the needs of the pregnancy, and provides nutrient support for the developing fetus. In many animals (such as the sheep) the fetus sends a signal to the mother when maturity has been reached which precipitates labour at the appropriate time. There is no evidence of any such mechanism in human pregnancy though it is such an attractive mechanism in biological terms that it is unlikely to have been lost completely with evolution. Only a small percentage of women (4%) will deliver on the calculated date of delivery, with the majority being distributed within a period of 2–3 weeks around this date. The mechanisms governing the exact timing of birth are not known, though it is unlikely that they are designed to be specific to any 24-hour period as the preliminary processes of labour occur over a matter of weeks.

The term parturition refers to the process of giving birth. The process of labour is not well understood. It involves cervical ripening, uterine activity and membrane rupture. The processes that occur to result in labour are outlined below. They occur in parallel to allow the cervix to 'give way' and convert the uterus from one which has incoordinate uterine contractions to coordinated regular contractions of greater amplitude and with greatly increased response to contractile stimuli.

Prior to the onset of labour, cervical ripening occurs; this involves softening of the substance of the cervix, the cervix assuming a more anterior position in the vagina, shortening of the cervix and dilatation. The leading part of the fetal head tends to descend with increasing ripeness of the cervix, a scoring system for which has been devised (the 'Bishop score'), which reflects the proximity of labour. The scoring system is outlined in Box 2.

Clearly the higher the score, the more likely that labour is imminent and the easier it would be to induce labour. Whilst this scoring system is easy to use, it may be that some scores do not give adequate value to certain characteristics of the cervix, e.g. dilatation.

When natural labour occurs in the absence of ripening, or premature attempts are made to induce labour without ripening the cervix, this has been described as akin to driving a car with the brakes on. Compliance of the cervix to the process of labour is pivotal in ensuring a good outcome and avoidance of prolonged and difficult labour.

Box 2 Bishop score for ripeness of the cervix

Score	0	1	2	3
Position of the cervix	post	mid-cavity	anterior	–
Dilatation (cm)	0	1–2	3–4	5+
Station	−3	−2	−1–0	1–2
Consistency	Firm	Medium	Soft	–
Length (cm)	3	2	1	0

With the onset of labour, the woman may notice the following:

- a 'show' – a normally bloody mucous plug passed vaginally
- spontaneous rupture of the membranes
- the onset of regular uterine contractions.

Passage of a show depends on the process of cervical ripening and it is often the first sign of labour. With cervical ripening the substance of the cervix becomes softer due to biochemical breakdown of connective tissue substances. This results in the gradual shortening of the cervix characteristic of effacement. In nulliparous labour, effacement clearly precedes dilatation. In multiparous labour, effacement and dilatation often coincide. Membrane rupture normally occurs in early labour, but this is variable and may not necessarily occur until delivery – i.e. it is not essential to the delivery process.

Uterine contractility

The uterus contracts throughout pregnancy. Prior to labour commencing the contractions are irregular, of low amplitude and do not result in cervical dilatation. At the onset of labour they become high amplitude, more intense, and are accompanied by cervical effacement and/or dilation.

Many mechanisms for the onset of labour have been proposed, but none proven in human pregnancy. They include:

- withdrawal of progesterone resulting in uterine activity at term. This appears to be unlikely in the human as, in contrast to some animals, human plasma progesterone concentrations increase toward term
- activation of the uterus in late pregnancy resulting in increased responses to agents such as oxytocin or prostaglandins
- prostaglandins as possible mediators of uterine activity in labour, though evidence for a causal role is lacking.

Uterine activity is dependent upon contraction of individual myometrial fibres. These contract in response to elevations in intracellular calcium, which mediates the interaction of myosin and actin, which causes the myometrial fibres to shorten.

It must be stressed that the 'cause' of labour is unknown and is the subject of much ongoing research. It is anticipated that increased knowledge in this area will translate into more effective ways of preventing pre-term labour and improved methods of induction of labour.

Self-assessment: questions

Multiple choice questions

1. Regarding normal pregnancy:
   a. Pregnancy lasts on average 40 weeks from conception
   b. If a woman has a long menstrual cycle, the expected date of delivery should be extended to reflect this
   c. Most women will deliver on the expected date of delivery
   d. Fetuses may be considered independently viable from 20 weeks' gestation
   e. The puerperium lasts approximately 10 days

2. Regarding physiological change in pregnancy:
   a. The plasma volume increases in pregnancy but the red cell mass does not. This results in a fall in the haemoglobin concentration
   b. Pregnant women are at risk of venous thromboembolism, but only in the third trimester
   c. Platelet counts fall in pregnancy
   d. The thrombin time is increased in pregnancy
   e. Contraction of the uterus is the most important mechanism to prevent postpartum haemorrhage

3. Regarding physiological change in pregnancy:
   a. Cardiac output increases by 40%
   b. Peripheral vascular resistance falls
   c. Blood pressure should be measured with the woman lying flat
   d. Oxygen consumption falls
   e. The ureters can appear dilated

4. Regarding the pregnant uterus:
   a. The major change is myometrial hypertrophy
   b. Uteroplacental blood flow is 500 ml/min at term
   c. Cervical ripening occurs rapidly within 48 hours of the onset of labour
   d. The placenta is composed mainly of trophoblastic tissue and fetoplacental blood vessels
   e. Trophoblastic tissue helps in the development of a low-resistance circulation on the maternal side of the placenta

Short notes

1. Discuss the implications for pregnancy in a woman presenting to her first antenatal clinic appointment with a history of asthma.

2. Describe the functions of the placenta, including some description of their clinical relevance.

Data interpretation

The following blood results were returned to the antenatal clinic for review by the junior medical staff. The laboratory puts an asterisk beside those values that are outside of their normal range. What action needs to be taken?

Full blood count
Hb = 10.4 g/dl	*	(11.4–14.2)
WCC = 12.01 10^9/L	*	(3.10–11.2)
Platelets = 130 10^9/L		(120–400)

Renal and liver profile
Sodium = 139 mmol/L		(135–145)
Potassium = 4.4 mmol/L		(3.5–5.5)
Creatinine= 105 mmol/L		(60–110)
Albumin = 27 g/L	*	(33–47)
Alk Phos = 216 IU/L	*	(30–130)
AST= 20 IU/L		(0–31)

Self-assessment: answers

Multiple choice answers

1. a. **False.** Pregnancy lasts 40 weeks from the first day of the last menstrual period in a 28-day cycle, or 38 weeks from conception.
   b. **True.**
   c. **False.** Only a small percentage will deliver on the expected date. Most deliver within a 2–3 week period of the calculated expected date.
   d. **False.** A fetus may be independently viable from 22 weeks' gestation. This is very rare, however, and most clinicians would consider the limit of viability to be 23 weeks. Between 23 and 26 weeks neonatal outcome is still uncertain and handicap rates appear to be very high. Approximately 50% of babies born at 26 weeks' gestation will survive.
   e. **False.** While many of the physiological changes of pregnancy are reversed within 10 days, some are not and 6 weeks is the traditional length of the puerperium.

2. a. **False.** There is a 20% increase in red cell mass in pregnancy. This is proportionately less than the 40% increase in plasma volume, however, resulting in a fall in haemoglobin concentration.
   b. **False.** There is an increased risk of venous thromboembolism throughout pregnancy. This is especially important when considering antithromboembolism prophylaxis as this may be required from the first trimester on in the presence of risk factors.
   c. **True.**
   d. **False.** Pregnancy is, however, associated with an increased coagulant activity. Any prolongation of the thrombin time suggesting a coagulation defect requires urgent attention.
   e. **True.**

3. a. **True.**
   b. **True.**
   c. **False.** Blood pressure should be measured with the woman sitting upright or semi-recumbent. When lying flat, the uterus can compress the vena cava causing falsely low blood pressure readings, i.e. the supine hypotensive syndrome.
   d. **False.** Oxygen consumption increases by 15% to meet the increased needs of the mother and fetus.
   e. **True.**

4. a. **True.**
   b. **True.**
   c. **False.** Cervical ripening occurs over weeks.
   d. **True.**
   e. **True.**

Short notes answers

1. Asthma is a common clinical problem in women of this age group. It is important that both the patient and her doctor understand that it should be treated just as vigorously during pregnancy as outside pregnancy. Medications such as oral and inhaled steroids and sympathomimetics are not known to have serious fetal side-effects. The potential for harm as a result of fear of using such medications is greater, resulting in serious maternal morbidity and occasionally mortality. For this reason the patient should be managed by both a physician with an interest in medical problems in pregnancy and her obstetrician from an early stage of pregnancy. This allows an opportunity for patient education, a review of inhaler technique, reassurance regarding medication and pregnancy outcome.

   The patient should be able to cope with attacks of asthma as these are not likely to be exacerbated by the pregnancy itself and there is normally substantial respiratory reserve. It is only in exceptional circumstances that this is not the case, such as with acute severe pneumonia or cystic fibrosis. In contrast with respiratory problems, cardiac disorders represent a more serious threat to maternal well-being as there is very little cardiac reserve.

   With any serious medical disorder the questions which must be asked include:

   1. How does the underlying physiology change in pregnancy?
   2. Is there a substantial risk of inheritance and does the issue of prenatal diagnosis arise?
   3. Will pregnancy or the puerperium alter the severity of the disease?
   4. Are the relevant medications safe in pregnancy? Do they need to be reviewed prior to conception?
   5. Who are the appropriate people to provide care during pregnancy and what should the arrangements for care be?
   6. Is increased fetal surveillance required?
   7. Are there specific risks attributable to mode of delivery?

8. What management problems may be anticipated with labour, delivery, or the immediate postpartum period?
9. What are the anaesthetic implications of the disorder and should the anaesthetist see the patient during the antenatal period?
10. Might a deterioration be expected in the puerperium?
11. Have the paediatricians been informed of any potential implications for the newborn baby?

2. Functions of the placenta
   - Respiratory
     Because of the role of the placenta in ensuring oxygenation of the fetus, any event which may cause shearing of the placental surface from the uterine wall, such as placental abruption (see p. 23), may result in deoxygenation of the fetus and potentially serious fetal morbidity. Because of the respiratory function of the placenta, there is no dependence on the fetal lungs in utero. This results in sudden and complete dependence on respiratory function at the time of delivery, and congenital respiratory malformations may only become apparent at this time.

     As a result of the lack of fetal pulmonary blood flow in utero, maternal antibiotic administration may not result in good tissue levels of antibiotics in fetal lungs in the presence of infection in the amniotic cavity. This results in a predisposition to pulmonary sepsis which again may only be apparent following delivery.
   - Endocrine
     The placenta is a site of both steroid and peptide hormone production. The fetal adrenal gland provides a rich supply of C_{19}-steroids which can then be converted to oestrogen by the syncytiotrophoblast. There is also a maternal contribution to placental hormone production as it supplies cholesterol as a precursor to progesterone synthesis. The placenta produces a huge variety of endocrine substances and pregnancy-specific proteins which cannot be listed exhaustively here. They include human placental lactogen which may play a role in lipolysis and as an anti-insulin; human chorionic gonadotrophin, the detection of which is the basis for most 'pregnancy tests'; corticotrophin-releasing hormone; and thyrotrophin-releasing hormone.
   - Immunological
     The placenta has an immunological function in ensuring that the conceptus, which may express paternal genomes, is not rejected by the mother. The precise mechanism by which this alteration in immunity is achieved is uncertain.
   - Barrier
     A transport or barrier function is also described. Calcium is transported actively to meet fetal demands. Many viruses, however, can also pass across the placental barrier, resulting in congenital viral infections such as with rubella and CMV.

Data interpretation

1. The haemoglobin level is consistent with the haemodilution of pregnancy. It can often be argued that some fall is a good reflection of the vascular adaptation to pregnancy and therefore a positive finding. On the other hand, the further the haemoglobin falls (and certainly with falls below 10 g/dl) the more one needs to exclude iron and folate deficiency.
2. White cell counts rise modestly with the changes of pregnancy and this count should not cause any concern.
3. Platelet counts tend to fall during pregnancy and therefore modest falls are often seen especially towards term. It is worth checking the original count at the beginning of pregnancy. A fall from $400 \times 10^9/L$ to this level requires action to exclude platelet consumption (such as with pre-eclampsia) whereas a fall from $150 \times 10^9/L$ does not.
4. Sodium and potassium concentrations rarely cause concern during pregnancy other than in the management of renal failure or in the differential diagnosis of hypertension.
5. A serum creatinine of 105 mmol/L is not normal for pregnancy. It falls within the normal range of the laboratory for the non-pregnant state and therefore is not asterisked. This level is high and pre-eclampsia and renal impairment need to be considered.
6. This albumin level is lower than normal but is acceptable for the pregnant state and is explained at least in part by the haemodilution of pregnancy.
7. Alkaline phosphatase levels are raised in pregnancy because of the placental contribution. It is seldom useful in pregnancy unlike the cellular liver enzymes (AST and ALT) which can be raised with pre-eclampsia, obstetric cholestasis and hepatitis. On this occasion the AST is normal.

Conclusion: The only test result that definitely requires action is the serum creatinine measurement and it is notable that this is not highlighted by the laboratory. Caution is therefore required in the assessment of blood results in pregnancy and knowledge of the underlying physiological changes is required.

2 Antenatal disorders

Overview

Disorders specific to pregnancy occur from the first trimester onwards. Hyperemesis gravidarum represents a florid manifestation of the nausea that accompanies the diagnosis of pregnancy. Pre-eclampsia is a risk from the late second trimester onwards and manifests as a widespread disruption of organ blood flow resulting in consumptive coagulopathy, cerebral complications, renal failure and problems secondary to poor placentation. This is sometimes accompanied by retroplacental bleeding (placental abruption). Placenta praevia is the other main cause of genital tract bleeding during the antenatal period and requires delivery by caesarean section often at premature gestations. Spontaneous premature delivery can also occur though the mechanisms underlying it are poorly understood. There is currently no treatment strategy that prevents preterm labour.

Introduction

Obstetrics differs from other medical specialties because two patients require consideration whenever a decision is made, the mother and fetus. The major difficulties encountered by the mother during pregnancy include problems such as pre-eclampsia which are particular to the pregnancy, and problems which may be incidental to the pregnancy such as cardiac disease, but where the physiological changes of pregnancy complicate management. This classification is useful both in practice and in audit of maternal outcome as described in Chapter 9.

Common minor disorders affecting the different systems are described in Chapter 3. During pregnancy a variety of physiological events occur which serve to accommodate the growing fetus and prepare the pregnant woman for labour. These changes can make pregnancy an unpleasant and painful experience for some but are not indicative of any serious problem. One of the problems arising from such non-specific symptoms, however, is that they may complicate the task of the attending doctor when trying to decide if complaints warrant serious investigation or intervention. All that is usually required is simple explanation and reassurance to the woman that the symptoms may be a normal aspect of pregnancy and that there is no serious underlying problem.

2.1 Hyperemesis gravidarum and vomiting in early pregnancy

Learning objectives

You should:

- understand the predisposing factors
- have a clear plan for treatment of the condition

Hyperemesis gravidarum is defined as persistent nausea and sickness in the first trimester requiring hospital admission. Most pregnant women experience some sickness in early pregnancy, and indeed it is often the first symptom, prompting a formal pregnancy test. Only a minority of women experience it to such an extent that hospital attention is required. The threshold for specialist referral is influenced by many factors including pre-existing medical conditions, social background and cultural factors.

Management includes:

- exclusion of electrolyte imbalance and anaemia
- exclusion of other causes of vomiting, e.g. urinary tract infection, appendicitis
- intravenous hydration with saline
- vitamin supplementation, including thiamine

- advice on diet; frequent small snacks, avoiding spicy and fatty foods, etc.
- psychological support
- antiemetic treatment.

Psychological support is very important in this condition as early pregnancy is a time of great emotional strain. The use of antiemetic treatment is subject to the advice that all drugs should be avoided in the first trimester whenever possible. Benzamides (such as metoclopramide) and phenothiazines and derivatives (chlorpromazine, promethazine) have been shown to be effective in the treatment of nausea in pregnancy. In the first instance oral antiemetics are tried. If oral treatment is not tolerated, a suppository such as prochlorperazine may be tried. If the patient remains unwell despite this, hospitalisation is warranted for parenteral administration and intravenous fluids. Clinical signs of dehydration and the presence of ketonuria are the best guide to this. If vomiting proves resistant to the above measures or is particularly severe or prolonged, the diagnosis must be reconsidered and possible medical and surgical causes excluded.

Predisposing factors must be sought:

- multiple pregnancy
- hydatidiform mole.

For this reason an ultrasound assessment is advisable. This may also help to reassure the woman regarding fetal well-being.

In the second trimester, urinary tract infection is the most common cause of vomiting, but vigilance is required to ensure an incidental diagnosis such as pancreatitis, cholecystitis or appendicitis is not missed. This is also true in the third trimester, though symptomatic pre-eclampsia must always be excluded as this can result in abdominal pain and vomiting.

Women must be reassured that pregnancy outcome is not impaired by the presence of hyperemesis. Indeed, it may reflect better implantation resulting in higher than average hormone levels, and improved outcome. Because of the association with molar and multiple pregnancy, 'pregnancy hormones' and in particular HCG have been implicated in the aetiology of hyperemesis gravidarum.

Associated gastrointestinal complaints such as gastroenteritis, pancreatitis, appendicitis and intestinal obstruction, also arise in pregnancy and these also should be considered in the differential diagnosis of hyperemesis. Heartburn is more common in late pregnancy. It arises because of the effect of increased pressure of the intra-abdominal contents on the oesophageal sphincter resulting in reflux. It is treated with antacid therapy.

Common minor disorders

Urinary frequency is a common problem in pregnancy, usually arising because of the effect of the intra-uterine contents pressing on the bladder. Exclusion of infection and reassurance is all that is required.

Pelvic, back and lower limb pain may all arise in pregnancy due to the combined effects of increased intra-abdominal pressure and of hormones on the joints of the pelvic girdle. There is little that can be done for these symptoms, though advice on posture and occasional recourse to analgesia may be helpful.

Candida vaginitis is a frequent complaint during pregnancy. It is thought to arise because of alterations in immunity. Though it is unrealistic to attempt to eradicate it during pregnancy, symptomatic bouts can be treated without harm to the fetus, and the imidazoles appear to be more effective than nystatin.

Constipation is a frequent problem in pregnancy, and is thought to be due to the smooth muscle relaxation effect of progesterone on the bowel. Dietary manipulation is favoured over medical treatment, and added fruit or fibre usually helps.

It must be stressed that with many of the above symptoms, all that is required is a simple explanation and reassurance that the symptoms may be a normal aspect of pregnancy and that there is no serious underlying problem.

2.2 Pre-eclampsia and hypertension

Learning objectives

You should:

- understand the pathophysiology of pre-eclampsia
- appreciate how this differs from essential hypertension
- and how this then affects your management strategy
- understand which anti-hypertensive agents can be used in pregnancy

High blood pressure in pregnancy has a variety of causes (see Box 3), and affects approximately 5–10% of pregnancies, affecting nulliparous more than multiparous women. The quoted incidence is variable because of variation in the definition used and the populations under study.

Definitions

Hypertension is usually determined by measuring the blood pressure in the semi-recumbent position (to avoid supine hypotensive syndrome), and may be defined as two or more diastolic readings of 90 mmHg or more, or an isolated diastolic reading of 110 mmHg.

Pregnancy-induced hypertension refers to hypertension developing during pregnancy, labour or the puerperium in a previously normotensive non-proteinuric woman. The term pre-eclamptic toxaemia (PET) refers to the above category with added proteinuria or abnormal blood tests, suggesting other organ involvement. Superimposed pre-eclampsia refers to the onset of proteinuria, or other systemic manifestations of PET in a woman with essential hypertension in pregnancy. Eclampsia refers to the onset of convulsions in the presence of hypertension or proteinuria.

In pre-eclampsia and pregnancy-induced hypertension, the high blood pressure usually arises in the second half of pregnancy, continues to rise until delivery, and reverts to normal afterwards. There is, however, much individual variation and pre-eclampsia may sometimes not become apparent until after delivery. Blood pressure of 140/90 or greater is considered high in pregnancy. However, the degree to which the blood pressure is elevated above a baseline reading is also important. Essential and secondary hypertension may have been diagnosed prior to pregnancy, evident from the blood pressure reading when the woman first attends, and will persist beyond the puerperium. It must be stressed that while it is important to distinguish between pregnancy-induced hypertension and other categories of hypertension, in practice this is not always possible until the pattern of blood pressure in the postnatal period is evident.

Pre-eclampsia is a multi-organ condition. Hypertension is just one aspect and all major systems can be affected. Simple measurement of blood pressure is therefore not necessarily a reflection of the severity of the disease.

Box 3 Causes of hypertension in pregnancy

Common
- Pregnancy-induced hypertension
- Pre-eclampsia
- Essential hypertension

Uncommon
- Renal disease

Rare
- Vasculitic conditions, e.g. systemic lupus erythematosus
- Endocrine causes
  — Phaeochromocytoma
  — Cushing's disease
  — Conn's syndrome
- Coarctation of the aorta

Pre-eclampsia

Pathophysiology

Pre-eclampsia is thought to arise within the placenta. This is because:

- it arises only in pregnancy and is cured shortly after delivery of the placenta
- it can also arise in the presence of a hydatidiform mole, suggesting that it is not fetal in origin (see p. 236).

In pregnancies complicated by pre-eclampsia, there is widespread vascular damage. This is thought to arise because of the effect of a product of placental origin on the maternal vascular endothelium.

Predisposing factors

Pre-eclampsia is more likely to arise:

- in primigravid women, 6 times more frequently than in multiparous women
- where there is a past history of pre-eclampsia
- in the presence of a family history in a mother or sister
- with pre-existing essential hypertension
- in a multiple pregnancy
- in the presence of medical problems such as diabetes, auto-immune disorders or renal disease and other disorders associated with increased blood clotting. It is often difficult in these circumstances to know if there is truly superimposed pre-eclampsia or an exacerbation of the underlying medical problem.

Clinical features

Many of the clinical and pathological features of pre-eclampsia arise from either the direct vascular damage characteristic of the disease or features of tissue hypoperfusion secondary to this.

Direct vascular damage

- Hypertension
- Oedema
- Platelet aggregation and disseminated intravascular coagulation (DIC)
- Cerebral haemorrhage
- Increased incidence of deep vein thrombosis.

Platelet aggregation is increased in pre-eclampsia. Furthermore, platelet counts fall and some patients become thrombocytopenic. This is thought to be due to excessive activation and consumption within the placental intervillous space and the systemic vasculature. If DIC occurs, this is reflected in raised fibrinogen degradation products (FDPs), low fibrinogen and prolonged thrombin time.

Secondary effects

Secondary effects may occur, with the following results:

- kidney – proteinuria
- brain – eclampsia, cerebral vascular damage
- liver – dysfunction, haemorrhage.

In addition to the maternal effects there are manifestations of the disease process within the uteroplacental unit. These are listed in Box 4.

One of the earliest events is failed trophoblastic invasion of the maternal uteroplacental spiral arteries. This gives rise to impaired placental perfusion and hence intra-uterine growth retardation due to poor oxygen and nutrient transfer to the fetus. In Chapter 1, the physiological process of trophoblastic invasion in the maternal uterine spiral arteries was described. In pre-eclampsia, the invasion does not occur consistently. This results in the spiral arteries retaining their smooth muscle medium, thereby retaining vascular tone and impairing the blood supply to the uteroplacental vascular bed. Oligohydramnios also occurs, which may be partly due to reduced urine output in the compromised growth-retarded fetus.

The presentation is variable:

1. Pre-eclampsia most commonly presents as a result of the organised screening programme which is part of routine antenatal care (Box 5). The blood pressure is measured and the urine tested for the presence of protein as part of the routine antenatal visit. These tests are the most important part of the visit.
2. The disease may present with maternal symptoms such as headaches and abdominal pain in the second half of pregnancy.
3. The maternal disease may first be noted following detection of growth retardation in the fetus.

Regardless of how it is first detected, subsequent management will involve a period of assessment to allow estimation of severity of the disease, blood tests to help exclude associated problems such as thrombocytopenia, exclusion of underlying medical problems and full assessment of the fetal condition.

Thus, hypertension is most commonly detected for the first time at a routine check in the antenatal clinic. If a woman has a blood pressure of 150/95 she should be

---

Box 4 Pre-eclampsia: uteroplacental effects

• Uteroplacental arteries	abnormal flow patterns, abnormal invasion (see below)
• Fetus	intra-uterine growth retardation
• Liquor	oligohydramnios

Box 5 Pre-eclampsia: presentation

Symptoms	Signs
• headache	• hypertension or proteinuria
• visual disturbances	• clonus, hyperreflexia
• abdominal pain (hepatic, uterine)	• abdominal tenderness (hepatic, uterine)

---

admitted to hospital, or an alternative form of intensive monitoring of blood pressure arranged. Specialised day care units are frequently used for this. If proteinuria is accompanied by hypertension, immediate hospital admission is warranted. If hypertension is confirmed, delivery should be considered if at term.

Investigations are helpful in assessing the severity of the disease, and in excluding other underlying causes of hypertension (Box 6).

Prevention

There has been considerable investigation into the use of low-dose aspirin prophylaxis (60 or 75 mg/day) in the prevention of pre-eclampsia. Current consensus of opinion suggests that there is no clear beneficial effect of aspirin, though it may be of value in women deemed at very high risk of early onset pre-eclampsia (i.e. before 32 weeks). It appears likely that any benefit may be con-

---

Box 6 Pre-eclampsia: tests and possible abnormalities

Tests	Possible abnormalities
• Full blood count	Thrombocytopenia
• Blood film	Haemolysis (rare)
• Renal function	Elevated urea or creatinine (rare) Impaired creatinine clearance
• Uric acid	Elevated
• Liver function	Hypoalbuminaemia Abnormal cellular enzymes
• 24-hour urinary protein	Elevated > 0.5 g in 24 hours
• 24-hour urine for catecholamines	Raised in phaeochromocytoma
• Tests of fetal well-being	Impaired growth (IUGR – see p. 55) Oligohydramnios (see p. 61) Abnormal placental blood flow (reduced or absent EDF on Doppler – see p. 59)

fined to a reduction in incidence of pre-eclampsia at very early gestations. Such an effect would of course be of considerable clinical significance. There appears to be no major effect on bleeding in the fetus or mother. For women deemed at high risk of early onset pre-eclampsia it seems sensible to commence treatment early in gestation, i.e. from the first trimester onwards.

Treatment

This condition is cured only by delivery of the fetus and placenta.

Aims of screening and treatment are:

1. to diagnose pre-eclampsia sufficiently early to allow the woman to be admitted to hospital for supervision and treatment
2. to avoid unnecessary premature delivery of women suffering from only mild pre-eclampsia
3. to allow optimal timing of delivery
4. to avoid any long-term morbidity from the maternal disease.

Delivery is indicated when hypertension is accompanied by symptoms attributable to pre-eclampsia, significant proteinuria or evidence based on laboratory testing of severe disease. Gestation will be the major influence on the timing of delivery.

The decision to deliver at premature gestations will be heavily influenced by the survival rates for the neonate at that gestation, balanced against the severity of the maternal disease and fetal condition (see Box 7).

At later gestations (34–37 weeks) the possibility of achieving a vaginal delivery after successful induction

Box 7 Pre-eclampsia: decision to deliver	
• 37 weeks onwards	Deliver if any proteinuria **or** unstable blood pressure **or** laboratory evidence of severe disease **or** fetal compromise
• 32–37 weeks	Similar to the above, but with unequivocal evidence of severe disease to support the decision to deliver
• 28–32 weeks	Deliver if severe disease after steroid administration and in-utero transfer if appropriate (steroids are given to promote fetal lung maturity)
• 23–27 weeks	Deliver if maternal well-being threatened in the presence of very severe disease

increases. Delivery may be necessary for maternal or fetal reasons. In the absence of an acute problem, vaginal delivery is generally aimed for.

Prior to 34 weeks, uncontrollable blood pressure, marked proteinuria, development of coagulopathy, HELLP syndrome, renal or cerebral complications or symptoms may all indicate that delivery is necessary in the maternal interest. (HELLP syndrome is a term used when the maternal condition is dominated by Haemolysis, Elevated Liver enzymes and Low Platelets). Cardiotocograph abnormalities would necessitate delivery in the fetal interest. It is likely that conservative management rather than aggressive early recourse to delivery will result in fewer neonatal complications prior to 30 weeks gestation.

In parallel with treatment by delivery or prior to it, the obstetrician must aim to prevent some of the potential complications of this condition.

Hypertension

Blood pressure readings of the order of 170/110 are associated with maternal cerebral complications such as haemorrhage and generally reflect serious underlying disease. The incidence of cerebral haemorrhage is strongly related to blood pressure control and good control is therefore essential. Generally a blood pressure of 130/90 is considered satisfactory. Cerebral complications also include eclampsia which is not dependent on blood pressure alone, and which may be influenced by the severity of the underlying disease, cerebral perfusion and cerebral autoregulation. In the acute phase, treatment may be with:

- an oral dose of nifedipine 10 mg. This will take effect within 30 minutes
- intravenous hydralazine, in 5 mg increments (slowly) every 15 minutes
- intravenous labetalol with 50 mg slow i.v. stat followed by i.v.i increasing from 20 mg/hr to 160 mg/hr over 2 hours.

Maintenance treatment of hypertension in pregnancy

As will be outlined below, anti-hypertensive treatment of both essential hypertension and pre-eclampsia reduces the incidence of severe hypertension. There is less evidence, however, that it affects important outcome measures such as perinatal death.

Methyldopa is a centrally-acting drug. It may cause maternal drowsiness and depression. There is long-term follow-up data (to 7 years) suggesting it is a very safe drug in pregnancy and for this reason it is the most commonly used drug in the UK. It reduces the incidence of severe hypertension. Once the woman is delivered, treatment is converted from methlydopa to a less sedative drug such as atenolol or nifedipine.

Nifedipine is a vasodilator and thus will reverse some of the pathological changes of pre-eclampsia. It may result in a headache, confusing the clinical picture, but is generally well tolerated. Hydralazine is also a vasodilator and well tolerated.

Labetalol and β-blockers have similar effects to methyldopa, though they appear to have fewer side-effects upon the mother. Concern has been expressed regarding a possible association between β-blockers and impaired fetal growth. They are often used as a second or third drug with methyldopa and nifedipine.

Drugs to be avoided are as follows.

- Diuretics may cause a further fall in intravascular volume
- Angiotensin-converting enzyme inhibitors are contraindicated because of high fetal loss rates in animal studies.
- Sedation of the pre-eclamptic patient (as opposed to true fit prophylaxis) may only serve to mask signs of the disease, and cause respiratory depression.

Management of severe pre-eclampsia

1. Control the blood pressure. This is necessary to prevent cerebral complications such as cerebral haemorrhage. There is little evidence to suggest which anti-hypertensive agent is optimal in this situation. Current practice favours the use of calcium antagonists such as nifedipine, hydralazine or labetalol. Anti-hypertensive treatment in this situation must be monitored closely for hypotension as this may precipitate fetal distress.
2. Consider agents to prevent fits. Prophylaxis is necessary for the most affected patients, and magnesium sulphate is first-line therapy.
3. Deliver the fetus.

The following must be monitored:

- urinary output. If output <30 ml/hr, may have renal impairment
- oxygen saturations because of pulmonary complications
- blood clotting.

Following delivery the underlying disease may deteriorate further, especially problems in relation to urinary output and pulmonary complications. Close monitoring is therefore indicated for 48 hours in severe cases, at which stage substantial improvement should have occurred. It must be remembered that prevention of

thromboembolism is a priority following pre-eclampsia, the increase in risk arising because of:

- endothelial damage
- likelihood of antenatal hospital admission and bed rest
- high likelihood of operative delivery, especially caesarean delivery
- possible underlying vascular disease.

Eclampsia

Eclampsia is defined as fits in the presence of hypertension or proteinuria. The patient may suffer a fit before the hypertension or proteinuria are detected. This is an extremely distressing problem which requires immediate action to stop the fit, initially with intravenous diazepam. Magnesium sulphate should then be commenced as prophylaxis against further fits. There are several regimens for administration of magnesium sulphate and normally it is prescribed by way of an initial intravenous bolus dose over 20 minutes followed by an infusion for 24–48 hours. The patient must be monitored by way of respiratory rate, checking reflexes and sometimes magnesium levels (normal range 2–4 mmol/L). This is to ensure that the patient does not develop toxic levels as reflected by loss of tendon reflexes and respiratory depression. The rate of infusion needs to be reduced in the presence of oliguria, rising urea or levels greater than 4 mmol/L. Should the patient become toxic, 10 ml of 10% calcium gluconate may be given intravenously if the clinical situation warrants this. Treating seizures in an eclamptic patient is an immediate priority, but it is equally important to treat any associated hypertension to prevent haemorrhagic cerebral complications.

Essential hypertension

The care of women suffering from essential hypertension must reflect their increased risk of pre-eclampsia and intra-uterine growth retardation. Anti-hypertensive medication prescribed to women with essential hypertension entering pregnancy minimises the incidence of severe hypertension and therefore may help avoid unnecessary premature delivery. Care for such women will require:

- hospital-based care
- good control of blood pressure
- stopping ACE inhibitors; consideration of methyldopa
- consideration of aspirin prophylaxis
- monitoring fetal growth by serial scans
- consideration of delivery if signs of superimposed pre-eclampsia.

Many obstetricians will advise daily home testing of proteinuria in selected patients to allow early diagnosis of superimposed pre-eclampsia. It is imperative that underlying causes of hypertension are considered at all times to ensure that such life-threatening conditions are not missed.

2.3 Antepartum haemorrhage

Learning objectives

You should:

- understand the differential diagnosis of genital tract bleeding in pregnancy
- understand how the management of retroplacental bleeding and bleeding from placenta praevia are managed

Antepartum haemorrhage (APH) is defined as bleeding from the genital tract in the second half of pregnancy, prior to delivery of the fetus. It occurs in up to 3% of pregnancies and is associated with increased perinatal and maternal mortality.

The causes of antepartum haemorrhage are listed in Box 8.

In the latest triennial report on maternal mortality, there were 12 deaths directly due to haemorrhage. Five deaths were due to postpartum haemorrhage (see Chapter 6); of the remainder four were due to placental abruption and three to placenta praevia. Haemorrhage was implicated in other deaths though not thought to be directly the cause. The risk of death from haemorrhage appears to increase with increasing maternal age.

Antepartum haemorrhage can be a sudden event with potentially serious consequences and must be antici-

pated. Antenatal services must have protocols in place for the treatment of anaemia, and determination of blood group and antibody status so that in the event of haemorrhage the woman is in optimal condition to cope with it and blood grouping is known to the laboratory. Disseminated intravascular coagulation is always a risk, and labour ward protocols for management of sudden acute haemorrhage, which include the availability of senior anaesthetists and a haematologist, must be in place reflecting this. Two major subtypes of antepartum haemorrhage, placental abruption and placenta praevia, will now be described, but it must be stressed that there is not always a clear clinical picture suggestive of one type.

Placental abruption

Placental abruption (also termed accidental haemorrhage) refers to the separation of a normally sited placenta from the uterine wall resulting in maternal haemorrhage into the intervening space. If this space communicates with the external os of the cervix, the haemorrhage will be revealed. If not, the haemorrhage will be concealed (see Fig. 4). Concealed haemorrhage may result in delay in diagnosis, and underestimation of blood loss, which in turn increases the likelihood of coagulopathy and maternal morbidity. In the presence of massive abruption, blood tracks under pressure back into the myometrium, and may be visible

---

Box 8 Antepartum haemorrhage: causes

- Vulval and vaginal lesions (rare)
- Cervical lesions (< 5%)
  — cervical erosion
  — cervicitis
  — cervical carcinoma (rare, but must be excluded)
- Placental bed bleeding (majority)
  — placental abruption
  — placental edge bleeding
  — placenta praevia
- Uterine bleeding
  — lower segment scar rupture (rare)
  — rupture of other scars (myomectomy)
- Fetoplacental
  — vasa praevia (very rare)

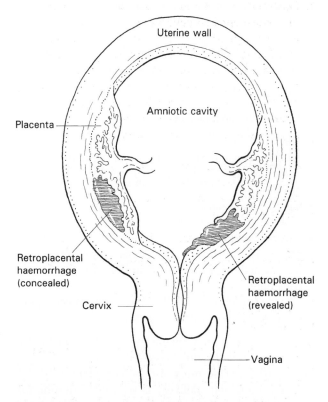

Fig. 4 Retroplacental bleeding may be concealed (left) or revealed (right).

beneath the uterine serosa at caesarean section. This appearance is referred to as a 'Couvelaire uterus'. Fetal bleeding can occur with placental abruption, though it is rare. It can be detected by a Kleihauer test which detects fetal haemoglobin in the maternal circulation and can be a clue to retroplacental bleeding in cases of trauma.

Placental abruption occurs in approximately 0.4% of all pregnancies, and is associated with a high perinatal mortality rate. This is a result of the sudden loss of placental exchange over the site of separation. As perinatal mortality from other causes has fallen, fetal death from placental abruption remains difficult to prevent, resulting in 15% of perinatal deaths in recent series.

Cause

The underlying mechanism of placental abruption is unknown. It is associated with pre-eclampsia, increasing age and parity, pre-term premature rupture of the membranes, maternal trauma (such as in a road traffic accident), cigarette smoking, cocaine abuse and retroplacental fibroids.

Clinical presentation

This will vary depending on how acutely it arises and the extent of the placental surface involved. The symptoms may be very non-specific and difficult to differentiate from similar symptoms arising in most healthy pregnancies. They include:

- abdominal pain, discomfort, or 'hardness'
- vaginal bleeding
- backache
- decreased fetal movement.

Signs include the following.

- The fetus may manifest no distress in the presence of substantial haemorrhage, or conversely may be dead in the presence of minimal or absent vaginal bleeding.
- Signs of maternal shock may be present even if there is no blood loss per vaginam.
- Uterine contractions may be the sole manifestation of placental abruption. In any case of pre-term uterine activity, placental abruption must be considered.
- Uterine tenderness. This, however, is not a very good guide to the size of the abruption.

In the presence of pre-term uterine activity and fetal distress, there is a substantial possibility of placental abruption (cord prolapse must also be considered). In this situation immediate delivery is warranted despite the prematurity of the fetus. Ultrasound is not useful in the diagnosis of placental abruption; it may be used, how-ever, to exclude placenta praevia, and confirm normal fetal growth.

Differential diagnosis

Differential diagnosis is indicated:

1. in any cause of antepartum haemorrhage
2. in the absence of bleeding, uterine fibroids undergoing degeneration, uterine rupture, acute intraperitoneal haemorrhage and other surgical causes of an acute abdomen.

Complications of abruption include coagulopathy and renal failure. A major complication of placental abruption is consumptive coagulopathy, manifest as hypofibrinogenaemia, raised fibrinogen degradation products (FDPs) or thrombocytopenia. Renal failure may rarely complicate placental abruption and is usually reversible. Placental abruption in the presence of pre-eclampsia is most likely to lead to renal failure. Adequate fluid replacement and resuscitation may help prevent both coagulopathy and renal failure.

Management

The management is outlined in Box 9. It is clear that management depends greatly upon the severity of the abruption, the presence or absence of a fetal heart, and the maturity of the fetus.

Fetal distress and demise is multifactorial. Contributory causes include maternal hypovolaemia, maternal anaemia, reduced maternal–placental exchange area due to the separation, reduced uteroplacental perfusion secondary to uterine contractions, and fetal haemorrhage. The major factor is reduced maternal–placental exchange area; as this is suddenly and irreversibly lost in the presence of abruption, there is no option but to deliver immediately in the presence of fetal distress. Urgency is

---

Box 9 After diagnosis of abruption

- **Fetus dead**
  Induce vaginal delivery
- **Fetus alive and < 36 weeks**
  Fetal distress: immediate caesarean
  No fetal distress: Observe closely
  Steroids
  No tocolysis
  Threshold to deliver depends on gestation
- **Fetus alive and > 36 weeks**
  Fetal distress: immediate caesarean
  No fetal distress: deliver vaginally

required as the area of abruption could extend at any time, causing fetal death.

Management depends on the severity of the abruption. If severe, care must be delivered with urgency and be coordinated between the different specialties involved. The steps involved in the management of a massive abruption are outlined below, and should be modified in less severe cases.

1. Summon help. The services of other specialists including anaesthesia, haematology, blood transfusion, midwives and porters are required.
2. Deliver the fetus and placenta.
3. Arrange blood grouping and cross-match (2–6 units depending on the degree of haemorrhage). Special caution is required because of the increased likelihood of post-partum haemorrhage. This is due to associated coagulopathy, the presence of FDPs inhibiting uterine contractility and the effect of haemorrhage tracking into the myometrium. Remember, myometrial contraction is the primary defence against postpartum haemorrhage.
4. Coagulation studies should be performed immediately. The priority is the assessment of platelet count and thrombin time. Other tests that may be performed less urgently include levels of FDPs and fibrinogen.
5. Two large bore (not less than 14 gauge) intravenous cannulas should be inserted, and central venous pressure (CVP) monitoring arranged to ensure appropriate volume replacement.
   In practice many of these steps are performed in unison, i.e. the appropriate bloods are taken as the first intravenous cannula is inserted.
   A display of intra-arterial pressure is also useful in severe cases.
6. The next step is to restore normovolaemia and tissue perfusion. This involves the immediate administration of 1–2 units of a colloid (modified fluid gelatin or hydroxyethylstarch solutions such as haemaccel), and 1–2 litres of crystalloid such as Hartmann's solution. Following the colloid and crystalloid, blood should be available. In the absence of cross-matched blood, and faced with the need for blood transfusion, group compatible uncross-matched blood can be given. Should this not be available, blood group O rhesus negative blood may be used.
7. In severe cases compression cuffs and blood warming equipment are useful. If more than 40% of blood volume is replaced with plasma reduced blood, additional crystalloid is necessary. 10% calcium chloride is given only if there is evidence of calcium deficiency.
8. Fresh frozen plasma (FFP), cryoprecipitate and platelet concentrates should be used as clinically indicated, i.e. in the presence of massive transfusion, fibrinogen deficiency or a platelet count of less than $40\,000 \times 10^9/L$.
9. Monitor pulse, blood pressure, central venous pressure, blood gases and acid–base status and urinary output. To allow monitoring of this intensity, consideration must be given to transfer to an intensive care bed.

Administration of anti-D should be considered.

There appears to be an increased risk of placental abruption in subsequent pregnancies, and there is little that can be done to prevent this. Folic acid is sometimes used and low-dose aspirin is considered if there is thought to be poor placentation.

Coagulation failure

Placental abruption is one of many causes of coagulation failure in obstetric practice. This normally manifests as disseminated intravascular coagulation (DIC), in which there is activation of the coagulation mechanism to such an extent that fibrinogen and platelets become depleted. Other causes are listed in Box 10.

Diagnosis of DIC is made by measurement of the thrombin time (prolonged), fibrinogen level (low), level of fibrin degradation products (high) and platelet count (low).

Placenta praevia

A placenta praevia is a placenta lying wholly or partly in the lower uterine segment (Fig. 5). Separation of such a placenta may result in antepartum haemorrhage, and accounts for approximately one third of cases.

Clinical features

1. Classically, placenta praevia is associated with painless vaginal bleeding. There may be pain present, however, if the patient is in labour, either term or pre-term, or if there is some concealed haemorrhage behind a low-lying placenta.

Box 10 Causes of coagulopathy in pregnancy

- Placental abruption
- Pre-eclampsia
- Severe haemorrhage due to other causes
- Sepsis
- Amniotic fluid embolism
- Retained dead fetus

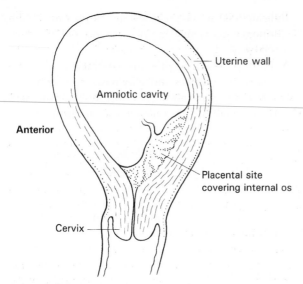

Fig. 5 A placenta praevia which extends from the posterior uterine wall across the internal cervical os preventing normal delivery of the fetus.

2. A placenta praevia is also associated with a high presenting part or an unstable lie, as the placenta displaces the presenting part from the pelvis.
3. The uterus is soft and non-tender.
4. Maternal shock.

There is usually no evidence of fetal compromise when bleeding occurs from a placenta praevia. However, the fetus must be monitored as fetal distress may arise with maternal hypovolaemia or if there is a significant amount of placental separation (unusual).

Classification

A placenta praevia may be classified as major or minor, depending upon the relationship to the internal cervical os:

- major if it covers the os or is within 2 cm of the os as measured by ultrasound scan
- minor if it does not cover the os. Consideration may be given to vaginal delivery in the presence of a minor degree of placenta praevia. If the distance between the leading edge of the placenta and the cervical os is greater than 5 cm on vaginal ultrasound, or the head is engaged, vaginal delivery is likely to be successful.

If a placenta is found to be low-lying in the uterus early in pregnancy approximately 90% will no longer be low-lying when the scan is repeated at 32 weeks. This is due to the development of the lower segment with relative movement of the placenta towards a more fundal position. When the initial scan suggests that the placenta is covering the os, or that the placenta is posterior, the

repeat scan at 32 weeks is more likely to demonstrate persistence of the low placental site. The scan may be repeated at 34 or 36 weeks, with vaginal ultrasound if it is necessary to measure the distance from the cervix to determine mode of delivery. The patient is admitted from 34 weeks to ensure prompt resuscitation in the event of bleeding, though admission will be required prior to this in the event of bleeding.

Management

The diagnosis is made by ultrasound, or at the time of caesarean section. If a placenta praevia is suspected, vaginal examination should be avoided so as not to provoke further bleeding. The patient must be advised of the need for hospitalisation until delivered. The blood group must be checked to determine if anti-D is required. 2 units of cross-matched blood should be kept continuously available for the patient.

Whenever possible patients are managed conservatively until the clinician is confident of viability, or the haemorrhage is severe and/or life-threatening. Elective delivery in the absence of severe bleeding will be by caesarean section at 38 weeks.

Risk of postpartum haemorrhage

The normal mechanism to prevent postpartum haemorrhage involves contraction of the myometrial tissue adjacent to the placental site, thereby compressing the blood supply. If the placenta is situated over the lower segment of the uterus, this contraction is less efficient because of the reduced myometrial fibre content of the uterus in the lower segment, and this predisposes the patient to postpartum haemorrhage.

It is recommended that any caesarean section for placenta praevia is performed or directly supervised by a senior obstetrician. This is especially necessary when a placenta praevia is present with a previous caesarean scar, when haemorrhage may be particularly difficult to control at delivery, and hysterectomy is occasionally required.

Other causes of antepartum haemorrhage

If there is a history of previous caesarean delivery or myomectomy, the integrity of the scar on the uterus must be considered in the presence of antepartum haemorrhage, whether or not there is accompanying pain. Cervical lesions are the next most common cause of vaginal bleeding during pregnancy and for this reason it is necessary to inquire of every patient whether the bleeding may have been post-coital. Cervical carcinomas rarely present with bleeding in pregnancy and thus a speculum examination of the cervix must be performed, normally once an ultrasound examination has excluded a placenta praevia. Vasa praevia is a rare cause of bleeding. It must be considered, however, whenever there is blood loss vaginally following rupture of the membranes, especially if accompanied by fetal distress.

2.4 Pre-term labour and rupture of the membranes

Learning objectives

You should:

- have some understanding of the mechanisms underlying pre-term labour

- understand how preterm labour is assessed clinically

- understand how preterm premature rupture of the membranes is managed

Pre-term delivery

Pre-term delivery is the major cause of perinatal mortality and morbidity despite huge advances in neonatal care over recent decades. While much of this is due to pre-term labour (75%), a substantial proportion is due to pre-term delivery for obstetric reasons such as pre-eclampsia. A substantial number of babies are also delivered because of fetal compromise such as intra-uterine growth retardation, discussed in Chapter 4. Up to 10% of all deliveries may be pre-term, the exact incidence varying between populations, depending upon socioeconomic and other conditions.

Causes of pre-term labour

The cause of pre-term labour is rarely known with certainty, and may be multifactorial (Box 11). It is defined as labour prior to 37 completed weeks of pregnancy. Delivery after 32 weeks, however, is associated with low levels of morbidity, whereas delivery after less than 28 weeks is associated with major morbidity.

When pre-term uterine activity arises, it may be idiopathic or due to placental abruption or intra-uterine sepsis. A large proportion of cases labelled as idiopathic may be associated with an altered vaginal bacterial flora. While it is clear that pre-term uterine activity associated with progressive cervical dilatation is pre-term labour, the diagnosis in practice is not always easy. The most difficult situation arises when the uterine activity is not associated with cervical change initially. It may be difficult to distinguish this from Braxton Hicks contractions. These are irregular and painless uterine contractions which are normal in the antenatal period and not associated with cervical change.

Cervical incompetence

Cervical incompetence (Box 12) is the term used to refer to a cervix which is intrinsically unable to resist the pressure of the intra-uterine contents. It is assumed that this is due to a loss of connective tissue substance giving rise to structural weakness.

The diagnosis is difficult to make. It is most commonly made on the basis of a history of relatively painless cervical dilatation in the midtrimester followed by spontaneous rupture of the membranes. It is occasionally made on the basis of a hysterosalpingogram, or loss of cervical resistance when examined under anaesthetic. The diagnosis is often complicated, however, by the presence of some uterine activity and intra-uterine sepsis. It is often uncertain whether or not the sepsis has arisen as a result of cervical dilatation or vice versa.

Treatment of cervical incompetence

This involves the insertion of a cervical suture in an attempt to increase the structural integrity of the cervix. The suture is most commonly inserted at a vaginal operation as in Figure 6, and the operation is normally performed under general anaesthesia. The timing of insertion is to ensure that fetal viability is confirmed, and that any problems related to structural weakness have not begun, i.e. at 12–14 weeks. The suture chosen is usually Mersilene tape or an inert suture material such as nylon.

Occasionally when a vaginal cervical suture has failed, a suture may be inserted abdominally during or

---

Box 11 Causes of pre-term delivery

- Pre-term labour
  — idiopathic
  — sepsis
  — abruption
- Cervical incompetence
- Elective delivery
  — pre-eclampsia
  — haemorrhage
  — fetal compromise

Box 12 Causes of cervical incompetence

- Previous cervical surgery
  — cone biopsy
  — cervical tear, i.e. with dilatation
- Associated with congenital uterine abnormalities
- Idiopathic

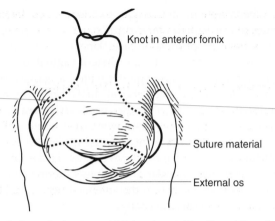

Fig. 6 A cervical suture which involves taking three bites of the cervix to provide support and which is then tied anteriorly.

prior to the next pregnancy to ensure that it is inserted at a level approximate to the internal os. Table 2 outlines the suggested benefit from cervical cerclage.

It can be seen that most benefit is derived when the patient is at highest risk, and though the benefit is not huge in absolute terms, it is of major importance to women with such bad obstetric histories. Problems relating to cervical sutures include a two-fold increase in the incidence of puerperal infection, and cervical tearing and bleeding when uterine activity commences when the suture is still in situ. Cervical sutures are generally removed without anaesthetic at 37 weeks.

If a woman presents in the midtrimester at 18–26 weeks, with relatively painless dilatation of the cervix, a diagnosis of cervical incompetence can be made. It is uncertain whether inserting a suture at this time is beneficial, though it is often considered. The main concern in this clinical situation is that the suture is not inserted with subclinical infection present as the suture may then exacerbate the underlying problem.

Causes of pre-term labour

True cervical incompetence contributes only a very small percentage of pre-term delivery. Pre-term labour may also result from:

- placental abruption (a minority)
- clinical intra-uterine sepsis
- subclinical sepsis/decidual activation
- idiopathic causes.

Increasingly attention is being focused on the possibility that activation of decidual cells prompts the initiation of labour. The decidual layer is strategically placed to release proteases that are capable of contributing to cervical softening and membrane degradation. It is also strategically placed to allow production of agents such as oxytocin and prostaglandins that can interact with the underlying myometrium to cause uterine contractions. It is suspected that haemorrhage into the decidual layer is capable of such activation and thereby precipitating pre-term delivery. Bacterial pathogens in the vaginal flora and bacterial vaginosis are also associated with pre-term delivery and therefore have been implicated as potential activators of the decidual layer.

Prevention of pre-term labour

As the cause of pre-term labour is multifactorial and poorly understood, there has been a variety of different attempts to prevent it. Such attempts have had low success rates. These are outlined in Table 3.

It is difficult to be certain of benefit in relation to any of these techniques. The problem is further exacerbated by the difficulty in predicting who is at risk of pre-term labour; those with one previous episode have a 66% chance of a successful outcome in a future pregnancy without intervention. β-mimetic agents such as ritodrine and salbutamol are widely used. They work by preventing smooth muscle contraction, but fail in the prevention of pre-term labour as it is difficult to maintain levels that suppress uterine contractions without unacceptable side-effects, and also because the body develops tolerance with time. There is evidence that progestogens work and this is thought to be mediated by a non-specific effect as a smooth muscle relaxant.

Table 2 Cervical cerclage: benefits to patients

	All	High risk*	Low risk
Delivery < 33 weeks	?↓	?20% reduction	–
Perinatal loss	?↓	?20% reduction	–
Puerperal pyrexia	↑		

*High risk equates to a past history of second trimester miscarriage or pre-term delivery. Women with a history of three or more early deliveries are especially likely to benefit from cervical cerclage.

Table 3 Prevention of pre-term labour: techniques, proposed benefits

Technique	Proposed benefit
Cervical sutures	Some benefit in high risk cases
Medications	
— β-mimetics	No benefit
— progestogens	May be of benefit
— antibiotics	May be of benefit in specific subgroups
Bed rest	No benefit
Intensive antenatal surveillance	Possibly some benefit, mechanism uncertain

Clinical presentation and diagnosis

Pre-term labour can present in a variety of ways (Box 13). The most common presentation is with regular lower abdominal pains. On occasions the history is less clear, with backache, non-specific abdominal discomfort and vaginal discharge or a show. Therefore there must always be a low threshold of suspicion when faced with such symptoms. The diagnosis is dependent on demonstrating cervical changes in association with uterine activity. Most episodes of pre-term labour occur with intact membranes.

Clinical assessment in pre-term labour must consider possible precipitating causes and complications (see Box 14).

Chorioamnionitis refers to infection within the amniotic cavity. It usually arises as a result of ascending infection from the vagina in the presence of ruptured membranes. It can also arise from transplacental spread in the presence of a maternal bacteraemia, or following maternal instrumentation such as amniocentesis. It is an extremely serious condition which causes pre-term labour or miscarriage, and can result in maternal death. If the presence of infection in the uterine cavity has not been sufficient to cause pre-term labour, then labour should be induced, or caesarean section considered.

Box 13 Pre-term labour: symptoms and signs

Symptoms	Signs
● Abdominal pain	● Uterine contractions
● 'Tightness'	● Uterine irritability
● Backache	● Cervical dilatation
● Vaginal loss (fluid or discharge)	● Confirmed ruptured membranes

---

Box 14 Pre-term labour: tests

Test	Purpose
Maternal temperature	? chorioamnionitis ? systemic maternal infection
Cardiotocograph	Determine frequency of uterine activity Confirm fetal well-being (? abruption, or infection)
White cell count	? chorioamnionitis (usually unhelpful)
High vaginal swab	? chorioamnionitis ? Group B Strep carriage
Ultrasound	Examine liquor volume Fetal lie and well-being

Emptying the uterine cavity of the infected contents is necessary to treat the mother effectively, as antibiotics will be insufficient without this.

Pre-term rupture of the membranes

Rupture of the membranes may occur in the absence of pre-term labour (occurs prior to 37 weeks in 1% of all pregnancies). It is not certain why this occurs, though infection may play a role. It can also occur in the presence of an incompetent cervix.

Risk factors for pre-term premature rupture of the membranes include:

● cervical incompetence
● polyhydramnios
● multiple pregnancy
● prior pre-term premature rupture of the membranes
● amniocentesis.

The priority therefore is to exclude chorioamnionitis, though it is thought that there is some ascending infection of the amnion in a third of cases.

Clinical sequelae of pre-term premature rupture of the membranes include:

● chorioamnionitis
● endometritis
● neonatal pneumonia and sepsis
● placental abruption
● cord prolapse
● pulmonary hypoplasia (see section on oligohydramnios, p. 61).

In the presence of uterine activity and ruptured membranes, there is little evidence to say whether or not tocolysis is beneficial to the baby. The priority in this situation is to detect intra-uterine infection or placental abruption, as this would exclude tocolysis. Steroid administration in this clinical setting is associated with a significant reduction in the incidence of hyaline membrane disease in the neonate without evidence of any substantial increase in neonatal infection.

Induction of labour should always be seriously considered therefore, following rupture of the membranes after 34 weeks. Between 34 and 37 weeks' gestation, prostaglandin induction of labour will result in less chorioamnionitis and endometritis, does not increase the caesarean rate, and does not appear to affect neonatal outcome. Prior to 34 weeks, the hazards of premature birth are thought to outweigh the advantages of delivery, and conservative treatment with steroids is appropriate.

Treatment

Tocolysis is the term given to medical treatment to suppress contractions. It is unclear that any form of treatment to suppress uterine contractions in pre-term labour is beneficial. Nonetheless, most obstetricians would elect to suppress pre-term labour up to 28 weeks' gestation as survival increases for the neonate by approximately 2% with each extra day of maturity. Beyond 28 weeks most would aim to suppress pre-term labour in the first instance to allow the administration of steroids to the mother to enhance fetal lung maturity, and allow in-utero transfer if necessary. Beyond 32 weeks' gestation there would appear to be no benefit from administering tocolysis, though steroids may of course be given. It is uncertain if steroids are beneficial beyond 34 weeks. If tocolysis is considered, fetal well-being must be confirmed and intra-uterine sepsis and abruption excluded as far as possible. Conditions for tocolysis are listed in Box 15.

If the decision is made to suppress the uterine contractions, there are a variety of agents available to do this. These are:

- β-mimetics
- cyclo-oxygenase inhibitors
- oxytocin receptor antagonists
- calcium antagonists
- progesterone.

Treatment of the woman in pre-term labour may be divided into treatment aimed at suppressing uterine activity and other measures. The efficacy of agents used to suppress pre-term labour is outlined in Table 4.

β-mimetic treatment with agents such as ritodrine, salbutamol, terbutaline and isoxsuprine has been eval-uated to determine their benefit in pre-term labour. These agents are of proven value in delaying delivery for either 24 hours (reduced by two thirds) or 48 hours (50% reduction) but have not been shown to have any impact on serious neonatal morbidity or mortality despite their effect on prolonging pregnancy. This may be because patients beyond 32 weeks had little to gain by prolongation of gestation, and also because in some pregnancies undiagnosed subclinical abruption or chorioamnionitis may have meant that delaying delivery was not in the fetal interest. They are likely to be most valuable prior to 28 weeks when survival is highly dependent on gestational age, or when the delay to delivery is used to administer steroid treatment or arrange an in-utero transfer. Side-effects include maternal tachycardia and pulmonary oedema which can be fatal. Fetal tachycardia can also arise, confusing cardiotocograph interpretation.

β-mimetics are very commonly used and because the side-effects include maternal pulmonary oedema, their administration must be carefully monitored (see Box 16). Particular care is required in the presence of diabetes to ensure that the patient does not become hyperglycaemic, as both steroids and β-mimetics are gluconeogenic. Blood glucose must be monitored and an insulin infusion considered in a diabetic patient.

Box 15 Conditions for tocolysis

- Indication
  < 28 weeks
  28–31 weeks while awaiting steroids or pending in-utero transfer
- Fetal well-being
- Placental abruption excluded
- Intra-uterine sepsis excluded

Box 16 Administering β-mimetics

- Clarify the indication
- Check there is no cardiovascular or respiratory compromise
- Administer in low volumes of normal saline, via syringe pump driver
- Maintain accurate fluid balance recording
- Discontinue if maternal pulse > 130
- Discontinue if any symptoms or signs suggestive of pulmonary oedema
- Continue beyond 48 hours in exceptional circumstances only

Table 4 Pre-term labour: suppressive agents

Agent	Benefit	Side-effects
β-mimetics	No improvement in fetal outcome Possible benefit if steroids given, or in-utero transfer arranged	Pulmonary oedema Maternal tachycardia
Indomethacin	Prevents pre-term delivery	Closure of the ductus arteriosus causing pulmonary hypertension in the neonate No fetal side-effects with < 48 hours' usage, < 32 wks –
Calcium antagonists	Insufficient experience	–
Oxytocin receptor antagonists	Delay in delivery	–

Cyclo-oxygenase inhibitors may also be used to suppress pre-term labour. Indomethacin is the most popular agent. It has been shown to be effective in reducing the incidence of delivery within 24 and 48 hours and of overall pre-term delivery rates, but again there is no evidence that overall perinatal outcome is improved. Side-effects include premature closure of the ductus arteriosus in the fetus resulting in pulmonary hypertension in the neonate, though this does not appear to be a major problem at the more premature gestations with short-term (<48 hours) use.

Oxytocin receptor antagonists have been shown to delay delivery. They do not appear to have significant maternal side effects though concern still exists about the overall effect on perinatal outcome.

Calcium antagonists are also effective in treating pre-term uterine activity though there is little clinical experience at present. There is no role for progesterone, ethanol or magnesium in the treatment of active pre-term labour on current evidence. Oral β-mimetic treatment may minimise the risk of recurrent episodes. There is no proven benefit in such treatment for the fetus, though it may be reasonable to consider this at gestations such as 24–28 weeks.

Antenatal steroid administration (betamethasone or dexamethasone 12 mg in two doses over 24 hours) reduces the risk of respiratory distress syndrome by approximately 50%, intraventricular haemorrhage, necrotising enterocolitis and early neonatal death by 40%.

2.5 Multiple pregnancy

Learning objectives

You should understand:

- zygosity and chorionicity
- how this affects risk with twin pregnancy
- how to manage twin pregnancy

The incidence of spontaneous twin pregnancies in the UK is approximately 1:80, and of triplets $1:80^2$. A disproportionate number of perinatal deaths occur in twins and higher order births. There is a variety of reasons for this, and attempts to reduce complications must be based on a sound understanding of the different types of twinning.

Zygosity and chorionicity

Zygosity refers to the genetic make-up of the twins. Monozygous twins are identical and dizygous are nonidentical. Monozygous twins (one third of the total) result from the division of one fertilised egg, dizygous twins (two thirds) from separate though coincidental fertilisation of separate eggs by two different spermatozoa. The relationship between zygosity and chorionicity is shown in Figure 7. Monozygous twins may be

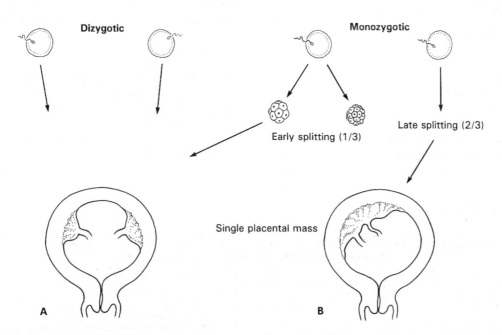

Fig. 7 Twins can develop from **(A)** fertilisation of separate ova resulting in dizygotic twins with two separate placental masses on a first trimester ultrasound scan, or **(B)** fertilisation of a single ovum resulting in monozygotic twins and a single placental mass in two thirds of cases.

monochorionic or dichorionic. If monochorionic, they will have anastomoses between their placental circulations and this will increase their risk of perinatal loss 2–3-fold relative to dichorionic twins. All dizygous twins and one third of monozygous twins will be dichorionic (have two separate placentas).

Predisposing factors to twinning (dizygotic) include:

- genetic/racial (increased in blacks)
- increased by ovulation induction techniques used for infertility treatment
- family history.

Diagnosis is almost universally by way of ultrasound in conventional practice in the UK. However, it may be prompted by a family history, infertility treatment or the presence of:

- hyperemesis
- larger than expected uterine size
- excessive fetal parts on palpation (more than two fetal poles)
- persistent fetal parts following delivery of the first twin.

When a woman presents for the first time in labour, without having had an ultrasound assessment in the current pregnancy, a second twin must be excluded following the delivery of the baby prior to the use of any oxytocic agent. If oxytocin or ergometrine is given without detection of a twin, fetal hypoxia and acidosis will occur due to the tetanic uterine contraction which will follow.

It can be seen that almost all complications of pregnancy are increased with twins (see Box 17). Furthermore, all symptoms which are normally related to the pressure of the intra-uterine contents within the maternal abdomen will be increased, such as urinary frequency and backache.

Management

All the above risks argue strongly for a high level of supervision of twin pregnancy in a hospital environment. Twin pregnancies should ideally be managed by obstetricians who take a special interest in such prob-

---

Box 18 Twin pregnancy: management

First trimester
- Prenatal diagnosis (nuchal fold thickness)
- Scan to determine chorionicity (separate placentas most easily seen in the first trimester)
- Iron and folic acid supplementation
- Consider reducing to twins if higher order multiple pregnancy

Second trimester
- Anomaly scan (increased incidence of anomalies)
- Serial assessment of monochorionic twins for FFTS (feto–fetal transfusion syndrome)
- Prenatal diagnosis (serum screening inappropriate)

Third trimester
- Watch for pre-term labour and pre-eclampsia
- Problems related to mode of delivery

Labour
- Problems with monitoring both twins
- Problems with delivery of the second twin
- Risk of postpartum haemorrhage

Puerperium
- Feeding difficulties
- Emotional and social support

---

lems (see Box 18). Specific problems need to be addressed in the different trimesters.

Feto–fetal transfusion syndrome arises in the presence of placental anastomoses in monochorionic twins; one twin becomes volume overloaded and develops marked polyhydramnios, and the second twin becomes oliguric and stuck in an amniotic cavity with minimal liquor ('stuck twin syndrome'). Perinatal mortality is very high because of the underlying condition, and as a result of pre-term labour and delivery secondary to the polyhydramnios.

Twins present in the following order:

- cephalic and cephalic
- cephalic followed by a breech (80% fall into the above categories)

Box 17 Problems increased by multiple pregnancy

- 3-fold increase in stillbirth rate
- 8-fold increase in early neonatal death rate
- Hyperemesis
- Pre-term labour ($\times$ 2–3)
- Pre-eclampsia ($\times$ 2)
- Anaemia

- Congenital abnormalities
- Intra-uterine growth retardation
- Malpresentations/cord prolapse
- Problems with monitoring in labour
- Increased late neonatal and infant death rates
- Increased incidence of cerebral palsy

- breech followed by cephalic (10%)
- cephalic and transverse
- breech and transverse
- both transverse.

Caesarean section is often performed for twin pregnancies because of the difficulties in monitoring both twins in labour and because of occasional problems with the delivery of the second twin. If the leading twin is cephalic then vaginal delivery is considered optimal. Caesarean section tends to be performed routinely if the leading twin presents by the breech. Because of the increasing safety of caesarean birth in general, there is a very low threshold for caesarean delivery with twins, and most obstetricians would not object if the parents expressed concerns regarding a possible traumatic delivery of the second twin. The issues surrounding vaginal delivery of twins are discussed in Chapter 7. Higher order multiples (triplets, quadruplets) are almost always delivered by caesarean in modern obstetric practice.

Problems following delivery include:

- postpartum haemorrhage
- increased problems related to operative delivery
- greater neonatal and infant morbidity, and therefore
- greater difficulty with coping on going home (ensure that patients are put in touch with all support services).

Self-assessment: questions

Multiple choice questions

1. In hyperemesis gravidarum:
   a. Antiemetics should be avoided if possible
   b. Thiamine deficiency can result in cerebral complications
   c. There is an increased incidence of multiple pregnancy
   d. A pyrexia occurs
   e. Colicky abdominal pain is characteristic

2. In pre-eclampsia:
   a. Platelet counts can rise due to haemoconcentration
   b. The haemoglobin concentration can be high due to haemoconcentration
   c. Renal failure is rare in the absence of other complications
   d. Uric acid is increased
   e. Alkaline phosphatase is mildly elevated

3. Regarding pre-eclampsia:
   a. It occurs more frequently in smokers
   b. It can cause upper abdominal pain
   c. Proteinuria is often due to coexistent urinary tract infection
   d. Detection of proteinuria in the antenatal clinic in the absence of hypertension is not serious
   e. It is never serious unless proteinuria is severe

4. Regarding eclampsia:
   a. It almost invariably occurs prior to delivery of the fetus and placenta
   b. Proteinuria is always present at the time of fitting
   c. Hypertension is always present at the time of fitting
   d. Magnesium sulphate should be used to prevent further fits
   e. Cerebral imaging should be considered if the clinical picture is atypical

5. In antepartum haemorrhage:
   a. Maternal deaths are caused equally by placental abruption and placenta praevia
   b. Cervical carcinoma can be excluded if there is a history of a negative smear test in the past year
   c. Management can be conservative at 41 weeks as it is likely to be due to a 'show'
   d. Fetal mortality is unusual with a placenta praevia
   e. Ultrasound is helpful in deciding the cause

6. With regard to placenta praevia:
   a. It is described as minor if vaginal bleeding has not occurred
   b. Intercourse should be avoided to reduce the risk of further bleeding
   c. Diagnosis is more difficult if the placenta is posterior
   d. Investigation with vaginal ultrasound is generally safe
   e. Bleeding from a placenta praevia does not require anti-D administration as there is never any fetomaternal haemorrhage

7. Placental abruption:
   a. Is associated with intra-uterine growth retardation
   b. Is associated with pre-eclampsia
   c. May be diagnosed with the help of the cardiotocograph
   d. May be a cause of pre-term labour
   e. May be conservatively managed at 32 weeks if the diagnosis is certain and blood transfusion can be arranged to treat maternal shock

8. Regarding cervical incompetence:
   a. It causes a high proportion of all pre-term delivery
   b. It is characteristically associated with pain
   c. It should not be considered if pre-term delivery is preceded by a clear history of spontaneous rupture of the membranes
   d. Treatment is by cervical cerclage
   e. Cervical sutures should be removed at 32 weeks to prevent cervical trauma from pre-term labour

9. Pre-term labour:
   a. Can be caused by intra-uterine growth retardation
   b. Is associated with bacterial vaginosis
   c. Should always be treated with ritodrine or salbutamol in the first instance
   d. Requires administration of steroids to enhance fetal lung maturity
   e. Often settles without any specific treatment

10. Regarding twins:
    a. Most are monozygotic (identical)
    b. Monozygotic twins face the greatest risks
    c. Pre-term labour is a major cause of mortality
    d. Infant mortality rates are higher for twins than for singletons
    e. There is an increased incidence of pre-eclampsia

True/false questions

Are the following statements true or false?

1. Vitamin supplementation is never required in hyperemesis because it is self limiting.
2. In the presence of preeclampsia the fetus never achieves normal growth.
3. The risk of post-partum haemorrhage is increased in the presence of placental abruption.
4. The incidence of pre-term labour is falling.
5. Fetal distress in one of twins puts the other twin at increased risk.

Short notes

1. Write notes on the issues you would raise in counselling a woman about to be delivered at 28 weeks gestation after a placental abruption.

2. Describe the management of a patient presenting at 38 weeks' gestation complaining of abdominal pain, a headache, and with severe hypertension and proteinuria.

3. What should be discussed with parents following a pregnancy complicated by severe midtrimester pre-eclampsia?

4. Discuss the side-effects and complications associated with the drugs used to treat pre-term labour.

Self-assessment: answers

Multiple choice answers

1. a. **True**, though antiemetics are required in severe cases.
   b. **True.** Wernicke's encephalopathy has been described in severe cases.
   c. **True.**
   d. **False.** In the presence of a pyrexia an alternative cause of the illness must be sought.
   e. **False.** If colicky abdominal pain occurs other causes should be sought.

2. a. **False.** Platelets fall.
   b. **True.** This means that those women with the highest haemoglobin concentration are the least tolerant of blood loss at the time of delivery.
   c. **True.**
   d. **True.**
   e. **False.** This is a normal finding in pregnancy.

3. a. **False.**
   b. **True.** Urinalysis and blood pressure should always be checked with unexplained epigastric pain.
   c. **False.**
   d. **False.** This must be taken seriously.
   e. **False.**

4. a. **False.** Many cases of eclampsia arise in the first 48 hours after delivery.
   b. **False.** Up to 20% may have no proteinuria immediately prior to fitting.
   c. **False.** – as for b.
   d. **True.**
   e. **True.** If the fits are resistant to treatment or atypical in presentation, CT or MRI should be considered to help exclude alternative diagnoses.

5. a. **True.**
   b. **False.** A negative smear does not exclude cervical carcinoma. This diagnosis must always be considered and speculum examination is necessary to allow direct visualisation of the cervix.
   c. **False.** If it is possible that a bleed is due to retroplacental haemorrhage at term, the safest management is to deliver.
   d. **True.**
   e. **True.** It will help exclude a placenta praevia.

6. a. **False.** It is described as minor if the placenta is 2 cm or more from the cervical os.
   b. **True.** If the diagnosis is clear and bleeding has already occurred.
   c. **True.**
   d. **True.**
   e. **False.** Fetomaternal haemorrhage is difficult to detect. It is safest to administer anti-D and repeat at 6-weekly intervals if needed.

7. a. **True.**
   b. **True.**
   c. **True.** In a woman with unexplained abdominal pain, a cardiotocograph finding of uterine activity and fetal compromise strongly suggest retroplacental haemorrhage.
   d. **True.**
   e. **False.** Conservative management would never be considered with such a significant retroplacental bleed at this gestation. Blood transfusion can be used to prolong a pregnancy where the diagnosis is placenta praevia.

8. a. **False.** Only a very small proportion is due to cervical incompetence.
   b. **False.** A diagnosis is usually made when there is painless midtrimester cervical dilatation with or without early rupture of the membranes.
   c. **False.**
   d. **True**, though this may cause further cervical trauma and exacerbation of any local infection.
   e. **False.** These are normally removed at 37 weeks, when the fetus is almost fully mature. The likelihood of spontaneous labour prior to this is low.

9. a. **False.**
   b. **True.**
   c. **False.** A decision to treat is dependent on careful exclusion of retroplacental bleeding and possible chorioamnionitis. Only a proportion of cases will be suitable for tocolytic therapy.
   d. **True.** This is the most important aspect of treatment.
   e. **True.**

10. a. **False.** Two thirds are dizygotic.
    b. **True.**
    c. **True.**
    d. **True.** All categories of perinatal and infant mortality rates are higher for twins.
    e. **True.**

True/false answers

1. **False.** Thiamine supplementation is appropriate as deficiency has been associated with Wernicke's encephalopathy.
2. **False.** Some babies seem to thrive in utero despite severe maternal disease.
3. **True.** Relevant factors here include the potential for coagulopathy, increased risk of operative delivery and the potential for increased uterine atony.
4. **False.** There is no evidence that this is the case.
5. **True.** This is particularly true in the presence of monochorionic twins if twin–twin transfusion syndrome arises. It is also true however with dichorionic twins as both can be affected by maternal disease and growth retardation.

Short notes answers

1. Is delivery necessary?
   Delivery would be indicated in the presence of cardiotocograph evidence of fetal compromise due to retroplacental haemorrhage. Conservative management would certainly result in fetal death. Immediate caesarean delivery gives the baby a chance of survival. If conservative management was pursued there would also be a risk of a deterioration in the maternal condition and of a coagulation disorder developing.

   Can the baby survive?
   Survival at 26 weeks' gestation is approximately 50–60% and at 28 weeks 80%. However, where there are signs of fetal compromise a more pessimistic view should be taken.

   Is there a risk of handicap?
   Yes. The risk is highest for those babies delivered between 23 and 26 weeks' gestation. At 28 weeks the risks are of neurodevelopmental delay and chronic lung disease. Most survivors, however, will do well.

   These are difficult issues to discuss with prospective parents, especially in an emergency situation such as placental abruption. It is helpful for all concerned if a paediatrician can be involved in counselling whenever possible, as this helps to ensure that the parents are given the most up-to-date and accurate information and establishes some rapport between the paediatric staff and the parents.

2. The diagnosis is pre-eclampsia, and this would be described as fulminating in view of the presence of symptoms and unstable blood pressure. The management problem is to see that the blood pressure is controlled, the patient is delivered without delay, and that no complications ensue.

   The care of such a patient requires a combined approach from several different specialties, and therefore senior members of staff, including an anaesthetist must be alerted immediately. The person in charge of the labour ward must coordinate services to ensure a dedicated midwife cares for the woman and that back-up services are available. In the first instance a wide bore cannula should be sited, allowing blood tests to be performed at the same time. This allows intravenous access immediately in case of a fit, will allow access for preloading for a regional anaesthetic and permit administration of anti-hypertensives. The blood tests to be performed will include (* denotes tests which should be performed urgently):

   - a full blood count — to detect thrombocytopenia* Evidence of haemolysis may be evident on a blood film
   - urea and electrolytes — creatinine will rise with renal impairment*
   - clotting screen — thrombin time prolonged if DIC*
   - save serum — necessary if caesarean indicated
   - liver function — abnormal if hepatic complications
   - albumin — may alter threshold for albumin administration.

   The first priority is to control the blood pressure. This may be achieved by the administration of hydralazine by either bolus or intravenous infusion depending on hospital preference. The major concern in this situation is a hypotensive response precipitating fetal distress. Therefore some would recommend the use of colloid such as Haemaccel prior to vasodilator treatment to prevent this. Labetalol is an alternative to hydralazine. The objective is to ensure a stable blood pressure with a maintenance infusion.

   Magnesium sulphate is the agent of choice in preventing further seizures in women who have suffered an eclamptic fit. It is also clear, however, that it is worth administering magnesium prophylactically in severe cases. Observations will include blood pressure monitoring, and ongoing fluid balance assessment. This will require an hourly urinary output, and also repeating the initial blood tests at intervals depending on the clinical picture.

   Delivery may either be through induction of labour or caesarean section. The decision as to which is appropriate will include consideration of cervical ripeness, parity, previous caesarean section, the degree of blood pressure control, patient symptoms and laboratory results. In general, the more severely affected patients will be delivered by caesarean. The advantages are immediate delivery whereas attempts at induction involve an uncertain timescale. The disadvantages include greater immediate morbidity should a coagulopathy develop in a patient who is predisposed to haemorrhagic complications; a subsequent increase in risk of thromboembolism; and finally the potential for the caesarean scar to complicate a future pregnancy. Regardless of mode of delivery, in the absence of a coagulopathy regional anaesthesia is optimal for such a patient.

Observations following delivery are similar to those pre-delivery. The major problem which arises is in relation to fluid balance. Women with pre-eclampsia tend to have excessive fluid retention. The fluid accumulates in the extravascular space resulting in oedema which can be marked, and this is accompanied by a depleted intravascular space. Management priorities therefore include:

- preventing further oedema
- ensuring an adequate intravascular volume
  — to prevent fetal distress prior to delivery
  — to ensure an adequate urinary output at all times.

In the absence of oliguria, it is reasonable to use intravenous Hartmann's equivalent to a litre over 12 hours. In the presence of oliguria, administration of Haemaccel will increase intravascular filling. A CVP line may be necessary to allow fine tuning of fluid administration in the presence of continued oliguria, as these patients are at increased risk of pulmonary oedema. Further management may require renal dose dopamine. Diuretic treatment is generally contraindicated, unless pulmonary oedema is present, as the intravascular space is already depleted and diuretic treatment may exacerbate this.

Women suffering from severe pre-eclampsia require intense supervision in a high dependency area for 24–48 hours following delivery. If there is marked difficulty in controlling blood pressure, recurrent seizures despite magnesium sulphate, or pulmonary complications, intensive care facilities will be needed.

3. Women who suffer from severe midtrimester pre-eclampsia experience a life-threatening illness and have no certainty of taking home a healthy baby. There are many issues that require clarification following delivery as this group of women are at risk of recurrent obstetric problems.

Many such women will have been delivered by caesarean section and will be concerned about mode of delivery in a future pregnancy. If a classical caesarean was performed via a vertical uterine incision, a repeat caesarean will be advised because of the increased risk of scar dehiscence. If a transverse lower segment incision in the uterus was used, then she may be allowed to deliver vaginally on the next occasion. However, such a patient is at increased risk of complications in a future pregnancy and any recurrence of pre-eclampsia may prompt a further caesarean. If the outcome of her recent pregnancy has not been favourable (neonatal death or morbidity) she may wish to avoid any risk associated with the process of labour in a future pregnancy and opt for a caesarean.

Women who have suffered from pre-eclampsia are at increased risk in a subsequent pregnancy especially if it has occurred in the midtrimester. The disease may fall into a number of categories:

- 'pure' pre-eclampsia which does not recur
- 'pure' pre-eclampsia which will recur, though the gestation cannot be certain
- essential hypertension with recurrent superimposed pre-eclampsia
- renal disease with recurrent superimposed pre-eclampsia
- anticardiolipin syndrome.

Following delivery, it is worth reviewing all clinical aspects of the case so that underlying renal disease and essential hypertension may be excluded. Clinical examination and urinalysis are important as persistent proteinuria or hypertension would warrant further investigation. It is also worth determining if the patient is positive for anticardiolipin antibodies or lupus anticoagulant as this also would increase the risk of recurrence in a future pregnancy, and prompt specific treatment.

The overall risk of recurrence will depend on which category she falls into. She must be reassured that recurrence of pre-eclampsia is not likely to be a major problem unless it recurs at gestations of less than 32 weeks, and most especially less than 28 weeks.

In a future pregnancy, the patient should be advised to have hospital-based care in a unit capable of offering ongoing fetal assessment as well as facilities to care for a very pre-term infant. She will require regular visits, with the added option of home urine testing. Early confirmation of gestational age is indicated and regular assessment of fetal growth from 24–28 weeks. She will probably be advised to take a low dose of aspirin, 75 mg, daily from the first trimester. This appears to reduce the incidence of subsequent severe midtrimester pre-eclampsia.

4. Because the benefits of prolonging pregnancy in a patient in pre-term labour are not clear, it is important that women are not exposed to undue side-effects from the treatment. While side-effects may arise from direct use of the tocolytic agents, it must be considered also that maternal and fetal morbidity can result from inappropriate attempts to suppress uterine activity. For example placental abruption and chorioamnionitis both represent a threat to fetal and maternal well-being which is best removed by prompt delivery of the uterine contents vaginally. In the presence of these pathologies, the intra-uterine environment may be so hostile that the fetus is best delivered despite a lack of maturity. These arguments support the practice of proceeding with tocolysis only when the clinician is happy that it is truly beneficial to prolong pregnancy.

β-mimetic treatment has been most associated with maternal side-effects probably because it is used more often than any other drug. Side-effects include:

- maternal tachycardia
- maternal discomfort, tremor
- hypokalaemia
- hyperglycaemia
- pulmonary oedema.

Pulmonary oedema has received most attention as it is life-threatening. Analysis of fatalities suggest that certain factors are associated with the development of pulmonary oedema. These include:

- administration with large volumes of crystalloid, particularly dextrose solutions
- failure to monitor fluid balance
- failure to exclude underlying cardiac disease
- prolonged administration
- administration in the presence of sepsis.

Therefore if β-mimetic treatment is to be considered, it must be given in accordance with guidelines, and withdrawn promptly if there is any suspicion of pulmonary complications.

Cyclo-oxygenase inhibitors such as indomethacin are the next most frequently used agents to suppress pre-term uterine contractions. The potential side-effects relate to inhibition of prostaglandins involved in the regulation of vascular tone and renal function, including:

- premature closure of the ductus arteriosus (resulting in pulmonary hypertension in the newborn)

- renal side-effects in the fetus (contributing to oliguria)
- renal side-effects in the mother.

For this reason treatment is normally of short duration (less than 48 hours) and used only at gestations of less than 32 weeks. If treatment is considered for longer periods than 48 hours, fetal urine output (reflected in liquor volume) and fetal haemodynamics (using Doppler ultrasound) may be monitored. The maternal side-effects are not normally a problem unless the drug is used in the presence of a contraindication. Occasionally the renal side-effects become a problem if maternal sepsis is not revealed until treatment has commenced and the patient then becomes hypotensive. This confirms the ongoing need to exclude such complications prior to suppression of uterine activity. Despite the above concerns, cyclo-oxygenase inhibitors remain the class of drug which has been shown most clearly to prevent pre-term delivery. There is a clear biological basis to their use in that prostaglandins are potent at initiating uterine contractions and at causing cervical change. The problems inherent in their use stem from the lack of specificity of their action on endogenous prostaglandin production, though this problem may be addressed in future through the use of specific cyclo-oxygenase (COX) inhibitors for the type 1 and 2 COX isoforms.

The agents discussed above are those most frequently used and are clearly lacking specificity of action. Calcium antagonists such as nifedipine are also used to suppress uterine contractions and again their action will not be specific to the uterus. It is not yet clear if there will be substantial side-effects from their use. The main concern must centre on potential cardiovascular side-effects, and therefore the potential for a hypotensive response and fetal distress in the presence of an undiagnosed abruption. Oxytocin receptor antagonists are, however, specific. Experience with these agents in treating pre-term labour to date reveals few maternal side effects.

In summary, there are major problems in treating pre-term labour. The greatest is in selecting those patients in whom treatment is truly worthwhile and the benefit to the fetus is clear. The next major problem is the lack of specificity of action of many of the agents currently used to treat pre-term labour, resulting in undesirable side-effects. New agents are currently being investigated to circumvent these problems.

Medical and surgical problems in pregnancy

Overview

Medical disorders can cause concern in pregnancy and pre-pregnancy counselling can alleviate this concern and ensure that patients do not enter pregnancy on teratogenic medication. This is particularly important with anti-epileptic medication, warfarin and ACE inhibitors. The embryo is also at risk from a hyperglycaemic environment and therefore diabetic control must be optimal in the first trimester. Other women suffer from renal disease or have past histories of thrombosis and they must be counselled about risks of pre-eclampsia, deterioration of renal function and about thromboprophylaxis. Serious cardiac disease in the mother can be life threatening and requires a team approach for successful management.

Introduction

While pregnant women are generally healthy, some suffer from particular medical disorders which may influence the course of pregnancy. Furthermore, pregnancy may have a deleterious effect on the natural history of certain diseases. Therefore aspects of care of particular relevance to pregnancy will be outlined in this chapter.

3.1 Pre-pregnancy counselling

Learning objectives

You should:

- understand which medical conditions are a problem during pregnancy
- know how to approach such a consultation

Any discussion of pre-pregnancy counselling may be divided into general considerations which may apply to any woman, and others specific to women with particular gynaecological, obstetrical or medical problems. Pre-pregnancy counselling will usually involve the general practitioner for those women without any previous complications, and often arises when contraceptive requirements are being reviewed. A thorough review of the past medical history is indicated to ensure that there are no medical conditions of relevance to pregnancy; some examples are given in Table 5.

These conditions will be described in greater detail later. A review of the family history is also important, to establish any possible genetic diseases which may require counselling and prenatal diagnosis. Gynaecological history is important and disorders such as surgery or damage to the cervix may require special attention during pregnancy. A cervical smear should be obtained prior to conception if due so that any treatment which may be necessary is undertaken prior to pregnancy. Women with a history of ectopic pregnancy or congenital malformations of the genital tract may require specific counselling.

Advice on the use of medications in pregnancy is appropriate, and any medications which the woman is being prescribed should be reviewed. Pregnancy is an ideal time for women to consider cessation of smoking

Table 5 Medical conditions which may require attention prior to conception

Condition or disease	Action
Recurrent urinary tract infection	Consult renal physician as appropriate
Renal disease	Check baseline renal function
Cardiac disease	Consult cardiologist? risk of serious deterioration in pregnancy
Rheumatic disorders	Ensure disease quiescence prior to conception Review medications (to avoid teratogens)
Hypertension	Review medications Establish optimal control Check renal function
Diabetes	Ensure good control prior to conception Exclude/treat retinopathy Assess renal function

Box 19 Topics in preconceptual counselling

- Past medical history
- Family history, e.g. genetic disorders
- Gynaecological history, e.g. cervical smear, previous ectopic
- Medications, e.g. anticoagulants, anti-hypertensives
- Review of previous obstetric problems
- Advice on prenatal diagnosis
- Folic acid supplementation
- Rubella immunity and rhesus status
- Smoking and alcohol
- Diet and travel

to ensure long-term reduction of any smoking-related morbidity, and also because the presence of the fetus provides additional motivation. Advice on excessive alcohol intake is also appropriate.

Women who have a previous child affected by a chromosomal abnormality or congenital malformation should be referred to a genetic counsellor or specialist in fetal medicine. It is currently recommended that women should take 400 µg of folic acid for 3 months prior to conception and continue this increased intake until approximately 12 weeks, to reduce the risk of neural tube defects. The relationship between the aetiology of neural tube defects and folic acid intake is not clear, however, despite the fact that folic acid is of proven value as prophylaxis. Women with a history of a previous pregnancy affected by a neural tube defect should, however, take a higher dose, i.e. 5 mg daily.

Women who have had serious obstetric problems in the past such as pre-term labour or severe pre-eclampsia may benefit from consultation with their obstetrician prior to pregnancy to discuss risk of recurrence, likelihood of success of the pregnancy, the possibility of damage to the long-term health of the woman and any therapeutic options to reduce risk.

It is optimal to discuss prenatal diagnosis prior to conception. This will ensure that prospective parents will have time to clarify their wishes with respect to the different screening options, and understand the importance of timing in relation to tests such as nuchal fold thickness. Rubella immunity should be checked and women should be aware of their rhesus group and antibody status. Dietary advice may be sensible. This would include attempts at weight reduction in those that are

obese, and specific advice regarding diet in pregnancy to reduce the risk of listeriosis. It is also sensible to counsel women on the best time to travel in pregnancy (<24 weeks) as this is often their last chance of a holiday prior to the arrival of a baby.

The general principles of preconceptual counselling are to consult with specialists in the field regarding specific problems and to ensure that the possibility of problems presenting during the pregnancy are minimised. A summary of points of relevance to preconceptual counselling is given in Box 19. It must be remembered that women of this age group are generally healthy, and that this information and counselling should be presented within a framework of ensuring optimal outcome to the pregnancy, rather than being excessively problem-orientated.

3.2 Diabetes

Learning objectives

You:

- must understand the importance of good glycaemic control in the first trimester

- must understand the importance of checking renal function and for retinal disease

- should have a clear plan for care during diabetic pregnancy

Diabetes in pregnancy is associated with many complications and a perinatal mortality 2–3 times average. However, when managed in optimal fashion it is generally associated with a good outcome. Tight control of blood glucose is central to good outcome, so the optimum management of diabetes in pregnancy uses a team approach with a physician/endocrinologist advising on alterations of insulin dosage, advice from a dedicated dietician, involvement of a specialist nurse adviser and the obstetrician. Problems that may arise in the course of pregnancy in a diabetic woman are summarised in Box 20.

This discussion will focus on management of diabetic women who become pregnant and will then address the issue of gestational diabetes, a condition in which intolerance of glucose is diagnosed for the first time during the course of the pregnancy.

The importance of advice prior to conception has already been stressed. It is imperative that the woman is confident in the management of her diabetes and that any improvements in education and dosage are in place prior to conception. The woman must understand that in diabetes there is a 2–3-fold increase in incidence of congenital malformation but that this can be reduced by ensuring optimal blood glucose control. The risk of congenital malformation is related to the concentration of haemoglobin A_{1C} in the first trimester, a marker of glucose control over a period of weeks. It is also important that other issues such as renal function, hypertension and need for laser treatment for retinopathy are assessed.

During pregnancy the diabetic woman should be reviewed every 2 weeks or even weekly depending upon the stage of the pregnancy and the control of blood sugar. Certain physiological changes occur during pregnancy that may affect carbohydrate metabolism.

- Insulin concentration increases due to increased demand and the antagonistic action of placental hormones, i.e. human placental lactogen.
- Blood glucose concentration does not change in normal pregnancy.

Box 20 Diabetic pregnancy: management problems

• Preconception	Ensure optimal control of blood glucose Investigate and treat any associated hypertension, renal or retinal disease
• First trimester	Tight control of blood glucose Congenital malformations Ophthalmology consultation
• Second and third trimester	Prenatal diagnosis Urinary tract and other infection Pre-term labour and pre-eclampsia Unexplained stillbirth Timing of delivery
• Delivery	Risk of dystocia Risk of shoulder dystocia
• Postpartum	Reduced insulin requirement Long-term counselling

- Glycosuria is more likely to occur as there is a lower renal threshold for glucose.

In the first trimester, insulin requirements will increase with the pregnancy. This is thought to be due to the antagonistic action of hormones of placental origin on the effect of insulin. Much effort is therefore directed at controlling blood glucose tightly in the first trimester. The alterations in insulin dosage and the control that is aimed for may expose the woman to a risk of hypoglycaemic attacks, and her tolerance of these will be much improved if she understands the objectives of the treatment.

Appropriate control of glucose concentrations will usually require bolus doses of short acting insulin with each meal, and one or two doses of intermediate acting insulin. Home monitoring using one of many blood glucose monitoring systems is necessary. Any oral hypoglycaemic agents must be stopped prior to conception, changing to insulin in view of the need for optimal control and the concern regarding adverse fetal effects. Renal function should be checked at the time of the first visit. An ultrasound scan should be arranged to check viability and dates. This is especially important in the diabetic pregnancy as there is an increased risk of pre-term delivery. Referral for retinal assessment should be arranged as retinopathy can deteriorate in pregnancy.

In the second trimester, the first concern is to ensure that issues in relation to prenatal diagnosis have been fully discussed. Congenital malformations that arise with greater frequency in diabetes include cardiac, CNS, skeletal and renal malformations. Sacral agenesis is very rare, but is more common in the diabetic population. Serum screening for trisomy 21 cannot be relied upon in diabetes and therefore nuchal fold scanning is preferred. An anomaly scan should be arranged with specific attention to the fetal heart.

Once the pregnancy progresses beyond 20 weeks' gestation, attention is increasingly focused on risks of serious urinary tract infection, pre-term labour and hypertension-related problems such as pre-eclampsia. Urinary tract infection requires prompt treatment in view of its association with pre-term labour, and the risk of glucose instability. Occasional ketotic episodes arise in poorly controlled diabetics. These require intensive management and pose a significant risk to the fetus. Pre-term labour is also more common: this may be related to overdistension of the uterus from polyhydramnios. The incidence of pre-eclampsia is thought to be increased two-fold in the diabetic population. This is often a difficult diagnosis in a population that has an increased incidence of hypertension and renal disease.

In the third trimester the main problems are the risk of polyhydramnios and fetal macrosomia. These complications can be reduced by tighter control of blood glucose. Serial ultrasound assessment is usually arranged to allow early diagnosis.

There is an increased incidence of respiratory distress in babies born to diabetic mothers. Unfortunately there is also an increased incidence of sudden intra-uterine death in the later third trimester which complicates management. Such intra-uterine deaths can be minimised by attempting to deliver early, i.e. 36–37 weeks. The problem is that this is not appropriate for most fetuses and early delivery will be associated with high caesarean section rates and neonatal respiratory distress. Therefore most patients are managed by awaiting spontaneous labour until approximately 39 weeks in the presence of good control and no complications. If there were significant concerns regarding glucose control or complications, delivery would be undertaken at 37–38 weeks.

In labour insulin is given via an infusion pump. Blood glucose is checked hourly, and the infusion rate adjusted accordingly. Post partum, the insulin requirement will fall immediately to the pre-pregnancy level and insulin doses can be reduced accordingly.

Neonatal risks from maternal diabetes include:

- prematurity
- congenital malformation
- respiratory distress
- polycythaemia
- hypoglycaemia
- birth trauma, including brachial plexus injury.

Gestational diabetes

Gestational diabetes is said to arise when the pregnant woman cannot control her blood glucose when faced with the stress of placental hormones. The exact definition varies between centres, though levels of fasting glucose of 7 mmol/L and 2-hour levels of 11 mmol/L after a 75 g oral load are certainly abnormal, and equate to maturity onset diabetes. Some units screen for this condition at critical stages of pregnancy such as 28 weeks either by a single glucose reading or by a modified glucose tolerance test. Other units diagnose this condition by selective screening in the presence of the following:

- a family history of diabetes in a first degree relative
- a previous unexplained stillbirth
- fetal macrosomia, or a previous baby >4 kg
- polyhydramnios.
- multiple pregnancy

Management during pregnancy is essentially the same as for those women with true diabetes. Control of blood glucose is achieved by diet alone with some patients, and through the use of insulin in others. Post partum, insulin should be avoided and the blood glucose monitored to ensure it reverts to normal.

3.3 Haematological disorders

Learning objectives

You should:

- understand the issues surrounding screening for haemoglobinopathies
- understand the arguments for iron supplementation in pregnancy

Iron and folic acid deficiency

Iron deficiency anaemia is the most common haematological problem in pregnancy. Many women enter pregnancy with their iron stores already depleted and the extra maternal and fetal requirements exacerbate this. This problem is largely preventable through a programme of iron supplementation in pregnancy, i.e. 60–100 mg daily. Iron deficiency is diagnosed by measurement of the serum ferritin concentration which reflects iron storage. Many women also experience folate deficiency in pregnancy and occasionally this is severe enough to cause a megaloblastic anaemia. Folate supplements of 100 µg daily are often given alongside iron supplementation for this reason.

Haemoglobinopathies

These conditions, thalassaemia and sickle disease, involve genetic defects of haemoglobin and its synthesis. Screening for these conditions in pregnancy is performed in many units in the UK and is most important for thalassaemia where there is an Asian, Greek, Cypriot or Italian community. Advice on prenatal diagnosis is then offered to anyone found to be a carrier of thalassaemia or sickle.

Haemoglobin electrophoresis will also allow detection of sickle trait and, if both parents are carriers, ensure that women at risk of giving birth to a child with sickle disease have prenatal diagnostic tests available to them. Diagnosis of sickling syndromes is important for maternal health as crises can occur during the course of the pregnancy and the puerperium. Obstetricians must be vigilant in their prevention, recognition and treatment. Appropriate use of blood transfusion (a transfusion protocol), maintenance of hydration and prompt treatment of any infectious complications are the most important points of management.

Because of the difficulties of ensuring early attendance in pregnancy, attempts have been made to ensure that young women in communities at risk are aware of the issue of prenatal diagnosis of these conditions, and that their partners will be prompt in attendance if partner testing is required for carrier status.

3.4 Venous thromboembolic disorders

Learning objectives

You should:

- understand why thrombosis is more common in pregnancy
- understand the diagnosis and treatment of thrombosis

Pregnancy increases the risk of thromboembolic complications as a result of the procoagulant changes in the clotting mechanism, risks of bed rest and operative intervention. There were 46 deaths from pulmonary embolus in the latest UK confidential enquiry into maternal mortality. 60% occur post partum and most of these arise after caesarean delivery. Deaths in the antenatal period mostly occur in the first trimester. Prophylaxis against thromboembolism must be considered in those with significant risk factors.

Risk factors

- Increasing maternal age
- Overweight
- Operative delivery
- Pre-eclampsia
- Family history or previous history of thromboembolism
- Lower limb paralysis
- Restricted mobility (including prolonged bed rest)
- Thrombophilia.

Diagnosis

It is important that thromboembolism in the antenatal period is diagnosed accurately. Clinical diagnosis is unreliable and, if not confirmed by appropriate investigation, will lead to unnecessary treatment in some cases. Suggestive symptoms of chest pain or breathlessness must be investigated. The diagnosis is often made clinically as a result of leg swelling, calf pain or tenderness. It should be confirmed non-invasively by Duplex ultrasound scanning of the leg veins and Doppler ultrasonography. If the diagnosis is still in doubt, further investigative procedures undertaken should be designed to minimise exposure of the fetus to radiation, especially in the first trimester. Limited venography may be performed with abdominal shielding, though a negative result does not exclude an iliac vein thrombosis.

A clinical diagnosis of pulmonary embolism may be made on a history of dyspnoea, chest pain, cough or haemoptysis. Oxygen saturation and arterial gases may help. A chest X-ray is sometimes required to exclude other conditions which may present with similar signs and symptoms, such as pneumonia. The diagnosis is confirmed by the use of perfusion scanning. This may be performed antenatally as the procedure exposes the fetus to only a very low dose of radiation.

Treatment

Immediate treatment involves intravenous heparinisation of the patient. In the antenatal period, this can then be converted to a subcutaneous form of heparin, rather than warfarin for the reasons outlined below. In the puerperium, either heparin or warfarin can be used.

Prophylaxis

Because of the increased risks associated with pregnancy, specific prophylaxis against thromboembolism is required for women at high risk, as follows:

- Previous history of thromboembolism in pregnancy or the puerperium
  —low-dose aspirin (75 mg) may be given antenatally
  —requires heparin prophylaxis in the puerperium
- Multiple episodes of thromboembolism in the past
  —require heparin during the pregnancy and in the puerperium
- After caesarean delivery
  —heparin if moderate or high risk.

Warfarin crosses the placenta and may cause serious side-effects in the fetus. Problems with organogenesis due to warfarin arise between 6 and 12 weeks, and for this reason heparin should be used during this period. The embryopathy due to warfarin comprises problems related to bone and cartilage formation. Later in pregnancy warfarin may give rise to fetal intracranial haemorrhage, possibly leading to developmental delay. Warfarin is generally stopped 4 weeks prior to delivery because of the risk of fetal intracranial haemorrhage at delivery.

Heparin does not cross the placenta, and risks associated with its use are confined to the mother. The major risk is of osteopenia, though this is a rare complication. While changes in bone density may be reversible, there are occasional serious complications due to fractures. Other potential complications include thrombocytopenia and haemorrhagic problems. Heparin should be administered during pregnancy as in the non-pregnant patient.

The use of fibrinolytic agents is generally contraindicated in pregnancy because of the risk of bleeding from the placental site. This risk persists for a number of days following delivery. Surgery is occasionally necessary to perform an embolectomy or to insert a caval filter in the presence of free-floating ileofemoral thrombus.

3.5 Renal disorders in pregnancy

Learning objectives

You should:

- understand why infection is more common in pregnancy
- understand the principles of care for women with established renal disease

Serious renal disease is not common in pregnancy, but there is a small population of young women with renal compromise who require a high level of care. These patients suffer from renal failure of varying degrees, occasionally with diabetes, and some undergo renal transplantation. Problems in relation to urinary infection are much more common.

Urinary infection occurs in pregnancy due to the relaxant effect of progesterone on ureteric tone, which results in urinary stasis. The pregnant uterus also causes some pressure on the urinary tract and further predisposes to urinary stasis and some dilatation of the urinary tract. These physiological changes should not be confused with more serious pathology which occasionally arises in pregnancy. The principles of care of renal patients in relation to pregnancy are outlined in Box 21.

In general most renal patients do well in pregnancy. Prognosis is related to serum creatinine, with a very good outlook for those with a normal creatinine, and a very guarded outlook when creatinine is elevated above 180 μmol/L. Pyelitis in pregnancy should be treated vigorously in view of the associated risk of premature labour:

- strict measures to reduce any pyrexia (paracetamol and sponging)
- intravenous antibiotics guided by culture and sensitivities when available
- intravenous hydration
- check for cervical dilatation, and vaginal carriage of organisms.

Box 21 Renal patients in pregnancy: principles of care

- Prenatal diagnosis; nuchal fold
- Review of medications, especially antihypertensives (see p. 22)
- Serial checks for urinary infection (urine dipstix and MSU)
- Monitor intensively for hypertensive complications
- Serial growth scans from 24 weeks
- Anticipate some early fall in serum urea and creatinine
- Anticipate some increase in proteinuria
- Deliver no later than 37–38 weeks
- Avoid cyclo-oxygenase inhibitors

The diagnosis of pre-term labour is not always easy in patients with confirmed urinary infection, and suspicion of chorioamnionitis should be maintained if the temperature fails to settle with treatment.

3.6 Cardiac disease

Learning objectives

You should:

- understand why cardiac reserve is reduced in pregnancy
- understand the principles of management of cardiac disease in pregnancy

The pattern of cardiac disease in pregnancy has changed greatly in recent decades, with the shift away from rheumatic valvular disease to other conditions such as ischaemic heart disease and surgically corrected congenital heart disease. Cardiac disease will always be a serious concern, however, in view of the magnitude of change in cardiovascular status in pregnancy, relating to the increased intravascular volume. There are certain principles in relation to care of cardiac disease in pregnancy:

- hospital-based
- combined care between the cardiologist and obstetrician
- prenatal counselling, and specific fetal cardiac anomaly scan ($\uparrow$ risk of fetal malformations if maternal congenital disease)
- screen for intra-uterine growth retardation (especially with R $\rightarrow$ L shunts as $PO_2\downarrow$)
- inform anaesthetist in advance of delivery
- arrange antibiotic prophylaxis as appropriate
- avoidance of ergometrine at delivery as leads to hypertension

- watch for cardiac failure in the immediate post-partum period (↑ circulatory volume following uterine contraction)
- low threshold for thromboprophylaxis (especially if haematocrit increased).

The greatest concern centres on patients who have pulmonary hypertension such as with Eisenmenger's syndrome. In this situation, they are at risk of reversal of the right to left shunt and sudden collapse. This condition carries at least a 30% risk of mortality in pregnancy, so patients must be counselled prior to conception.

3.7 Thyroid disorders

Most women suffering from severe hyperthyroidism are infertile. Women with mild disease do become pregnant and their medication requires careful monitoring. Carbimazole or propylthiouracil may be used, with the dosage tailored to the results of the free thyroxine level. This ensures minimal fetal exposure to the drugs, which cross the placenta and can cause fetal goitre and hypothyroidism. Neonatal thyroid function should therefore be checked at birth. Hyperthyroidism may be diagnosed during pregnancy. If untreated it is associated with high perinatal loss rates. It should be suspected clinically when there is failure to gain weight or inappropriate tachycardia. Hypothyroidism should be treated during pregnancy with thyroxine replacement.

3.8 Hepatic and gastrointestinal disease

Causes of jaundice in pregnancy include:

- infectious hepatitis
- gallstones
- intrahepatic cholestasis of pregnancy
- acute fatty liver of pregnancy
- HELLP syndrome (see p. 21).

Infectious hepatitis

Viral hepatitis is the most common cause of jaundice in pregnancy. Hepatitis B may be detected by an antenatal screening programme. This allows the infant of the carrier mother to be protected against the risk of perinatal infection. A combination of active (vaccine) and passive (immunoglobulin) prophylaxis at birth gives very high levels of protection against vertical transmission.

Intrahepatic cholestasis of pregnancy

This rare but potentially serious condition is specific to pregnancy. It is more common in Scandinavia and Chile. There is a clear genetic predisposition. The clinical features include generalised pruritus, jaundice and fetal compromise. The pruritus dominates the clinical picture, can be impossible to control and is cured only by delivery. Steatorrhoea and dark urine may occur.

Investigations reveal:

- a conjugated hyperbilirubinaemia
- raised AST and ALT
- viral hepatitis screen negative
- autoantibody screen negative
- serum bile acids are raised
- ultrasound to exclude gallstones
- the condition of the fetus.

Fetal compromise with meconium staining of the liquor may occur and necessitate early delivery. Vitamin K should be prescribed orally to the mother. Ursodeoxycholic acid can be used to treat the mother, and often reduces the itch. The timing of delivery is most important and cardiotocograph evidence of fetal distress may prompt premature delivery. If the diagnosis is made at 37 weeks or later, the woman should be delivered immediately. This condition is likely to recur in subsequent pregnancies and can recur with use of the oral contraceptive pill.

Acute fatty liver of pregnancy

This rare condition may cause maternal death; it gives rise to:

- abdominal pain
- nausea and vomiting
- jaundice
- +/− signs of associated pre-eclampsia.

Hypoglycaemia, coagulation failure, liver and renal failure may all occur. Liver function tests are markedly abnormal, with the AST elevated up to 10 times normal. Histological examination of the liver reveals extensive fatty infiltration and necrosis. Management involves control of any hypertension, correction of clotting failure, and delivery.

Gastrointestinal

Misoprostol should not be used for the treatment of peptic ulceration in pregnancy. It is a prostaglandin analogue and can cause abortion; anecdotal reports of congenital abnormalities add to the concern. Antacids and ranitidine are thought to be safe.

3.9 Epilepsy

Epilepsy is a serious concern in pregnancy because of the possible teratogenic effect of anti-convulsant medication, and the need to ensure optimal fit prophylaxis during pregnancy. The risk of fetal malformation appears to be increased in a mother with epilepsy even if she is not on medication, but it is further increased, to twice the population risk, if she is on medication. Most malformations are minor, however, though cleft lip and palate, neural tube defects (NTDs), cardiac anomalies and diaphragmatic hernia do occur. Sodium valproate and carbamazepine both increase the risk of NTDs. Valproate may also cause neurodevelopmental problems and should be avoided if at all possible. Phenytoin and phenobarbitone both appear to increase the risk of congenital heart disease and cleft palate. In view of these concerns, preconception counselling should aim to stabilise the epilepsy with monotherapy wherever possible.

A plan for care of the pregnant woman with epilepsy

- Preconceptual alteration in treatment, ideally to monodrug therapy and to avoid valproate
- Folic acid prophylaxis
- Neural tube defect screening (sodium valproate and carbamazepine)
- Congenital heart disease screen (phenytoin and phenobarbitone)
- Explain the importance of compliance (many women are tempted to discontinue treatment during pregnancy)
- Do not alter treatment in the presence of good seizure control
- Plasma concentrations of drugs alter because of
  —increased liver metabolism: (∴ drug level reduced)
  —reduced protein binding (∴ free drug level increased)
  —increased plasma volume (∴ drug dilution)
- Clinical status should primarily dictate dosage alterations
- Return to pre-pregnancy dose in the postpartum period
- Oral vitamin K from 36 weeks to prevent neonatal haemorrhagic disease.

Fits do not generally harm the fetus apart from the effect of falls, though any episode involving cardiovascular instability or desaturation must pose a theoretical risk. Fits need to be distinguished from fainting attacks in early pregnancy, and from eclampsia later on.

3.10 Systemic lupus erythematosus (SLE) and anticardiolipin syndrome

Systemic lupus erythematosus (SLE) is a serious condition in pregnancy because of poor reproductive performance, risk of hypertensive complications, and disease flares. Patients with this condition are often concerned about the teratogenic risk of their drugs but it must be impressed on them that though complete reassurance cannot be given, the priority is that they conceive when the disease is quiescent, and hence stay on their medication.

Pregnancy should be managed as follows:

- conception during disease quiescence
- combined care between physician and obstetrician
- screen for anticardiolipin antibodies
- early scan to ensure accurate dating (because of the possibility of severe early-onset intra-uterine growth retardation (IUGR))
- serial ultrasound assessment of growth and placental blood flow
- watch for hypertensive complications and disease flares
- consider increasing steroids post partum, because of risk of flare
- venous thromboembolic prophylaxis
- check for fetal congenital heart block.

The term antiphospholipid syndrome refers to the combination of:

- recurrent miscarriage including midtrimester fetal loss (fetal death) *or*
- thromboembolic complications *with*
- positive test for anticardiolipin antibodies or lupus anticoagulant.

Treatment is controversial, however, with low-dose aspirin (75 mg) and heparin being the possible options. Depending on the degree of risk, low-dose aspirin is usually prescribed with heparin reserved for the more high-risk cases. Intensive fetal surveillance is warranted with regular ultrasound assessment from 24 weeks.

3.11 Carpal tunnel syndrome

Symptoms of paraesthesia due to median nerve compression are common in pregnancy. They are generally worse at night and often affect both hands. Reassurance is often all that is required and an explanation that symptoms will disappear after delivery. Splinting of the wrists is effective though not acceptable to many patients unless the symptoms are severe. Local steroid injections may be considered and surgical division of the transcarpal ligaments for the most severe cases.

3.12 Infection

Learning objectives

You should:

- understand which infections pose a risk to the fetus
- understand the rationale for screening for certain infectious diseases

It is important that any infectious illness is thoroughly investigated, as:

- management may be complicated by the pregnancy (pneumonia)
- intra-uterine infection must be considered (chorioamnionitis)
- fetal death can occur (listeria)
- there may be problems of neonatal morbidity due to congenital infection.

Rubella

Rubella virus infection should be prevented by the current vaccination programme. Where this has failed and primary infection occurs in the first 16 weeks of pregnancy there is a risk of congenital abnormality. This is greatest in the earliest weeks of the first trimester. When there is concern about infection,

- the mother should have serial estimations of IgG and IgM rubella antibodies
- an ultrasound assessment of gestational age should be arranged
- termination may be offered if the risk of congenital abnormality is judged to be high.

Congenital rubella syndrome may cause cataracts, cardiac malformations, hepatosplenomegaly, and deafness.

Cytomegalovirus infection (CMV)

This virus is a major cause of neonatal handicap. It is not currently preventable, because maternal infection is often asymptomatic or mistaken for a flu-like illness. It can be transmitted to the fetus and can cause:

- intra-uterine growth retardation
- hepatosplenomegaly
- microcephaly
- deafness later in childhood.

Toxoplasma

Toxoplasmosis is important because it can cause serious congenital infection in the fetus or neonate. This follows primary maternal infection. The risk of serious fetal morbidity is greater with maternal infection in early pregnancy. Fetal and neonatal morbidity includes chorioretinitis leading to blindness, microcephaly and cerebral calcification, and epilepsy. Stillbirth and neonatal death can occur.

Screening for toxoplasma is performed during pregnancy in many continental countries where the prevalence of infection is high. It is not performed routinely in the UK because of the lower prevalence of infection and the small number of affected children born each year.

Genital herpes

Genital herpes infection can result in viral transmission to the fetus during delivery, which can cause serious morbidity. Caesarean section prevents this from occurring, providing membranes are intact or < 4 hours from rupture. Asymptomatic women with a past history of genital herpes or infection earlier in the pregnancy do not warrant caesarean section.

HIV

Pregnancy does not appear to have a major impact on the progression of HIV disease, but the virus can be passed on to the fetus. Transmission may occur during labour and caesarean section appears to be protective. Procedures involving the fetus (cordocentesis, scalp electrodes) should be avoided during the pregnancy as they may facilitate transmission of the virus from mother to fetus. The antiviral zidovudine taken antenatally, continued intrapartum and neonatally, greatly reduces the incidence of vertical transmission. Breast feeding should be avoided if possible.

Listeriosis

Listeria is rare but poses particular difficulties during pregnancy. Infection arises as a result of poor food hygiene, with soft cheeses and pâté posing particular risks. It is commonly misdiagnosed as urinary tract infection, reflecting its clinical presentation:

- feeling generally unwell
- backache
- abdominal or loin pain
- pyrexia.

Women are often given antibiotics on the basis of a diagnosed urinary tract infection (which may coexist) and then return manifesting signs of intra-uterine infection some weeks later. Intra-uterine infection can result in premature labour and fetal death. The diagnosis is made by specifically requesting listeria culture on blood cultures, urine specimens, placental specimens and vaginal swabs. Treatment involves high-dose ampicillin.

3.13 Medications, teratogenicity

Drugs may affect the fetus directly or indirectly through their effects on the mother. A drug is said to be teratogenic if when given to the mother during the development of the embryo it causes harm to the fetus, i.e. abortion, a congenital malformation or behavioural disorders. Examples include thalidomide and warfarin. Lipid-soluble molecules cross the placenta more easily than water-soluble molecules.

Prescribing in pregnancy must reflect concern about teratogenicity but must also consider the potential benefit of therapy to mother and fetus. Safe practice is to:

- review and alter medications prior to conception
- prescribe in pregnancy only when absolutely necessary
- prescribe well-known drugs with a good safety profile.

3.14 Drug abuse

Women who are abusing drugs pose specific risks during pregnancy (see Box 22). This may be due to poor socioeconomic background, failure to obtain medical and midwifery care, or specific side-effects of the drugs concerned. Alcohol is the most commonly abused substance and is associated with a specific syndrome of fetal

---

Box 22 Specific associations of commonly used drugs

- Alcohol — fetal alcohol syndrome
- Cannabis — premature delivery
  intra-uterine growth retardation
- Opiates — antepartum haemorrhage
  intra-uterine growth retardation
  increased perinatal mortality
  meconium staining
  premature delivery
  neonatal withdrawal syndrome
- Cocaine — retroplacental haemorrhage
  intra-uterine growth retardation
  congenital abnormalities
  pre-term delivery

---

abnormality when ingested in large volumes. The fetal alcohol syndrome comprises growth retardation, a characteristic facial appearance and mental retardation.

3.15 Surgical problems

Surgical problems arise in pregnancy usually as acute emergencies. The most common is acute appendicitis. This should be treated in the same manner as in the non-pregnant state. Problems can arise if the diagnosis is delayed or atypical due to the pregnant state. The appendix, and the site of tenderness, can be displaced upwards by the pregnant uterus, making the presentation atypical. Abdominal complications can cause peritonitis. This may result in uterine irritability, pre-term labour and delivery. This emphasises the importance of early diagnosis in minimising complications.

Self-assessment: questions

Multiple choice questions

1. Topics suitable for discussion at preconception counselling include:
   a. Alcohol intake
   b. Long-term warfarin usage
   c. Aspirin use in a nulliparous woman to prevent pre-eclampsia
   d. Rubella status
   e. Cervical cytology

2. Diabetes:
   a. Is associated with a decreased incidence of congenital abnormality
   b. Is associated with postmaturity rather than prematurity, resulting in increased birth weights
   c. Is associated with an increased incidence of respiratory distress in the neonate
   d. Is associated with a reduced insulin requirement in pregnancy
   e. Maternal hypoglycaemia can occur in the puerperium

3. Regarding thromboembolism:
   a. It seldom occurs after the first 48 hours of the puerperium have elapsed
   b. Heparin crosses the placenta
   c. Venography should always be avoided in pregnancy
   d. Warfarin is safe in the puerperium
   e. Risk is increased in older mothers

4. Regarding medical problems in pregnancy:
   a. Iron deficiency is common in pregnancy
   b. Iron supplementation saves babies
   c. Cardiac abnormalities may present in the puerperium
   d. Tocolysis with β-mimetics is contraindicated in the presence of serious cardiac disease
   e. Women should be advised of the need for caution in the use of inhaler treatment for asthma in pregnancy as β-mimetics can cause uterine relaxation

5. Perinatal mortality is increased in:
   a. Asthma
   b. SLE
   c. Anticardiolipin syndrome
   d. Iron deficiency
   e. Renal disease

6. Perinatal infection:
   a. With group B streptococcus can be prevented with intravenous penicillin in labour
   b. With primary herpes virus can be prevented by caesarean delivery
   c. With rubella virus after 20 weeks results in serious morbidity
   d. With CMV and toxoplasma can result in serious handicap
   e. Viral transmission may be exacerbated by the use of fetal blood sampling

7. In pregnancy:
   a. Pyrexial illness can cause pre-term labour
   b. Peritonitis can cause pre-term labour
   c. Renal infection can be associated with pre-term labour
   d. Carpal tunnel syndrome is a common problem
   e. Treatment of hyperthyroidism can affect the fetus

True/false questions

1. A lady with poorly controlled hypertension attends her GP immediately after performing a pregnancy test which is positive. The GP should stop her ACE inhibitor immediately.
2. A lady who suffers from acne wishes to continue using a topical retinoid during her pregnancy. Her doctor should insist that she stops using it immediately.
3. A lady has a confirmed diagnosis of obstetric cholestasis which has responded to ursodeoxycholic acid. She can be reassured that there is no fetal risk and therefore no rationale for early delivery.
4. Sodium valproate should be stopped if at all possible prior to conception.
5. Patients with pulmonary hypertension should be advised to avoid pregnancy.

Short notes

1. Write short notes on the assessment and management of diabetes in the first trimester.

2. Write notes on your management of a 15-year-old girl who is pregnant, whom you suspect of drug abuse.

Self-assessment: answers

Multiple choice answers

1. a. **True.** Women should be advised of any risk associated with maternal alcohol intake in pregnancy.
   b. **True.** Warfarin is extremely teratogenic and alternative therapies should be discussed in any woman planning a pregnancy.
   c. **False.** Aspirin may only be warranted for this purpose in a very specific subgroup at high risk of midtrimester pre-eclampsia.
   d. **True.** Rubella infection in the first trimester is associated with very high rates of congenital defect. Women at highest risk include those educated outside the UK or who for other reasons may not have been vaccinated in the established programme.
   e. **True.**

2. a. **False.** The incidence is increased and related to periconceptual control of the blood glucose concentration.
   b. **False.** Prematurity is increased in diabetes. Birth weight is increased, though not by postmaturity, which is unlikely to arise as most diabetic women are delivered between 38 weeks and term. It is thought that birth weight is increased due to the effect of high insulin levels in the fetus.
   c. **True.** This is more likely to arise due to prematurity, an increased incidence of hyaline membrane disease in infants of diabetic mothers, and occasionally a cardiomyopathy in the neonate.
   d. **False.** There is a substantial rise in insulin requirement to overcome the antagonistic effect of placental hormones.
   e. **True**, if insulin dosage is not reduced to levels approximating the requirement prior to pregnancy.

3. a. **False.** Women continue to be at risk for several weeks after delivery.
   b. **False.** Heparin does not cross the placenta.
   c. **False.** Venography can be safely performed in pregnancy, but ultrasound diagnosis should be attempted first.
   d. **True**, though many women prefer to stay on heparin subcutaneously.
   e. **True.** Increased maternal age is a major risk factor.

4. a. **True**, and can be prevented by iron supplementation.
   b. **False.** There is no evidence of benefit to the fetus or neonate.
   c. **True.** Cardiac abnormalities can occasionally be diagnosed for the first time in the puerperium, largely having presented with pulmonary oedema due to problems with fluid balance.
   d. **True.** β-mimetic agents cause a marked tachycardia and can result in deterioration of cardiac disease.
   e. **False.** There is no evidence that such inhaler treatment can do harm and women must be assured that they need to use inhalers just as they would in the non-pregnant state.

5. a. **False.** In general asthma does not pose a risk to the fetus.
   b. **True.**
   c. **True.** The precise reason for impaired fetal outcome in SLE and in the presence of anticardiolipin antibodies is not known.
   d. **False.**
   e. **True.**

6. a. **True.** Intravenous penicillin or amoxycillin should be administered in labour to known group B streptococcus carriers.
   b. **True.** Caesarean delivery may help prevent perinatal transmission if there are active lesions present in the genital tract.
   c. **False.** Rubella virus causes most harm in the first trimester.
   d. **True.**
   e. **True.** While this is not relevant to the vast majority of women, it is a concern in the presence of HIV or hepatitis B virus.

7. a. **True** Pyrexia should always be treated vigorously.
   b. **True.**
   c. **True.** Pre-term labour may be due to pyrexia, coincidental carriage of infective organisms and coexisting congenital uterine abnormalities.
   d. **True.**
   e. **True.** Antithyroid treatment can cross the placenta and cause hypothyroidism in the fetus and neonate.

True/false answers

1. **False.** She should be referred urgently to the relevant specialist. Her blood pressure still needs to be controlled and the ACE inhibitor needs to be withdrawn in carefully monitored fashion and as

peripheral resistance falls with the onset of vascular adaptation to pregnancy.

2. **True.** Systemic retinoids cause fetal malformations. There is little evidence of this with topical treatment at present but it is safest to stop the treatment. Unlike severe hypertension, the indication for treatment is cosmetic and abrupt withdrawal is not going to be harmful.

3. **False.** She cannot be totally reassured. Most practitioners would still opt for delivery at 37 weeks.

4. **True.** There are real concerns about its effect on neurodevelopmental outcome.

5. **True.** This poses one of the greatest risks to women in pregnancy. Mortality rates are 30–50% depending on the underlying diagnosis.

Short notes answers

1. The first objective is to establish what level of control of blood glucose is being achieved. This is best assessed by home glucose monitoring. The woman will measure her glucose concentration immediately on rising and then 2 hours after breakfast. Further measurements are then made according to need, most commonly 2 hours following her midday meal and again after supper. This regimen identifies specific times when control is not being achieved and hence is a guide to insulin dosage. A longer-term assessment is made by the measurement of the haemoglobin A_{1C} concentration. Elevated readings reflect suboptimal control in the preceding weeks, i.e. at the time of conception.

Insulin is usually prescribed as a basal bolus regimen with fast acting insulin before each meal, and intermediate acting in the mornings and evenings as needed. Some hypoglycaemic attacks will occur with tight control, and the patient must be forewarned and understand the reasons why tight control is necessary.

An early dating scan is advisable to demonstrate fetal viability and for reassurance that alterations in the insulin regimen are worthwhile. Some discussion of prenatal diagnosis is valuable at this point and arrangements should be put in place for a nuchal fold, anomaly scan or amniocentesis if necessary.

Management during the pregnancy should be discussed with the patient, any risks explained and the rationale for any hospital visits explained. She should be informed in advance of the increasing insulin requirement and the potential problems of polyhydramnios, macrosomia and need for delivery at 38–40 weeks. This will all help to ensure compliance and minimise complications throughout the pregnancy.

2. This is a high risk pregnancy. An accurate dating scan should be arranged as soon as possible as pregnancy is often concealed in this age group and presentation can be late. It is important that rapport is established from the first hospital visit, as default from care is a major problem in this group. This means that risk must be made clear whilst avoiding a patronising approach which may antagonise the patient.

Contact should be made with the family if possible. The social services department should be involved to ensure that help and support is available when the baby is born and that there is a satisfactory environment in which the baby can be cared for.

The question of drug abuse must be discussed openly with the patient and a urinary toxicology screen requested. The patient must understand that drugs can harm fetal development. If opiate abuse is confirmed she should be considered for a methadone support programme.

There is a high background risk of intra-uterine growth retardation, so serial ultrasound assessment of growth are indicated. This risk is increased in the presence of drug abuse. Risk of abruption is also high and the patient must be alerted to the symptoms which should prompt hospital attendance.

Screening for hepatitis and HIV should be performed with the patient's consent.

Overview

Intra-uterine growth retardation can arise because the placenta fails to provide sufficient nutrition to the fetus in-utero, or because the fetus is suffering from intra-uterine infection, a chromosomal disorder or a congenital abnormality. Growth retardation may be accompanied by a reduction in liquor volume. Excessive liquor volume can also arise either for fetal reasons such as neuromuscular disorders or congenital abnormalities affecting ability to swallow, or related to maternal diabetes. Rhesus disease causes haemolysis in the fetus/neonate and arises because of a maternal antibody to the rhesus antigen in the fetus. It is largely preventable with a programme of Anti-D prophylaxis. Invasive prenatal diagnostic techniques carry risks of miscarriage of approximately 1%.

Introduction

An overview of perinatal mortality as in Chapter 9 reveals that the fetus may be affected by many conditions. Although the major proportion relate to congenital malformations and inherited disease, they also include many medical and surgical conditions, as may occur in adult medicine. Some fetal disease, however, arises because of the very specific relationship of the fetus to the outside world, where the placenta (and not the lungs) is the respiratory exchange mechanism. The major condition of placental origin resulting in perinatal mortality is intra-uterine growth retardation (IUGR). Fetuses which fail to demonstrate growth comparable to the normal population are at significant risk of intra-uterine death and morbidity. Much of the screening effort in antenatal clinics is therefore directed to the detection of the small fetus.

Ultrasound

Many of the issues discussed below are highly dependent on the use of ultrasound examination of the fetus. Being scanned during pregnancy is clearly an enjoyable experience for most mothers and their families and it has been demonstrated that detailed explanation of the ultrasound examination has a positive psychological impact on the mother. It is much less clear, however, what effect abnormal or equivocal findings may have for the mother or her baby. There is no clear evidence of any physical harm to the baby arising from antenatal ultrasound use. School performance assessed in 8 to 9-year-olds who had had second and third trimester scans was no different from that in a control group who had had no scans. Nonetheless some caution is warranted and patients should not be scanned unnecessarily or for longer periods than required. It is also important that ultrasound examination is performed by adequately trained staff using good quality equipment.

Routine use of ultrasound in early pregnancy results in:

- more accurate assessment of gestational age
- earlier identification of multiple pregnancy
- determination of chorionicity in multiple pregnancy
- less induction of labour for apparent postmaturity
- detection of 60% of fetal malformations
- assessment of risk of aneuploidy
- diagnosis of placenta praevia.

It is estimated that in the absence of a routine screening programme, 70% of women would have a clinical indication for a scan at some time during their pregnancy.

4.1 Intra-uterine growth retardation (IUGR)

Learning objectives

You should:

- know how to assess uterine size

Learning objectives (*continued*)

- understand the causes of growth retardation
- understand the contrasting management of symmetric and asymmetric growth retardation
- be familiar with the methods of fetal assessment

Intra-uterine growth retardation (IUGR) refers to fetal growth which is significantly less than normal and implies underlying pathology. The diagnosis is important because the number of stillbirths in physically normal infants in this category is several times higher than when growth is appropriate to gestational age. Monitoring of the IUGR fetus and timely delivery results in improved perinatal outcome.

However, the criteria for making this diagnosis varies from hospital to hospital. At delivery IUGR is often said to exist if the birth weight is less than the tenth centile for gestational age. It is clear, however, that not all babies in this category are unwell, and many have achieved their growth potential in utero. If the fifth or third centile are used then a greater proportion of the neonates falling within the definition will have been exposed to some form of pathology. When deciding on the centile charts to be used, the population from which these charts have been derived must be considered, and ideally correction should be considered for factors such as sex, race and changes in birth weight with time.

The diagnosis is therefore not straightforward. Attempts to make the diagnosis in utero depend on clinical skills, and increasingly upon ultrasound evidence. Clinical evidence of IUGR may include:

- fundal height less than expected for the gestational age, by palpation
- symphyso-fundal height reading in centimetres less than expected
- oligohydramnios.

Fundal height is traditionally assessed by palpation according to Box 23.

Adjustment is then made according to gestation. Although this method is not ideal, it is likely to detect gross discrepancies in growth. A tape measure can be used in an attempt to make the judgement more objective. The distance from the upper border of symphysis pubis to uterine fundus is measured and the reading compared with gestational age, with the measurement roughly equivalent to the number of weeks in centimetres ± 2–4 cm:

- 20 weeks   19 cm ± 2 cm
- 28 weeks   27 cm ± 3 cm
- 36 weeks   35 cm ± 3–4 cm

While this has not been demonstrated to be definitively useful, such measurements are widely used as an adjunct to palpation. Tape measurements are inaccurate in the presence of maternal obesity, multiple pregnancy or a transverse lie.

Ultrasound evidence of IUGR is based upon calculated measurements of the fetal abdominal circumference and head circumference, and liquor volume assessment. Based upon the above readings a calculation of estimated fetal weight is made which can then be plotted on the appropriate centile charts. In cases of IUGR secondary to malnourishment of the fetus, the abdominal size is disproportionately reduced, similar to the effect of an enforced diet in an adult.

Causes of IUGR

There are many possible causes of intra-uterine growth retardation. In the first instance every effort must be made to ensure gestational age calculations are correct, preferably by ultrasound dating in the first half of pregnancy. If the gestational age is confirmed, then a list of possible causes must be considered. The fetus may be prefectly healthy, but fall within the definition used despite achieving its growth potential, i.e. 'small for dates' (SFD) but not growth retarded. Typically this fetus will have a normal ratio of head to abdominal circumference, a normal liquor volume, and normal umbilical artery Doppler waveform.

The fetus may, however, be truly growth retarded. In this situation it is not achieving its true growth potential because of some constraint (see Box 24). The commonest cause is 'placental insufficiency'. In this situation the head circumference will be disproportionately large in compari-

---

Box 23 Fundal height: assessment by palpation

- Approaching xiphoid   36 weeks
- Midway between umbilicus and xiphoid   28 weeks
- Umbilicus   20–22 weeks
- Suprapubic   12–14 weeks

Box 24 Causes of intra-uterine growth retardation

- **Fetal**   Chromosomal abnormalities
Congenital infection
Congenital malformations
- **Placental**   Placental dysfunction (most common)
- **Maternal**   Vascular disease, e.g. SLE
Maternal hypertension/pre-eclampsia

son with the reduced abdominal circumference, there may be associated oligohydramnios, and the umbilical artery Doppler waveform study may reveal reduced, absent or reversed end-diastolic flow through the placenta.

Such asymmetric reduction of abdominal circumference relative to head circumference is a reflection of the 'brain sparing effect' by which blood is diverted disproportionately to the brain at the expense of other areas of the body as a fetal response to stress. This results in poor growth of the liver and subcutaneous fat resulting in a lower abdominal circumference.

Intra-uterine growth retardation may also occur in the presence of a major congenital abnormality, as these fetuses grow less well. The diagnosis of abnormality is made on ultrasound examination in 60% of cases, and in the remainder it is made at birth. In this situation the liquor volume is usually normal, although it may be reduced in renal tract abnormalities or increased with some other abnormalities (see oligohydramnios, p. 60 and polyhydramnios, p. 61).

Impaired fetal growth may be the first sign of karyotypic abnormality, for example Trisomy 21 or 18. With a SFD fetus, therefore, markers of aneuploidy must be sought. The umbilical artery Doppler waveform analysis may be abnormal in this situation.

Intra-uterine infection is another cause of growth retardation. The most common infections include congenital CMV, toxoplasmosis and rubella. Diagnosis of these conditions is often difficult, though amniocentesis and cordocentesis may play a role looking for evidence of transplacental spread of infection and fetal immune response (see Box 25).

Box 25 Investigation of IUGR

- Maternal screen for hypertension or vasculitic condition (check for evidence of anticardiolipin antibody syndrome if severe midtrimester IUGR)
- Placental blood flow studies
- Fetal ultrasound examination
  — growth
  — liquor volume
  — confirm lack of congenital abnormality
  — look for markers of aneuploidy
  — look for markers of congenital infection
- Biophysical profile
  — fetal movement
  — fetal breathing
  — liquor volume
  — fetal tone
  — fetal heart rate test (CTG)
- Fetal karyotype (if suspicion of chromosomal abnormality)
  — amniocentesis
  — cordocentesis

Investigation

The investigation of IUGR is outlined in Box 25. Only selected tests will be appropriate for most cases, with resort to invasive measures such as cordocentesis reserved for only the most difficult. An overview of methods of fetal assessment and their value is necessary to explain which tests are appropriate in certain clinical circumstances.

Assessment of fetal well-being

The assessment of fetal well-being is dependent upon clinical awareness of risk factors for poor perinatal outcome, and the application of specific tests of fetal health. Traditional obstetrics has relied on the perception of risk factors for certain women such as hypertension, nulliparity or grand multiparity. This approach is still important, and the interpretation of the tests outlined below should take account of such factors.

Fetal movement counting

Women are routinely asked during antenatal visits if they are feeling fetal movements. This is to confirm that the fetus is indeed alive, and because reduction in fetal movement can indicate fetal hypoxia, acidosis or other form of stress in utero. Some units ask women to formally record their perception of fetal movement on a daily basis from 28 weeks' gestation on a 'count to ten' chart. On a day when she does not feel ten movements by a predetermined time she is requested to attend the hospital for a cardiotocograph (CTG) recording. However, such counting has never been formally shown to be of benefit. Problems include the fact that the maternal perception of movement is often inaccurate, and also that even if accurate this does not necessarily mean that delivery or intervention will improve the outcome for the baby. There is no evidence therefore that there would be a reduction in the number of intrauterine deaths, and it may result in increased demand on medical services and increase the number of operative deliveries.

Cardiotocography

While the presence of fetal movement or the fetal heart simply confirm fetal viability, they do not provide information regarding fetal well-being. Cardiotocography is a method of determining fetal well-being on a daily basis, and involves recording the fetal heart rate and uterine contractility over a period of time, usually 20–40 minutes. Criteria for fetal heart rate (FHR) normality include:

- a baseline of 110–150 beats per minute
- the presence of accelerations – temporary increases in FHR often associated with fetal movement, of 15 beats per minute, lasting 15 seconds

- the absence of decelerations – temporary reductions in FHR which may be related to contractions
- good 'beat to beat' variation – short-term changes in FHR of greater than 5 beats per minute
- baseline variability – longer-term changes in the baseline rate.

A typical normal antenatal CTG is shown in Figure 8. A normal FHR is reassuring that in the short term there is minimal risk of fetal morbidity or death within the next 24 hours. This does not apply if there is an acute problem in the interim such as placental abruption, chorioamnionitis or cord accident.

The CTG is not primarily a test of the fetal heart. It is a test to ensure that cerebral control of FHR variability through the autonomic nervous system is intact, reflecting absence of fetal cerebral acidosis. In assessing fetal well-being, therefore, the short term measures of fetal health on a daily basis include the maternal perception of fetal movement and the CTG. It is ideal that the fetus should not be exposed to hypoxia and acidosis and that fetal compromise should be detectable prior to an abnormal CTG. Such assessment is largely dependent on ultrasound.

It has been suggested that performing routine CTGs at intervals may help reduce perinatal loss, but there is no evidence that such practice helps to reduce the incidence of intra-uterine death in high risk pregnancy. It seems likely that a CTG gives reasonable reassurance over a 24-hour period that the fetus is well, but not for longer intervals.

Over the past 2–3 decades some hormonal placental function tests have been assessed to determine whether they have a role in diagnosing fetal compromise. Levels of placental products such as human placental lactogen and oestriol were measured and compared with controls. There was, however, too much overlap between the values in IUGR and control pregnancies and attention has subsequently moved to ultrasound-based techniques.

Ultrasound examination of fetal growth

This is performed when the clinician is concerned about fetal growth, or fetal movement, or there is a past history of IUGR, or a significant maternal problem such as pre-eclampsia.

Ultrasound involves measuring fetal growth, assessing amniotic fluid volume, and on occasions confirming that the fetus is structurally normal. There is a margin of error in assessing fetal growth of the order of 10%, and

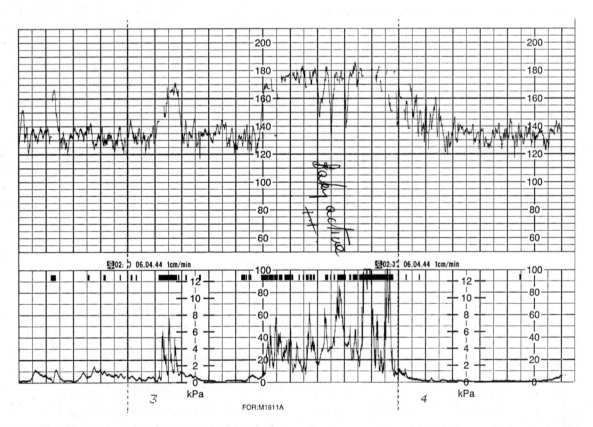

Fig. 8 A normal cardiotocograph recording showing a baseline reading between 120 and 140 beats per minute, accelerations, and a sustained acceleration associated with fetal movement. The fetal movement has resulted in altered pressure readings as shown at the bottom of the diagram. Clinicians should ensure that patient's name, date and time of recording are all clear.

therefore serial readings at 2-weekly intervals provide more reliable information than one isolated measurement. If ultrasound assessment suggests that the fetus is appropriately grown, it is unlikely that intra-uterine death will occur within the next 2 weeks.

Biophysical profile scoring

This involves ultrasound assessment of:

- fetal tone
- fetal body movements
- fetal breathing movements
- amniotic fluid volume
- FHR patterns.

A score is awarded if the factors above are present and therefore low scores represent fetal compromise. The role of such assessment is unclear at present because the criteria assessed do not have equal importance and the more important, i.e. amniotic fluid volume and FHR patterns, can be assessed much more quickly. It is not widely used at present.

Grannum grading of the placenta is a technique where placental appearance is assessed by ultrasound looking for calification and cotyledonary formation, these changes being associated with increased fetal risk. There is some evidence that routine use of this technique in late pregnancy may reduce perinatal death rates, by identifying cases of placental insufficiency that can be delivered early.

Doppler blood flow studies

Doppler blood flow studies are being increasingly performed in the hope that they will provide additional information concerning fetal well-being. The uteroplacental and fetoplacental circulations have been the subject of most study. In pregnancies complicated by hypertension, there is an increased incidence of abnormal waveforms in the uteroplacental circulation thought to be indicative of increased vascular resistance.

Doppler blood flow tests in obstetrics include:

- uteroplacental — prediction of hypertension and IUGR
- umbilical (fetoplacental) — fetal well-being
- fetal middle cerebral artery — cerebral redistribution of blood flow in IUGR.

Most major fetal vessels can be assessed with Doppler and there are occasions when this is useful, such as examination of renal blood flow in cases of possible renal malformation. The most clinically useful test, however, is the umbilical artery waveform analysis. The presence of normal end-diastolic flow is useful reassurance that the fetus is not compromised and the fetus, if growth retarded, falls into the 'small but healthy' category. If the end-diastolic flow is reduced it is possible that there is significant compromise. In the absence of end-diastolic flow, the risk of fetal death in utero increases and the patient needs daily assessment unless sufficiently far on in pregnancy to allow delivery. In the presence of reversed end-diastolic flow, immediate delivery is required for the fetus to have a realistic chance of survival. Current evidence suggests that clinicians' awareness of the results of Doppler studies leads to reduced perinatal mortality and stillbirth rates of the order of 35%.

Occasionally, invasive tests are required to aid in fetal assessment. Cordocentesis (see section 4.4 below) involves taking a blood sample from the cord or hepatic vein. The blood may then be tested for the degree of hypoxia and acidaemia and a normal karyotype confirmed. The test is useful only in exceptional circumstances, however, as it does not give information predictive of the fetal condition, and there is a procedure-related loss rate.

Screening

There is no evidence to support routine ultrasound screening for IUGR. It may even result in unnecessary intervention. Furthermore, despite the usefulness of Doppler studies in selected cases, there is no evidence of any benefit when applied as a screening procedure to the general population.

Management

If a diagnosis of IUGR is made by clinical and ultrasound assessment in the absence of any suggestion of infection, aneuploidy or congenital abnormality, i.e. placental insufficiency, then a management plan must be formulated to determine if delivery is required and when. The plan will ultimately depend on where the tests suggest the fetus is relative to the normal pattern of evolution of IUGR (Table 6).

Table 6 Evolution of IUGR

Onset of IUGR
↓
Relative malnutrition
↓
Cerebral redistribution   Development of asymmetry
↓
Asymmetrical growth; ? borderline umbilical artery Doppler
↓
Asymmetrical IUGR with absent end-diastolic flow

The tests as described above give reassurance for limited periods of time (Table 7). The time scales involved are not clearly defined, however, and therefore complementary tests are often performed in parallel depending on the degree of suspicion.

The decision to deliver will ultimately depend on gestation. There are no rigid guidelines and considerable variation exists between clinicians. At premature gestations much will depend on the survival figures locally and availability of special care cots. Box 26 gives a rough guide.

The mode of delivery needs also to be considered. As in the discussion on pre-eclampsia (p. 21), induction of labour prior to 34 weeks tends to be difficult, particularly in the primigravida, and if delivery is indicated, caesarean section is often the most appropriate. After 34 weeks induction of labour may be considered but only if it is felt that the fetus will have sufficient reserve to withstand the stress of labour. An attempt at induction would therefore be inappropriate with severe IUGR and absent umbilical artery end-diastolic flow, but may be appropriate with mild to moderate IUGR at term. Continuous fetal heart monitoring throughout induction and labour is essential.

The paediatric staff must be involved when delivery is planned to ensure that they are prepared for it. Recognised complications following delivery of growth-retarded fetuses include:

- asphyxia
- meconium aspiration
- hypoglycaemia in the first 48 hours
- complications of prematurity.

4.2 Disorders of amniotic fluid volume

Learning objectives

You should:

- understand the causes of polyhydramnios and oligohydramnios
- be familiar with the management options for these conditions

The liquor volume may be normal, increased (polyhydramnios) or decreased (oligohydramnios). Anhydramnios refers to the complete absence of amniotic fluid from the uterine cavity. Amniotic fluid volume may be assessed clinically and by ultrasound examination.

Polyhydramnios

Excessive amniotic fluid may be suspected clinically by:

- uterus being larger than expected for gestational age
- maternal discomfort and uterine irritability

Table 7 Tests of fetal well-being and their potential role

Test	Time of reassurance	Plan (guidelines)
Short term		
Fetal movement	Uncertain	CTG (more objective)
CTG	24 hours	No action if normal
		Deliver if abnormal
Longer term		
Fetal growth scan	2 weeks	Repeat in 2 weeks if normal
		Doppler if abnormal
Umbilical artery Doppler	3–4 days	Term: deliver if abnormal
Reversed end-diastolic flow	None	Deliver immediately
Absent end-diastolic flow	None	>32 weeks: steroids and deliver
		<32 weeks: CTG and steroids

Box 26 Indications for delivery in IUGR

- Term — Deliver if any clinical suspicion
- 32–37 wks — Deliver if clear diagnosis, with absent growth for 3–4 weeks or absent end-diastolic flow
- 28–32 wks — Deliver if CTG abnormal (includes ↓ beat to beat, etc. or reversed flow)

  Delivery may be indicated especially in 30–32 range if CTG is non-reassuring, there is absent flow on the Doppler study

  Steroids should be given if time allows
- < 28 wks — Deliver only if clearly decelerative CTG or reversed flow. Ensure steroids have been given

- fetal parts being difficult to palpate (normally palpable from 26–28 weeks in the presence of normal amniotic fluid volume)
- presenting part being unexpectedly high or the lie unstable.

The incidence of clinically important polyhydramnios is approximately 1% depending on the definition used.

Ultrasound assessment of amniotic fluid volume is usually by the amniotic fluid index (AFI). This assessment involves measuring the vertical depth of the largest pocket of fluid in each of the four quadrants of the uterus and expressing the result as the sum of the four measurements. There are some changes with gestation, but in general, measurements over 25 cm are excessive. Formal ultrasound assessment is arranged once polyhydramnios is diagnosed. Amniotic fluid may be assessed subjectively though increasingly the amniotic fluid index is measured. The causes of polyhydramnios are given in Box 27.

Congenital anomalies and fetal hydrops are sought on ultrasound, special care being taken to ensure that a twin pregnancy is not missed. Tracheo-oesophageal fistula and duodenal atresia may not always be apparent on scan. Karyotyping should be considered and discussed with the patient and a glucose tolerance test performed.

Complications include:

- those of the underlying disorder
- cord prolapse in the presence of membrane rupture
- unstable lie.

Management options are limited:

- amnioreduction, whereby amniotic fluid is aspirated via a spinal needle inserted directly into the uterus
- indometacin administration (reduces fetal renal output).

Amnioreduction and indometacin treatment should be considered when there appears to be a significant risk of pre-term labour or if there is maternal discomfort. It must be recognised that neither treatment is free of side-effects, and surveillance instituted for these. Indomethacin is associated with pulmonary hypertension in the newborn due to its effect on the ductus arteriosus. This is most commonly seen at gestations beyond 30 weeks and with usage for longer than 48 hours. Any woman with polyhydramnios should be advised to attend immediately with the onset of labour or rupture of the membranes. An unstable lie normally prompts admission from 36 weeks. The neonate should have a careful paediatric assessment at birth to exclude congenital abnormalities.

Oligohydramnios

Oligohydramnios refers to a deficiency of amniotic fluid and occurs in up to 5% of all pregnancies, though it is clinically important in approximately 1%. It can be associated with very poor perinatal outcome in certain clinical circumstances and always warrants thorough evaluation of the fetal condition.

Causes

Oligohydramnios or anhydramnios may occur for a variety of reasons:

- Ruptured membranes. This is not always clear from the history and a sterile speculum examination should be performed to look for liquor in the vagina.
- IUGR may be associated with oligohydramnios. This normally implies that there is a primary placental problem.
- Fetal renal abnormalities (also CNS, skeletal and cardiac) may cause oligohydramnios.
- Maternal treatment with non-steroidal anti-inflammatory drugs (such as indometacin) and angiotensin-converting enzyme (ACE) inhibitors may cause reduced urine output in the fetus and oligohydramnios.
- Twin pregnancy (4%).

Lack of amniotic fluid makes performance and interpretation of the ultrasound scan difficult. Some experts therefore infuse physiological solution into the uterine cavity to aid visualisation and allow more accurate assessments of fetal anatomy.

Complications

Adequate amniotic fluid is necessary for fetal pulmonary development. Pulmonary hypoplasia may arise if oligohydramnios is present at 18–24 weeks' gestation, a critical time in pulmonary development. If severe oligohydramnios or anhydramnios has been present

---

Box 27 Excessive amniotic fluid: causes

- Idiopathic (60%)
- Fetal causes (30%)
  — high urine output (macrosomia, twin to twin transfusion)
  — obstructed GI tract (oesophageal or duodenal atresia)
  — neuromuscular (poor swallowing)
  — CNS defects
- Maternal causes
  — diabetes (5% – may be higher depending on population)
  — Rhesus disease

over this time period, termination of the pregnancy should be discussed with the patient in view of the extremely poor prognosis. If there is an obstructive lesion in the fetal urinary tract, insertion of a shunt should be considered to divert urine to the amniotic cavity. Oligohydramnios in the midtrimester in association with vaginal bleeding also carries a very poor prognosis. Pressure deformities can complicate prolonged oligohydramnios, as can the formation of adhesions within the amniotic cavity ('amniotic bands').

4.3 Rhesus disease

Learning objectives

You should understand:

- when sensitisation may arise
- how to prevent it
- how the disease affects the fetus

This used to be called hydrops fetalis, and the description was of neonates with jaundice, anaemia and hydrops. Hydrops refers to an increase in total body water content, reflected in serous accumulations in the peritoneal, pleural and pericardial spaces. It is not always immune in origin, as in Rhesus disease. Causes of non-immune hydrops include congenital infections (CMV, parvovirus), congenital heart defects and arrhythmias, and genetic disorders. Immune hydrops arises because antibodies in the mother's (Rhesus type negative) blood cross the placenta and cause haemolysis of fetal red cells expressing the Rhesus D antigen if the fetus has inherited this from the father. For this to happen, a Rhesus negative mother must have been exposed to Rhesus positive antigens at some time. The potential times for this to occur are outlined under Prevention of Rhesus disease below.

Prevention of Rhesus disease

There are substantial risks once sensitisation has occurred and care is very costly. Ideally, the disease can be prevented, and the introduction of anti-D immunoprophylaxis since the 1960s has been very successful in this regard. Sensitisation can occur whenever a rhesus D negative woman is exposed to rhesus D positive blood. This can occur as follows:

- following a miscarriage (first or second trimester)
- following a procedure such as amniocentesis
- following an episode of bleeding in pregnancy

- following an episode of pain even in the absence of bleeding (retroplacental bleeding may occur in either of these circumstances)
- during the latter half of pregnancy even in the absence of the above symptoms – this is referred to as antepartum sensitisation.

Women should always receive anti-D in the presence of a possible precipitating event. Antepartum sensitisation is thought to occur as a result of a low level of leakage of Rhesus positive blood into the maternal circulation in the absence of any clinically apparent event. This therefore cannot be prevented by responding to clinical circumstances, but could be by a programme of anti-D administration to all Rhesus negative women at 28 and 34 weeks. The dose used in the latter half of pregnancy is generally 500 IU intramuscularly, and it lasts approximately 6 weeks in the maternal circulation. Hence the mother should be covered from 28 weeks onwards and clinical experience confirms the efficacy of this approach.

It is possible for antibodies to form to other paternally-inherited antigens and to cause haemolytic disease in the newborn. In general, the D antigen is the one associated with the most severe disease. Nonetheless, when atypical antibodies are found on screening, expert advice must be sought and referral to a fetal medicine practice arranged if necessary. Antibodies to the Kell antigen, for instance, cause 14% of fetal hydrops and antibody levels are again poorly predictive of the fetal condition.

Causes of sensitisation to Rhesus D antigen (1.5% of Rhesus negative mothers)

- Antepartum sensitisation
- Failure to administer anti-D prophylaxis
- Therapeutic failures
- Transfusion-related (incompatible blood transfusion)

A sensitised mother may suffer recurrent reproductive loss. Owing to prophylaxis the incidence of sensitisation has been greatly reduced. Nonetheless, for the sensitised mother it remains a serious problem.

The true fetal loss rate due to this disease is not reflected in the perinatal mortality figures, as many of the worst affected fetuses die prior to viability, and other pregnancies are terminated.

When the mother first attends for antenatal care, her blood group will be checked. At the same time the serum will be screened for antibodies. Should anti-D be detected, the level of antibody will need to be quantified, any past history consistent with Rhesus haemolytic disease identified, and a review undertaken of her recent care to determine when sensitisation occurred. Care should be managed with the help of a specialised fetal medicine service. Fetal blood sampling to detect fetal blood group and degree of anaemia may then be performed, or amniocentesis to measure the bilirubin level in the amniotic fluid. The amniotic fluid bilirubin level, measured by spectrophotometric measurement of the deviation in optical density at 450 nm (ΔOD450) reflects fetal haemolysis.

The effect on the fetus is variable and unfortunately is difficult to predict from antibody levels. The only way to measure objectively the degree of haemolysis is to take a blood sample from the fetus in utero. The timing of the first blood sample depends on:

- the past obstetric history
- a very high level of antibody or a sudden increase
- fetal ascites or hydrops on scan.

Should the fetus be found to be markedly anaemic, an intra-uterine blood transfusion can be performed at the same time, and arrangements made for serial sampling and transfusion as the pregnancy progresses. It must be remembered that fetal blood sampling carries a small risk for the fetus.

4.4 Genetic disorders and prenatal diagnosis

Learning objectives

You should:

- be familiar with invasive techniques and their complication rates
- understand the screening methods for Down's syndrome

Many parents are extremely anxious about the possibility of having to care for a handicapped child and for this reason there are a number of mechanisms whereby potential abnormalities are detected (see Box 28).

Box 28 Categories of congenital abnormality and detection

• Structural anomalies	Routine anomaly scan at 18–20 wks Investigation of poly- or oligohydramnios Incidental May only be discovered at delivery
• Abnormal karyotype	Amniocentesis Placental biopsy Cordocentesis May only be discovered at delivery
• Congenital infection	Clinical infection, with seroconversion Invasive tests

Counselling

Counselling patients about their risk of congenital disease and genetic risk in the antenatal period is a specialised field and extremely time-consuming. It is very important in counselling that the potential benefit of preventing handicap is not outweighed by doing harm through causing unnecessary anxiety. The ethical acceptability of different treatment options must be considered as this will vary considerably between individuals. Counselling must be honest and avoid giving the impression that some congenital defects are socially unacceptable. Parents must understand the objectives of the different tests and must feel able to decline tests according to their needs and ethics. It should not be assumed that parents would not want prenatal diagnosis because they would not consider termination of an affected pregnancy. Often parents change their minds when presented with greater information about the defects concerned, and even if they do not opt for termination they appreciate forewarning of the pending problem.

Detection of aneuploidy

Amniocentesis

In a low risk population there is a three-fold increase in the risk of miscarriage following amniocentesis at 16 weeks, i.e. an attributable risk of 1%. Other risks of amniocentesis at this gestation include low birth weight, neonatal respiratory distress syndrome, neonatal pneumonia, and Rhesus isoimmunisation.

Amniocentesis may be performed at 10–14 weeks' gestation. This will provide an early result for the parents but there are concerns regarding the effect of such a procedure upon fetal lung development and loss rates are higher than at 16 weeks.

Chorionic villus sampling (CVS)

Chorionic villus sampling (CVS) is performed earlier in gestation than amniocentesis. It can be performed between 8 and 12 weeks, though in view of the concerns regarding limb reduction defects with early procedures, it is generally performed at 10–12 weeks. Earlier results lead to fewer psychological problems for the mother and easier vaginal termination of pregnancy if appropriate. Comparison of CVS with amniocentesis performed at 16 weeks suggests that CVS is technically more demanding, more likely to provoke bleeding at the time of the procedure and carries a higher risk of diagnostic inaccuracy. Transcervical CVS also appears to be associated with a greater incidence of spontaneous miscarriage, pre-term delivery, IUGR, and pregnancy loss.

Furthermore, following CVS there appears to be a greater incidence of false positive diagnoses, mostly due to placental mosaicism. Placental mosaicism arises when abnormal chromosomal patterns have arisen in the development of the placenta but are not present in the fetus. Transabdominal CVS appears to be safer than the transcervical route, easier to perform and less likely to require a repeat procedure.

Screening for Down's syndrome

A decision to proceed to amniocentesis or CVS is a serious decision for prospective parents. In view of the increased miscarriage rate following such procedures, they are reserved for women at higher than average risk of carrying a baby with Down's syndrome. As risk increases with age, amniocentesis was traditionally offered to women over 35 years of age. This method, however, had little impact on the overall delivery rate of babies with Down's syndrome as the vast majority of births are to women below this age cut-off.

Recently, efforts have been made to assess individual women's risk of Down's syndrome more accurately, by:

- serum screening
- measurement of nuchal translucency.

Serum screening – done at 16 weeks
This refers to the measurement of:

- serum alfa-fetoprotein, lower in Down's syndrome
- human chorionic gonadotrophin, increased in Down's syndrome
- unconjugated oestriol, lower in Down's syndrome.

These serum markers provide prediction of Down's syndrome and are taken into consideration alongside maternal age. The risk can then be calculated for individual women and those at highest risk offered amniocentesis. Measurement of the above substances must be performed in relation to the gestational age as assessed by ultrasound scan: accurate dating of the pregnancy is essential for correct interpretation.

Nuchal translucency scanning – done at 12 weeks
This technique aims to calculate the risk of Down's syndrome by testing the fetus directly. An ultrasound assessment of a fluid collection behind the fetal neck is made. In the presence of chromosomal problems accumulation of fluid in this space is increased. Measurements of nuchal translucency greater than or equal to 3 mm increase the risk of trisomies 5-fold. This test can also help in the diagnosis of conditions other than Down's, such as cardiac abnormalities. A further advantage is that the woman may proceed to CVS and know the karyotype at a much earlier gestation than with serum screening.

Efforts are being made to refine the above techniques and to improve their accuracy. This is being achieved through the measurement of a fourth serum marker at 16 weeks, and by attempting serum screening at 12 weeks' gestation, as an adjunct to nuchal translucency scanning.

Cordocentesis

Cordocentesis refers to the procedure whereby fetal blood is taken from the umbilical cord. It is performed through a fine needle under ultrasound guidance in the late second and third trimesters. Complications can arise because of bleeding from the sampling site resulting in haemorrhage into the amniotic cavity or localised haematoma formation. Fetal loss rates from this procedure are approximately 1%, though they may be greater if there is already fetal compromise at the time of the procedure. The same procedure may be followed to allow fetal blood transfusion as in Rhesus disease. This technique has been extended to allow sampling of fetal blood from the intrahepatic vein. Indications for cordocentesis are relatively rare by comparison with amniocentesis or CVS and include determination of fetal karyotype or blood gases.

Preimplantation diagnosis

This refers to a procedure in which prenatal diagnostic tests are performed at the blastocyst stage. This can only occur in assisted conception cycles where tests are performed on individual cells taken from the blastocyst. It is reserved for couples at very high risk of serious genetic defects. It can allow sexing, such as in cases of muscular dystrophy, or screening for conditions such as cystic fibrosis.

4.5 Congenital malformations

Major congenital malformations occur in approximately 2% of all pregnancies. A large proportion of these are diagnosed antenatally by ultrasound scan and are followed by termination of pregnancy where legally permissible. Thus the proportion of babies delivered with major congenital malformations will depend upon the extent and quality of the local ultrasound screening programme. Major malformations may be diagnosed in utero as mentioned, at postmortem following a stillbirth, or for the first time in the days and weeks following delivery. For this reason, quoted perinatal mortality rates exclude major congenital malformations.

Many congenital malformations are the result of the interaction of multiple genes and environmental factors, while some result from single gene defects. Ultrasound imaging of the fetus is the major method of detecting structural congenital anomalies. The success of ultrasound varies with:

- different levels of skill among those performing the scan
- the risk status of the population
- because some defects are easier to detect than others
- the relative difficulty in detection of certain malformations, e.g. aortic coarctation.

Approximately 80% of lethal malformations are detectable, and up to 70% of all abnormalities. It is important that once an abnormality is identified, the patient has the opportunity to be re-scanned, and is offered specialist counselling. This is most commonly performed in fetal medicine centres where there will also be facilities for subspecialty consultations with urologists, paediatric cardiologists and geneticists. Following this the diagnosis will be amended in approximately one third of cases. There are occasions when the diagnosis may only become clear with serial scans over weeks.

It is important that the limitations of ultrasound examination are understood by the patient. It has been demonstrated that the use of an autopsy refines the diagnosis in 40% of cases when this information is available, and confirms the diagnosis in 50%. In 10–15% of cases the performance of an autopsy leads to a reappraisal of the recurrence risk. Ultrasound is much better at identifying some abnormalities than others, for instance neural tube defects are diagnosed with over 95% certainty whereas congenital heart defects are often not diagnosed antenatally.

Self-assessment: questions

Multiple choice questions

1. Features suggestive of IUGR include:
   a. Reduced liquor volume
   b. Maternal asthma
   c. Pre-eclampsia
   d. Plentiful fetal breathing movements
   e. Reduced end-diastolic flow on umbilical artery Doppler

2. Congenital malformations:
   a. Can present with polyhydramnios
   b. Can present with oligohydramnios
   c. Can present with intra-uterine growth retardation
   d. Can present with a breech presentation at term
   e. Are normally detectable on ultrasound

3. Amniocentesis:
   a. Can occasionally fail to provide the fetal karyotype
   b. Carries a 1% risk of miscarriage due to the procedure
   c. Involves culture of fetal cells from amniotic fluid which means a 6-week delay in providing the result
   d. Should be performed under ultrasound guidance
   e. Can be performed in the third trimester

4. Oligohydramnios:
   a. Can be caused by amniocentesis
   b. Can be associated with 'postmaturity'
   c. Can be caused by diabetes
   d. Can cause hypoxic damage to the fetal heart
   e. Makes the fetus more susceptible to trauma

5. Regarding Rhesus disease:
   a. It is still a common cause of fetal death
   b. It arises when a Rhesus positive mother develops an antibody which causes haemolysis in the fetus
   c. Father's blood group is of no importance
   d. It can occur even when the mother has had anti-D prophylaxis at all appropriate times
   e. It can cause fetal hydrops

True / false questions

1. A clinical diagnosis of intrauterine growth retardation should be confirmed on ultrasound.
2. Patients with polyhydramnios should always be admitted because of the risk of cord prolapse.
3. The incidence of rhesus disease has steadily declined.
4. Anti D prophylaxis should be considered after road traffic accidents.
5. Nuchal fold assessment should be offered to patients with diabetes and renal disease rather than serum screening for Down's syndrome.

Short notes

1. A patient is admitted at 32 weeks' gestation with intra-uterine growth retardation. Describe your management.

2. Explain the differential diagnosis of a small for dates (SFD) uterus and a large for dates (LFD) uterus.

Self-assessment: answers

Multiple choice answers

1. a. **True.**
   b. **False.** This is not associated.
   c. **True.**
   d. **False.** This is suggestive of fetal well-being.
   e. **True.** This strongly supports the diagnosis.

2. a. **True.** Abnormalities of liquor volume, either excess or reduction, may suggest congenital abnormalities.
   b. **True.**
   c. **True.**
   d. **True.** Assessment of the breech presentation at term includes ultrasound evaluation to exclude abnormalities such as neural tube defects/hydrocephalus.
   e. **True.**

3. a. **True.** Occasional culture failures arise (less than 1%) and the patient should be forewarned.
   b. **True.**
   c. **False.** Culture of fetal cells is required but takes between 2 and 4 weeks.
   d. **True.** This is to minimise the possibility of direct needle injury to the fetus, and to make the procedure easier and therefore less stressful to the mother.
   e. **True,** but the delay of 2–4 weeks for karyotyping makes it less useful for this purpose. In the third trimester it is more commonly performed for assessment of fetal lung maturity as manifest by the L/S ratio, or to provide symptomatic relief of polyhydramnios.

4. a. **True.** This could arise if the procedure precipitates pre-term premature rupture of the membranes.
   b. **True.** Liquor volume is reduced as the pregnancy is prolonged beyond the due date. This may indicate fetal compromise.
   c. **False.** Maternal diabetes is more commonly associated with polyhydramnios.
   d. **False.** Oligohydramnios does not cause any hypoxic damage. It may be associated with fetal hypoxia which rarely affects the fetal heart other than in the most severe cases.
   e. **False.** There is no evidence to support this.

5. a. **False.** This is now quite rare.
   b. **False.** It arises when a Rhesus negative woman develops an antibody to the Rhesus antigen.

c. **False.** The father in a particular pregnancy may determine the fetal blood group. The father must be Rhesus positive (most are) for the fetus to be positive and hence susceptible to the antibody.
d. **True.** The mother can become sensitised despite all appropriate precautions being taken, but this is increasingly rare.
e. **True.** The maternal antibody crosses the placenta and causes haemolysis of the fetal red cells resulting in fetal anaemia and hydrops.

True / false answers

1. **True.** Clinical diagnosis is not reliable. It may be reasonable at term to proceed to delivery if the obstetrician is very confident of the diagnosis.
2. **False.** The risk is real but is low in absolute terms especially at earlier gestations. Patients are admitted in this situation if the lie is unstable at term.
3. **True.** The programme of anti-D prophylaxis has been successful.
4. **True.** This is a potential indication. If there is any suspicion that there may have been retro-placental bleeding as a result of the trauma, anti-D should be given.
5. **True.** Serum screening is not reliable in the presence of renal failure or diabetes. These patients are high risk and are normally reviewed in the first trimester allowing time for the nuchal scan to be performed.

Short notes answers

1. 50% of clinical diagnoses of intra-uterine growth retardation are wrong. In the first instance the calculation of gestational age must be re-checked. Then ultrasound is used to assess fetal growth, and the estimated fetal weight is calculated based on the head and abdominal circumference. If both circumferences are reduced (symmetrical growth retardation), fetal abnormalities must be excluded, and evidence of intra-uterine infection such as intracranial calcification or microcephaly sought. Maternal serum may be taken to look for evidence of infection.

   Markers of aneuploidy must be sought and, if present, fetal karyotyping considered. This may involve amniocentesis, though the result may take 2–3 weeks. However, fetal loss is minimal from amniocentesis at this gestation, though there is a small risk of precipitating premature labour. Cordocentesis will provide a result within 48 hours, but carries a 1% risk of fetal loss. This is therefore only performed when there is high risk of aneuploidy or a rapid result is needed.

If the abdominal circumference is reduced relative to the head circumference, this is termed asymmetrical IUGR. This suggests a placental cause (placental insufficiency). In this situation further investigation is directed at detecting hypoxia and acidosis in the fetus.

At 32 weeks management would involve the administration of steroids to the mother to promote fetal lung maturity. The patient would be advised of what might be expected if her baby were to be born between 32 weeks and term. Surveillance would either be by serial ultrasound assessment of liquor and doppler twice a week, or CTG monitoring depending on the severity of the growth retardation. Oligohydramnios or absent flow on the Doppler would be sufficient to warrant delivery at this gestation if steroids have been administered.

2. A common clinical problem facing the obstetrician is to determine if the assessment of uterine size is consistent with the gestation of the pregnancy and, if not, why this may be so.

A uterus that appears small for dates (SFD) may well be so, but the obstetrician must first check that the dates are correct. This is done by re-checking the date of the last menstrual period, ensuring the woman had a regular menstrual cycle (a 35-day cycle may mean that a further week should be added when calculating the expected date of delivery), excluding the use of hormonal preparations such as the oral contraceptive pill, which make dating by the last menstrual period unreliable, asking the woman if she knows when she conceived, and determining the time when her pregnancy test was first positive. All these points may give valuable clues as to the accuracy of her dates. However, the best guide to expected date of delivery is ultrasound assessment of gestational age prior to 22 weeks, which has been shown to be more accurate than any of the above.

Ultrasound assessment of gestational age is best performed early in pregnancy (see Box 29).

When the gestation has been confirmed, other explanations for the uterus to be small must be sought. These include poor fetal growth and oligohydramnios. The differential diagnosis of intra-uterine growth retardation will include fetal causes (chromosomal abnormalities, congenital infection or malformation), placental dysfunction, and maternal vascular disease or hypertension/pre-eclampsia. If oligohydramnios is the cause, rupture of the membranes needs to be excluded, followed by assessment for structural abnormalities.

If the uterus is thought to be large for dates, the dates must be checked as suggested above, and ultimately ultrasound confirmation of gestation sought. Other explanations of a large for dates uterus include:

- fetal macrosomia
- undiagnosed multiple pregnancy
- polyhydramnios
- uterine fibroids.

Box 29 Ultrasound assessment of gestational age

Gestation

• 5 weeks post LMP	Visible sac on transvaginal sound (TVS)
• 6	Visible fetal heart on TVS
	Visible sac on abdominal scan
• 7	Visible fetal heart on abdominal scan
• 7–12	Crown–rump length measurement
• 14–22	Biparietal diameter measurement

5 Organisation of maternity services

Overview

Women are normally referred to a hospital clinic early in pregnancy. The first visit is termed the 'booking visit' and a plan is made for the rest of the pregnancy and Down's syndrome screening discussed if the patient wishes. Subsequent visits are performed at monthly intervals and then more frequently from 28 weeks. The main scan during the pregnancy is performed at approximately 20 weeks gestation and is designed to detect most major fetal abnormalities. In the third trimester women are encouraged to attend antenatal classes to prepare them for labour. Most women deliver in a hospital environment though approximately 1% choose to deliver at home. Following delivery, community midwifes are in contact with women for about 10 days prior to handing over responsibility to district nursing services.

Introduction

Learning objectives

You should:

- learn how the maternity services are organised
- understand the pattern of routine care which is offered to women
- understand the rationale behind many of the routine tests in pregnancy

The aims of preconceptual counselling were outlined in Chapter 3. There is, however, no formal arrangement for pre-conceptual care in the community in the UK. Certain groups of patients are likely to have access to such care through a variety of mechanisms, as outlined in Box 30.

It is clear that the delivery of such care is patchy. For this reason young women from socioeconomically disadvantaged backgrounds are those most likely not to be seen prior to conception. Education through schools and family planning clinics is a potential mechanism to increase awareness of issues such as rubella immunisation in this population.

5.1 Antenatal care

Antenatal care is currently delivered through a combination of general practitioner-based services, district midwives, and hospital-led consultant and midwifery care. Care is initiated following the attendance of the woman to her GP. The GP, having confirmed the pregnancy, then

---

Box 30 Referral pattern for pre-conceptual counselling

• History of congenital abnormality	Genetic counsellor/ paediatrician
• Previous pre-term labour	Obstetrician
• Known renal or hypertensive disease	Physician/obstetrician
• Family history of inherited disease	Genetic counsellor

writes to the hospital to request that the patient is booked for care, and the hospital responds by arranging a 'booking visit'. The GP will ensure that at the time of referral the woman is aware of advice concerning folic acid supplementation, and that the referral allows sufficient time to ensure appropriate prenatal diagnosis.

The 'booking' visit serves the following purposes:

- to familiarise the woman with the hospital at which she may deliver
- to allow the woman to meet some of the midwifery staff who may subsequently be responsible for her care
- to allow a member of the obstetric staff to assess the woman and determine whether she falls into a high risk category
- to determine the most appropriate type of care throughout the pregnancy
- to instigate screening for diseases relevant to the pregnancy
- to allow referral to associated medical specialists
- to allow referral to social services departments as necessary.

The booking visit includes a discussion with a midwife, followed by history taking and examination by the doctor. The history must ascertain the expected date of delivery, any relevant medical history and address any current problems in the pregnancy. The patient is then examined with specific emphasis on the points listed in Box 31.

The blood tests normally performed at the first booking visit are summarised below in Table 8.

In addition to the above, patients may be referred for ultrasound assessment of gestational age (normally by biparietal diameter) if serum screening for Trisomy 21 is planned or the gestational age is uncertain. An anomaly scan is usually performed at 18–20 weeks' gestation. At this examination a full assessment of the fetus is performed.

At the booking visit, a decision is usually made to deliver shared care with the GP or a midwife working

Box 31 Booking visit: examination	
● Blood pressure	Baseline reading for the pregnancy
● Cardiac	Exclude underlying cardiac disease
● Abdomen	Confirm fundal height appropriate
● Speculum examination	To allow smear test if necessary
● Vaginal examination	Normally only if there is a specific indication
(A vaginal examination used to be performed routinely, but is not now as the vast majority of women undergo an ultrasonic assessment to exclude significant ovarian pathology, etc.)	

from the practice. This form of care generally involves a hospital visit at booking, and at 41 weeks, with all other visits to the GP's surgery (see Box 32). These arrangements are amended according to local facilities, and ease of travel to the hospital. Women considered at risk of complications during the pregnancy will need hospital-based care.

This traditional pattern of antenatal care is unnecessary for most healthy women, who may wish to have the vast majority of their care with the midwife who will eventually deliver them in labour. Various arrangements of midwifery-led care are currently being evaluated in terms of the effectiveness of care delivered and acceptability to pregnant women. Some evidence exists that by ensuring continuity of care maternal satisfaction with the pregnancy is increased, less analgesia is required in labour, and waiting times in the clinic may be reduced. There is, however, insufficient data at present to say whether total care by the midwife is as safe as traditional hospital or shared care systems. Other methods used to ensure women feel more positively towards their pregnancy, and more in control, are the allocation

Table 8 Blood tests performed in early pregnancy: rationale

Test	Rationale
Full blood count	Exclude anaemia (p. 44)
Haemoglobin electrophoresis	Allows genetic counselling re haemoglobinopathies (p. 44)
VDRL/TPHA	Now controversial. Value dependent on community prevalence of syphillis
Blood group	Allows transfusion of group compatible blood in haemorrhagic emergency and entry to Rhesus programme if Rh −ve (p. 62)
Antibody screen	To detect pregnancies at risk of haemolytic disease
Hepatitis B screen	Allows neonatal immunisation if at risk (p. 47)
Rubella screen	Documents rubella status at onset of pregnancy. Serum often kept as a baseline screen for other infectious diseases in pregnancy
Serum screening for Down's	Allows assessment of risk status for Trisomy 21 in the pregnancy. AFP may serve as a marker for neural tube and other congenital defects
Toxoplasma screen test HIV	Neither of these tests is performed as a routine, but HIV is recommended and may be requested following counselling of the patient

Box 32 General pattern of care during pregnancy

● Booking visit at 12 weeks	Initial screening procedures as above
● Thereafter every 4 weeks to 28 weeks	Allows screening for early onset pre-eclampsia or intra-uterine growth retardation
● 28 weeks	Includes screen for anaemia and development of antibodies
● Every 2 weeks between 28 and 36 weeks	Further screening for PET and IUGR
● Every week from 36 weeks until delivery	Includes the above plus a check on presentation

of antenatal birth plans and allowing women to keep their own hospital case records during the pregnancy.

One of the major concerns in the third trimester is the detection of intra-uterine growth retardation (IUGR). There is little evidence to say which health care professional is likely to do this most efficiently. Symphysis–fundal height measurement is commonly used to screen for IUGR, though the only trial of its efficacy failed to show it to be of value. In addition, routine counting of fetal movement has not been shown to improve perinatal outcome.

5.2 Ultrasound services

Ultrasound provides a safe method of imaging the fetus in utero, and allows visualisation of some fetal abnormalities (see Ch. 4). It also provides information on fetal growth and well-being. Studies on the safety of ultrasound have failed to demonstrate any adverse effects. Table 9 outlines the aims of ultrasound assessment at different stages of pregnancy.

Routine ultrasound examination in early pregnancy improves the assessment of gestational age, allows earlier diagnosis of multiple pregnancies, and allows the detection of fetal abnormalities.

In the third trimester the priority is to ensure fetal well-being. However, there is no evidence that routine scanning in late pregnancy or routine use of Doppler ultrasound in healthy women improves pregnancy outcome. In high risk pregnancies or where there is clinical suspicion of IUGR, fetal growth is assessed and Doppler blood flow studies performed. There is evidence that grading of the appearance of the placenta during the third trimester allows improved detection of fetal compromise and fewer perinatal deaths.

5.3 Patient education

Much effort is directed towards ensuring that patients are educated about pregnancy and care during and after labour. This is done in an attempt to improve compliance with advice on issues such as smoking and diet during pregnancy, and helps to minimise fear of childbirth, reduce requirements for analgesia and render the whole experience more fulfilling. Such education is achieved through the media, notices in GP surgeries and family planning clinics, advice at the booking visit, patient education booklets and formal antenatal classes. Classes are usually held during the last trimester, and address issues that include posture and exercises during

Table 9 Rationale of ultrasound assessment at different gestations

First trimester	Confirm intra-uterine pregnancy	from 5 weeks (TV)
		from 6 weeks (TA)
	Confirm viability	from 6 weeks (TV)
	Assess gestational age	from 7 weeks (TA)
	Nuchal fold thickness	Crown–rump length (CRL) at 10–13 weeks
Second trimester	Assess gestational age	Biparietal diameter (BPD)
	Fetal anomaly scan	at 18–20 weeks
	Placental site	at 18–20 weeks
	Cervix	some high risk pregnancies 14–24 weeks
	Exclude early IUGR	high risk pregnancies only
Third trimester	Fetal growth	28 weeks–
	Liquor volume	
	Confirm presentation	36 weeks–
	Placental site	32 weeks–
	Doppler assessment	if suspicion of IUGR
	Placental appearance	if suspicion of IUGR

TA = transabdominal; TV = transvaginal; IUGR = intra-uterine growth retardation.

pregnancy, care and analgesia during labour, and infant feeding. Some mothers may require counselling and advice in different environments. This applies to high risk groups such as teenagers, who may be targeted by advice given in youth club settings or family planning clinics.

5.4 Social factors and diet

Socioeconomic background has a major influence on perinatal outcome, and there is little that health care professionals can do to alter this, although attempts can be made to direct health care towards those at greatest risk. There is some evidence that providing extra support for women from disadvantaged backgrounds during the perinatal period improves child health and reduces the risk of subsequent unwanted pregnancies. There is, however, no evidence that it influences outcome of the index pregnancy. The threshold at which investigations are performed to detect IUGR is altered by the risk status of the mother and this should be reflected in the pattern of antenatal care.

It is likely that pregnancy is a time when motivation to stop smoking is high and therefore a time when advice on smoking and strategies to reduce smoking may be effective. Effective smoking cessation programmes can increase mean birth weight, but their effect on perinatal mortality remains uncertain.

Aerobic exercise is not harmful during pregnancy and can therefore be encouraged. There appears to be no beneficial effect on labour duration. The effects of strenuous fitness training are largely unknown and any exercise associated with a risk of trauma should be avoided.

Dietary advice

There is no evidence that increasing either caloric or protein intake of a pregnant woman confers any benefit, and it may possibly be harmful. Protein/energy supplementation does appear to increase fetal weight. There is no evidence that caloric restriction in overweight women improves pregnancy outcome. Women should therefore be advised to eat a normal and balanced diet.

Routine iron supplementation in pregnancy raises the serum ferritin level and prevents anaemia in late pregnancy, but does not appear to affect pregnancy outcome. However, in high risk populations iron and folic acid supplementation is warranted.

Periconceptual supplementation with a multivitamin preparation including folic acid 0.8 mg per day reduces the incidence of neural tube defects, as discussed in Chapter 3. There may be a role for Vitamin D supplementation during pregnancy for women at risk, i.e. vegetarian women in countries with inadequate exposure to sunlight, such as Asian women living in Britain.

5.5 In-utero and ex-utero transfer

When a premature infant is delivered, or anticipated, special care or neonatal intensive care facilities may be needed. If these are not available on site, transfer to a unit with such facilities will be necessary. Transfer of women prior to delivery is referred to as in-utero transfer. Possible reasons may include:

- threatened pre-term labour, to a centre capable of care of the extremely pre-term baby, i.e. at 22–28 weeks
- threatened pre-term labour up to 34 weeks, if the hospital special care baby unit is full and cannot cope with another baby which may require ventilation
- if urgent delivery is being considered and there is a specific surgical condition requiring paediatric surgical facilities.

Ex-utero transfer refers to transfer after delivery. The disadvantage is that the neonate must be exposed to the ambulance journey at a time when stability is important. In general, in-utero transfer is therefore preferred, and neonatal outcome is better.

5.6 Care in labour and place of delivery

In most developed countries, care is provided in labour by a midwife and the place of delivery is the hospital. Chapter 6 outlines the duties of the midwife in the conduct of normal labour. There is much debate about the safest place for childbirth. Some argue that conducting childbirth in a hospital setting leads to an unnecessarily medical approach, resulting in high rates of intervention which in turn result in high rates of intervention which in turn result in high rates of iatrogenic morbidity.

Those in favour of hospital delivery argue that it is impossible to predict which women are at risk of sudden and serious complications requiring medical assistance or neonatal resuscitation.

There is currently no firm evidence to suggest which is the best place for delivery. Women at low risk of complications therefore are more likely to seek home delivery, though most women currently still deliver in a hospital setting. Efforts are being made to ensure that hospital facilities are user-friendly and not unlike a home environment.

5.7 The puerperium

Care in the puerperium is discussed in Chapter 8. During this time it is a legal obligation that a midwife sees the woman each day or is in contact with her on a daily basis for the first 10 days after delivery. Most problems arise in the first 48 hours after delivery and these are normally cared for in a hospital setting.

A visit to a doctor at approximately 6 weeks following delivery is traditional. The need for such a visit is now questioned though there is a need for contraceptive advice, preconceptual counselling, and for symptoms to be addressed. This visit is normally conducted by the GP, and the woman is seen in a hospital setting only if complications are anticipated.

Self-assessment: questions

Multiple choice questions

1. At 20 weeks' gestation:
   a. Serum screening for Down's syndrome should be discussed
   b. Assessing fetal growth is important
   c. An anomaly scan is often performed
   d. Placenta praevia can be diagnosed on this scan
   e. Fetal movements can be felt

2. Regarding tests performed at the booking visit:
   a. A full blood count should be performed
   b. A high vaginal swab is advised
   c. Blood group should be established
   d. Vaginal examination should be performed
   e. Screening for Down's syndrome should be discussed

3. Regarding hospital/home care and antenatal visits:
   a. Hospital delivery has been shown to be safer than home delivery in low risk cases
   b. Perinatal mortality has fallen in the past 4 decades due to hospital care
   c. Midwifery-based antenatal care is associated with failure to diagnose intra-uterine growth retardation
   d. Women are traditionally seen every week from 28 weeks
   e. Deaths from pre-eclampsia and eclampsia do not occur after 36 weeks because of the frequent checks which occur at this stage of the pregnancy

Short notes

1. Write notes on the rationale for women to attend for antenatal care at 20, 28 and 36 weeks.

Self-assessment: answers

Multiple choice answers

1. a. **False.** This is normally performed at 14–16 weeks' gestation.
    b. **False.** Problems with fetal growth seldom arise at 20 weeks, though they can do in very high risk pregnancies.
    c. **True.** The fetus can be assessed at this gestation and termination of pregnancy arranged if warranted.
    d. **False.** The placenta may be seen to be 'low-lying' on this scan. The term placenta praevia is used to refer to bleeding in later pregnancy in association with a 'low-lying' placenta or where it is still low after 32 weeks.
    e. **True.** Fetal movements are normally felt by 20–22 weeks in a nulliparous woman and 16–18 weeks in a multiparous woman.

2. a. **True.**
    b. **False.** This is reserved for specific indications.
    c. **True.**
    d. **False.** There is no indication for vaginal examination on a routine basis.
    e. **True.** This will require discussion of the implications of a positive screening result.

3. a. **False.** This is an area of dispute.
    b. **False.** Hospital-based care may have made a significant contribution but the major influence is likely to have been improvements in socioeconomic conditions.
    c. **False.**
    d. **False.** Every two weeks from 28 weeks and weekly from 36 weeks. Some obstetricians question the need to see women so frequently.
    e. **False.** This emphasises that any reduction in the level of care may be associated with increasing mortality from this condition.

Short notes answer

1. a. At 20 weeks' gestation:
    - check the results of all the blood tests performed at the booking visit
    - discuss any outstanding issues in relation to prenatal diagnosis
    - ensure that an anomaly scan is performed
    - ensure that a plan of care is documented for the rest of the pregnancy

    b. At 28 weeks' gestation:
    - check the blood pressure is normal and that there is no proteinuria
    - ensure that the fundal height is adequate for dates
    - check the fetal heart and fetal movements
    - check the fetal lie
    - excessive liquor may make the fetal parts difficult to palpate
    - check that glucose tolerance is tested if indicated
    - Check fetal blood count and antibodies: if Rhesus negative, administer anti D.

    c. At 36 weeks' gestation:
    - the presentation must be checked: if persistently breech, external cephalic version can be considered
    - blood pressure and urine are checked to exclude pre-eclampsia
    - fetal growth is checked
    - liquor volume is assessed
    - anaemia is excluded
    - antibody check is carried out
    - any anticipated problems in relation to labour must be discussed.

6 Labour

Overview

Labour is characterised by dilatation of the cervix and descent of the head. Successful labour depends on adequate uterine contractions, adequate pelvic capacity and favourable presentation and size of the fetus. Episiotomies are performed in selective cases to prevent excessive perineal trauma or tearing. Severe perineal tears are most likely with operative deliveries. If labour is slow, intervention with artificial rupture of the membranes can be performed, and oxytocin prescribed. The same procedures are used for induction of labour. When the cervix is not sufficiently dilated to allow rupture of the membranes, prostaglandin pessaries can induce favourable change to allow this. The fetus must be monitored in labour, and this should be with continuous electronic monitoring if high risk. Haemorrhage can occur immediately after delivery and is usually due to lack of uterine contraction.

Introduction

Labour is the process by which the contents of the pregnant uterus are expelled. Labour must overcome all the mechanisms which prevent premature expulsion of the fetus prior to maturation, and allow safe delivery of the fetus and full return to normal of the mother. Not surprisingly, nature does not always succeed completely in achieving the above objectives:

- premature labour and delivery is a major problem
- obstructed labour can cause maternal and fetal problems
- labour is a major contributor to maternal problems of prolapse and incontinence in later life
- there are risks of asphyxia, perinatal infection and trauma to the fetus.

However, most women will deliver normally and without any major immediate morbidity. Thus care during labour has to reflect this while at the same time ensuring vigilance for any complications.

Care during the course of normal labour is provided by a midwife, who is specifically trained to be able to recognise complications. If complications arise the midwife will inform a member of the medical staff. It is the midwife who provides on-going psychological and nursing support for the woman whether or not complications arise, and who is the person the woman will normally identify with regarding the birth.

Prior to the onset of labour women are encouraged to attend antenatal classes. Such classes provide prospective parents with advice on issues such as when to attend in labour. This will substantially reduce the number of women presenting to the labour ward with uncertainty regarding labour, etc. They also teach parents about hospital procedures in the event of complications and about the different options in relation to pain relief for the delivery. A guided tour of the labour ward area is also normally provided. All the above measures help provide reassurance for the woman prior to labour and help both her and her partner to feel more positively about the delivery process.

6.1 Normal labour and delivery

Learning objectives

You should:

- understand the mechanism of normal labour
- be familiar with the stages of labour
- be familiar with the basic care offered to a woman in labour

As mentioned, care during normal labour will normally be provided by a midwife. Great efforts are currently being made to ensure that the woman will have the opportunity to meet the midwife concerned prior to her admission to hospital in labour, though in practice this is difficult to achieve. Provision of continuous support throughout labour by a midwife is associated with improvement in outcome of labour and a more positive attitude towards the experience for the woman. Such psychological support appears to be more important than the effect of the environment in which the woman delivers. Nonetheless, efforts must be made to provide as 'home-like' an environment as possible within the hospital setting. Some births do occur on a planned basis at home, but the norm in the UK continues to be delivery in a hospital setting. For this reason the discussion below relates to hospital delivery.

The stages of labour

The process of labour is divided into three stages.

First stage

The first stage is characterised by dilatation of the cervix and lasts from the onset of labour until full dilatation (Fig. 9A).

The term 'latent phase' describes the progress of labour from 0 to 3 cm dilatation. The woman may present at this time feeling she is in labour, but these degrees of dilatation may occur during the process of cervical ripening prior to labour itself. Progress in terms of cervical dilatation can be slow in this phase in contrast with the active phase described below.

The 'active phase' is the term used to describe the progress from 3 cm to just before full dilatation. This phase is normally characterised by progress of at least 1 cm per hour and presents no difficulty in diagnosis.

Second stage

The second stage lasts from full dilatation to delivery of the fetus (Fig. 9B).

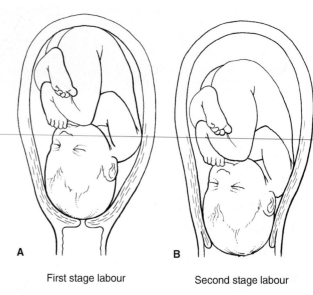

First stage labour   Second stage labour

Fig. 9   In the first stage of labour (**A**) the cervix can be seen to be effaced and dilating; the vertex is still high, though well applied to the cervix. In the second stage (**B**) the cervix is no longer visible and the vertex has descended.

'Passive second stage' refers to the period defined above but in the absence of pushing (normally to allow descent of the fetal head prior to pushing).

'Active second stage' refers to the active process of maternal pushing directed to achieving delivery.

Third stage

This extends from delivery of the baby to delivery of the placenta and membranes.

Diagnosis

Determining the true onset of labour can be very difficult, reflecting the fact that the onset is phased over a period of time rather than occurring at a specific moment. As outlined in Chapter 1, the processes preceding labour last weeks and are not always clearly distinguishable from the acute event. Diagnosis of labour is normally defined as follows: *the onset of regular painful uterine contractions associated with effacement and dilatation of the cervix.*

Difficulties can arise as a result of reliance on a definition such as that used above:

1. Some women complain of contractions in the absence of cervical change. These women are normally experiencing the latent phase of labour.
2. Not all women find the contractions painful (relatively rare).
3. Effacement of the cervix prior to dilatation is characteristic of primiparous labour rather than multiparous labour (Fig. 10).

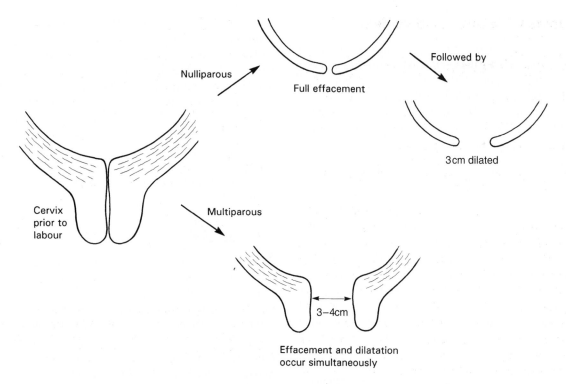

Fig. 10 The 'tubular' appearance of the cervix prior to labour. In the nulliparous woman the cervix shortens (effaces) prior to dilating, whereas in the multiparous woman both occur simultaneously in the early stages of labour.

Diagnosis of labour is not dependent solely on the above and most would accept the diagnosis if regular painful contractions are accompanied by spontaneous rupture of the membranes in the absence of cervical dilatation.

Duration of labour

As it is so difficult to define the onset of labour, it is often measured simply from the time of admission to hospital to the time of delivery of the placenta and membranes. Many women will already be 3–4 cm dilated at the time of admission in labour even in their first pregnancy, and long labours are seldom a problem in such women. Accordingly, almost 80–90% of women will be delivered within 10–12 hours of admission. Prolonged labour is traditionally defined as lasting longer than 24 hours.

The mechanisms of normal labour and delivery

Normal labour is one which starts spontaneously, where the presentation is cephalic, and where no intervention is required to augment progress or assist delivery. During the course of such normal labour the force generated by uterine activity and maternal pushing must overcome resistance to the delivery of the fetus through the birth canal.

It is traditional to consider the process of normal labour and delivery as being determined by the interaction of three major variables, the three Ps:

- the passages
- the passenger(s)
- the powers.

As can be seen from Box 33, resistance is overcome, and therefore progress towards delivery occurs over a number of stages. Some may be overcome by the force of uterine activity, but not exclusively so. This is important because it must be appreciated that increasing uterine activity will not necessarily overcome all resistance to delivery and may be dangerous. The bony pelvis, however, is the major obstruction to delivery.

Box 33 Resistance that must be overcome to allow delivery	
Stretching of the pelvic ligaments (mainly the sacroiliac joints and symphysis pubis)	prior to and during labour
Effacement and dilatation of the cervix	prior to labour and during the first stage
Compression of maternal soft tissues	first and second stages of labour

The pelvis

The pelvic inlet extends from the centre of the sacral promontory along the ileopectineal lines to the posterior aspect of the upper surface of the pubic bone (see Fig. 11). The longest diameter of the inlet runs transversely (see Table 10). The pelvic outlet extends from the tip of the coccyx to the ischial tuberosities and then to the lower border of the symphysis pubis. Between the outlet and the inlet the pelvis is shaped concavely towards the pubic bone. The levator ani muscles originate at the level of a plane which extends from the inferior margin of the symphysis pubis via the ischial spines to the tip of the sacrum. An obstetric 'mid cavity' lies between this plane and the pelvic inlet.

In the process of normal labour the fetal head enters the pelvis transversely at the level of the pelvic inlet, as this presents the least resistance. It descends in this position through the mid cavity until it reaches the level of the levator muscles. As a result of the shape of this muscular hammock internal rotation of the fetal head occurs

here, i.e. the head is rotated normally to the more favourable occipito-anterior position.

These measurements relate to the normal human female pelvis which is termed gynaecoid. It can be seen that the normal process of labour is one in which the natural mechanisms take advantage of the most favourable diameter at each level. The fetus must rotate and flex accordingly. There are variants of the normal shape of the pelvis which can impair descent as a result of lack of space, and which can encourage the head to descend in an unfavourable position such as with the occiput posterior (see Ch. 7).

The passenger

This term refers to the fetus, though it is clear that the placenta and membranes must also pass through the birth canal. At the beginning of normal labour the fetal head will lie over the pelvic inlet and be well flexed. This results in the vertex, i.e. the area between the biparietal eminences and the anterior and posterior fontanelles, entering the pelvis first. This means that the maximum diameter of the fetal head will be approximately 9.5 cm. This represents a tight fit and therefore if circumstances arise which prevent optimal engagement of the fetal head into the pelvis, problems can arise as described in Chapter 7.

Thus the passenger can also be important in determining progress in labour. Factors that relate to the fetus that may impede progress include:

- fetal weight; larger babies will have greater difficulty in passing through the pelvis
- adoption of an unfavourable position of the presenting part (occipito-posterior position); there is an increase in the relative diameter of the presenting part to the size of the pelvis
- some fetal abnormalities such as hydrocephalus.

It must be appreciated that the head is the least compressible part of the fetus and therefore provides the greatest obstacle to delivery. It is very rare for the size of any other part of the fetus to provide such an obstacle.

The powers

The powers refer to the force generated to ensure expulsion of the fetus from the genital tract. This force is generated by uterine activity alone for the first stage of labour and the passive second stage, and by uterine activity combined with maternal expulsive effort in the activity second stage.

Efficient uterine contractions produce progressive cervical dilatation but cause temporary impairment of fetal oxygenation by impairing intervillous blood flow.

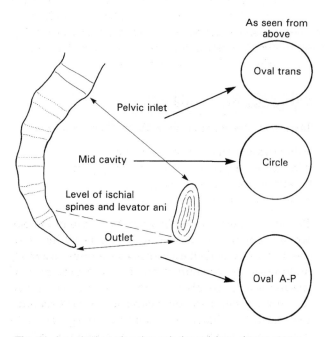

Fig. 11 A sagittal section through the pelvis to demonstrate the pelvic inlet, mid cavity and outlet. The corresponding shape of the pelvis as seen from above in cross section is shown to the right.

Table 10 Measurements of the bony pelvis		
Pelvic inlet	anteroposterior	11.5 cm
	transversely	13.6 cm
Mid cavity	all diameters	12 cm
Pelvic outlet	anteroposterior	12.5 cm
	transversely at the level of the spines	10.5 cm

Uterine activity can be assessed by palpation or by the use of an external pressure transducer on the abdominal wall overlying the uterus. Both methods give reliable information about frequency and duration of contractions but are a poor guide to their intensity. Pain levels are not a good guide to contraction intensity either as they are dependent on an individual's pain threshold. Uterine activity appears to increase as labour progresses, and is greater in total in nulliparous labour than in multiparous labour.

Procedure on admission

When a woman presents to the labour ward believing herself to be in labour, a midwife will be allocated to look after her. Her priorities at the time of admission will be:

1. to establish a rapport with the woman by showing that she is committed to caring for her and that she understands the importance of the occasion as a major life event for the woman and her partner. Being friendly and supportive is of major importance to the prospective parents, who will often be very apprehensive at this stage
2. taking a history to confirm that the reason for admission is consistent with early or established labour and to answer any questions she may have
3. performing basic observations such as temperature, blood pressure and urinalysis to provide reassurance that there is no underlying chorioamnionitis or pre-eclampsia
4. confirming fetal well-being, with or without the use of cardiotocography
5. examining the woman, including a vaginal examination in an attempt to confirm or refute a diagnosis of labour.

Once all the above issues have been addressed and the diagnosis confirmed, the midwife will usually then consider with the parents their wishes in relation to how the delivery is conducted (the birth plan) and discuss the issue of analgesia. Most women will have a pattern of contractions at this stage of approximately 2 to 4 contractions every 10 minutes, though there is considerable variation.

Midwifery care during a normal first stage of labour will usually include:

- pulse and blood pressure every 30 minutes
- temperature every 2 hours
- fetal heart auscultation every 15 minutes; this should involve continuous auscultation for 1 minute after a contraction or the use of the cardiotocograph
- monitoring of the urinary output and urinalysis
- vaginal examination at 2–4-hourly intervals depending on the rate of progress and parity.

Most women like to remain upright in early labour. There is no evidence that this does any harm and it results in less analgesia and augmentation. For this reason women should be allowed to adopt the posture of their choice in early labour. The use of technology which results in the woman being confined to a bed is frequently resented and this should always be remembered. Many women also find the use of a warm bath very comforting in the early stages of labour.

Advice regarding oral intake during labour varies substantially. Such advice reflects concern that if emergency anaesthesia is required, aspiration of gastric contents can result in substantial morbidity and even maternal death (Mendelson's syndrome). For this reason women are often requested to refrain from eating solids during the course of labour, though fluid intake is encouraged to maintain hydration. Routine administration of antacid treatment or cimetidine during labour will substantially reduce the number of women with a gastric pH of less than 2.5. This is not recommended for women other than those at high risk of requiring emergency anaesthesia (see Box 34). Furthermore, such a protocol does not protect totally against Mendelson's syndrome.

Traditional practices such as routine perineal shaving are not indicated and there is no evidence that routine enemas in early labour are worthwhile.

Progress in normal labour

During the course of normal labour, there should be:

- progressive dilatation of the cervix
- progressive descent of the presenting part
- satisfactory fetal well-being
- satisfactory maternal analgesia.

Progress is slower in nulliparous than in multiparous women. For uterine activity to be translated into progressive cervical dilatation, the uterus must contract, and then relax but with retraction – i.e. some length of the cervix must be taken up. There must also be a sustained relaxation between contractions of 1–2 minutes for intervillous blood flow and fetal oxygenation to recover. The contractions appear to arise in the upper cornual regions of the uterus, and so the midwife will normally palpate near the fundus if she wishes to detect

> **Box 34** Women at high risk of requiring emergency anaesthesia
>
> - Previous caesarean delivery
> - Breech presentation
> - Poor progress in labour
> - Twin deliveries
> - Persistently high head

the beginning of a contraction. Contractions then spread to the lower pole progressively.

Descent of the head

Descent can be assessed by both abdominal and vaginal examination. Abdominal examination prevents errors arising as a result of increasing caput and moulding which create the impression of descent on vaginal examination. The head will normally be engaged during the course of the latter stages of labour and failure of this to occur should prompt concern. The head is said to be engaged when the maximum diameter of the fetal head has passed through the brim of the pelvis.

Descent of the fetal head is usually assessed with reference to the ischial spines on vaginal examination. Variations in pelvic shape and depth prevent extrapolation from abdominal assessment to findings on vaginal examination. The station refers to the level within the pelvis to which the leading fetal part has descended.

The second stage

The second stage of labour begins when full dilatation is first recognised (see Fig. 9). Thereafter descent of the fetal head is the sole determinant of progress. The vertex will normally be at the level of the ischial spines or lower at the onset of the second stage. With maternal effort superimposed on the force generated by uterine activity, the vertex will emerge at the level of the introitus. At first it will recede between contractions, but when the level of the biparietal diameter has passed the pelvic outlet, the vertex will no longer recede and crowning is said to have occurred.

In the presence of an epidural anaesthetic it is advisable to avoid immediate pushing when full dilatation is reached until the vertex is visible at the introitus.

Immediate pushing is associated with an increased need for rotational forceps deliveries.

Episiotomy and tears

The term episiotomy is used to refer to the process of cutting the perineum with scissors or knife with the intention of widening the soft tissue diameter at the introitus in order to prevent tearing of the tissues at delivery. It is clearly only logical to do this if the tear which one is trying to prevent is likely to be worse than the episiotomy itself. This of course can be a difficult judgement to make. Episiotomy may also prevent damage to the supporting tissues at the level of the introitus due to excessive stretching.

Episiotomy is thought to result in less damage to the anal sphincter by way of third degree tears. A mediolateral episiotomy is normally used as midline episiotomies appear more likely to extend to the anal sphincter. In deliveries at high risk of sphincter damage (forceps) an episiotomy can therefore be recommended.

Episiotomy may also be used to shorten the second stage of labour and as such might be indicated if there was serious fetal distress. In the presence of premature delivery, episiotomies used to be performed routinely for this reason, but this is no longer the case as most pre-term deliveries occur without any undue delay.

Prevention of perineal trauma will therefore include the avoidance of liberal use of episiotomy, avoidance of unnecessary operative deliveries, and the use of ventouse in place of forceps when operative vaginal delivery is indicated.

Perineal tears (see Fig. 12) at delivery are classified as:

- first degree   confined to perineal or vaginal skin
- second degree   includes the deep perineal muscles
- third degree   includes the external anal sphincter.

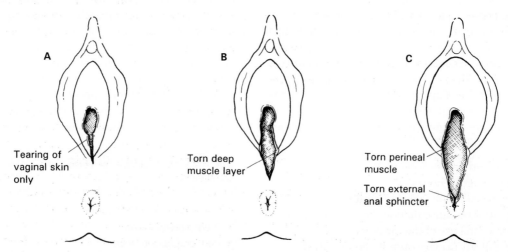

A   Tearing of vaginal skin only

B   Torn deep muscle layer

C   Torn perineal muscle
Torn external anal sphincter

Fig. 12   Perineal tearing: (**A**) a first degree tear with torn vaginal skin only, (**B**) a second degree tear with extension of the tear into the deep musculature and (**C**) a third degree tear with further extension involving the anal sphincter.

Some authors classify fourth degree tears as when the anorectal mucosa is also torn with the anal sphincter. In the UK these are all classified as third degree tears.

Technique of repair of episiotomy or tear

The vaginal incision is normally closed first with a continuous suture of absorbable material such as 2/0 polyglycolic acid. The deep muscle layers are then approximated using a stronger suture, again of polyglycolic acid. The use of a subcuticular suture for repair of the perineal skin is recommended and is associated with less short-term pain, though there is little difference with interrupted sutures in the long term. Interrupted sutures may be a better option if the perineal skin is very irregular or there is a problem with haemostasis. Absorbable suture materials are preferable as they result in less discomfort and less wound breakdown. Short-term pain appears to be 30–50% less likely if polyglycolic acid is used as opposed to chromic catgut. It also results in a reduced likelihood of wound breakdown resulting in re-suturing, though for some women it causes sufficient irritation to necessitate suture removal. In the event of wound breakdown, resuturing of the wound results in an earlier return to pain-free intercourse for the woman.

Long term there is no evidence that addition of salt or antibacterial agents such as Savlon affect either perineal discomfort or wound healing. The use of local steroid preparations does not reduce pain and may interfere with wound healing. Topical applications appear not to have a major impact on perineal discomfort. Ultrasound is used to alleviate perineal pain and while this is achieved in the short term, no longer-term benefits have been demonstrated.

Recently, the extent of anal sphincter damage with childbirth has been reassessed. It appears that much damage goes unrecognised at the time of delivery and that detected third degree tears may be only one manifestation of such damage. Long-term problems may also arise as a result of partial sphincter tears and denervation injury.

The third stage of labour

The third stage of labour extends from delivery of the baby to delivery of the placenta and membranes. The major risk at this time is of haemorrhage. This is as a result of bleeding from the placental bed where the maternal uterine vasculature is capable of delivering 500 ml of blood each minute. Once delivery has been completed and the placenta shears from the uterine wall, this blood flow must be stopped. The natural mechanism to achieve this is by uterine contraction, and as a result the myometrial tissue compresses the uterine vessels as they course through the wall. This is an extremely effective mechanism for reducing blood loss. Haemorrhage may still be a problem and so oxytocic drugs are used to augment this natural mechanism.

Oxytocic drugs are normally first given with delivery of the anterior shoulder of the baby in a singleton pregnancy. Their effects include 60% reduction in postpartum haemorrhage and 70% reduction in the use of therapeutic oxytocics. The relative merits of oxytocin and ergometrine are uncertain, though side-effects such as retained placenta, nausea and hypertension are much less likely with oxytocin than ergometrine. Syntometrine is a preparation containing 5 IU of oxytocin and 500 µg of ergometrine. Ergometrine appears to have an additional protective effect in comparison with oxytocin alone against postpartum haemorrhage. Because of the potential side-effects of ergometrine (especially nausea) oxytocin alone is normally preferred unless there are specific risk factors.

Active management of the third stage of labour involves early cord clamping, the use of an oxytocic drug and controlled traction on the cord. This management results in:

- a reduction in postpartum blood loss
- less anaemia postnatally
- reduced need for a blood transfusion
- decreased incidence of a high haematocrit in the neonate.

There is, however, some concern that this policy may result in an increased incidence of retained placenta.

Delivery of the placenta is normally achieved by using one hand to maintain and steady the uterine fundus in the suprapubic region. The other hand exerts traction on the umbilical cord. As the placenta shears off the wall of the uterus, traction on the cord is rewarded with descent of the placenta (referred to as combined cord traction).

Uterine inversion

It is important not to exert undue traction on the cord as the placenta can be abnormally adherent to the uterus. Traction will then result in inversion of the uterine fundus and its descent to the introitus.

Inversion can also occur rarely without morbid adherence of the placenta. This complication can result in extreme maternal shock and haemorrhage. The inversion should be replaced immediately if noticed before shock supervenes. Otherwise hydrostatic pressure within the vagina is required. This is best achieved through the instillation of warm physiological solution into the vagina under anaesthetic.

Premature rupture of the membranes

Premature rupture of the membranes refers to membrane rupture prior to the commencement of labour. When this occurs there is a risk of intra-uterine infection, and therefore induction of labour must be considered. From 37 weeks onwards active management by early induction may be associated with a higher caesarean rate, though there appears to be a lower risk of endometritis and a lower risk of neonatal infection than with a policy of expectant management. Expectant management is associated with a risk of serious perinatal infection. This is reduced by two thirds by active management, which in such cases involves induction of labour with oxytocin infusion alone or with prostaglandins followed by oxytocin as necessary. The use of prostaglandins is likely to reduce the possibility of eventual caesarean delivery, but there is some concern that it could be associated with a higher rate of serious perinatal infection as it results in some delay in effecting delivery. If < 37 weeks, see Pre-term labour, Chapter 2, page 29.

6.2 The partogram, and slow progress in labour

Learning objectives

You should understand:

- the causes of and the consequences of prolonged labour
- the measures that can be used to deal with slow progress

Normal labour has been described in the section above. While many problems can arise in labour the two most frequent are failure to progress and hypoxia and acidosis in the fetus.

Failure of the labour to progress

This arises in a minority of labours but is capable of causing serious morbidity to both mother and fetus, as outlined in Box 35.

When cervical dilatation fails to occur in the presence of uterine contractions, the fetus is exposed to the risk of hypoxia. Caput formation and moulding of the fetal head will also occur as the uterus attempts to 'squash' the head into the pelvis. Moulding refers to the process whereby the fetal skull bones begin to overlap. This presents a reduced diameter of the fetal head to the birth canal. Caput formation refers to the development of a localised area of oedema overlying the presenting part.

Box 35 Morbidity arising as a result of long labour

Maternal	**Fetal**
● Endometritis	● Congenital pneumonia/infection
● Dehydration	● Risk of hypoxia and acidosis
● Uterine rupture if severe	
● Fistula formation from gross pelvic damage if neglected	

In order to establish if progress is slow during the course of a labour, the midwife will plot the rate of cervical dilatation against time on a graph; this graph is referred to as a partogram. It is a graphic representation of progress over time during the labour. Most women will progress at at least 1 cm per hour and many midwives use this as a pointer for deciding whether action is required to speed up the progress.

If progress falls below this rate, the options are:

- to continue observation
- to rupture the membranes
- to use oxytocin.

There is no defined time limit by which a labour must end. Therefore action is not necessarily required if progress is slow, and the woman is happy with this, and there are no complications. In recent years there has been a trend towards assuring women that their labour will not last longer than a pre-defined length of time, the aim being to avoid the physical and psychological damage that can result from a long traumatic labour.

Amniotomy

The first step that is taken when faced with slow or absent progress in labour is to perform an amniotomy if the membranes have not already ruptured. This is performed by passing a sharp instrument through the cervix and tearing the membranes where they overlie the presenting part. Amniotomy is thought to hasten labour through local release of prostaglandins which augment the uterine contractions. In the course of a normal labour early rupture of the membranes results in a mean reduction in the length of labour of 1–2 hours. This of course means that it has no effect in some women, while in others it may have a marked effect on the duration of labour.

Oxytocin

Oxytocin can be used intravenously to augment uterine contractions and therefore to hasten progress in labour.

and onset of labour, which often take several weeks.

Box 36 Contrasting features of nulliparous and multiparous labour

Nulliparous	Multiparous
• Pelvis of unknown capacity	• Pelvis of proven capacity
• Longer duration	• Shorter duration
• Inefficient uterine action occurs	• Inefficient uterine action rare
• Oxytocin may be required	• Oxytocin rarely required

This may result in more painful contractions, so a careful explanation of the rationale for augmenting the labour is essential. The routine use of early amniotomy and oxytocin has not yet been shown to be effective in reducing caesarean section rates though it does result in labours of shorter duration.

Box 36 outlines some of the features of nulliparous women in labour compared with those who have already delivered a child vaginally. In a multiparous woman, if progress in labour is not satisfactory, it is rarely due to a lack of uterine activity and may be a sign that there is a problem with obstruction. Oxytocin is rarely indicated in this situation. In a nulliparous woman, the uterus may not contract effectively and may therefore respond extremely well to oxytocin administration, resulting in a normal delivery.

Ultimately if labour does not progress, caesarean delivery may be required to prevent the complications of long and neglected labour outlined above. Caesarean delivery would be required if there were failure to progress over a 4-hour period. In a nulliparous woman this would involve lack of progress over such a period despite oxytocin administration. Failure to progress in labour is the underlying reason for almost half the emergency caesarean deliveries in modern practice.

6.3 Induction of labour

Learning objectives

You should:

• understand the reasons labour may be induced

• be familiar with the methods of induction

• understand the disadvantages of induction

This refers to starting labour at a time of medical and social convenience. It is difficult to achieve reliably as one must mimic the natural process of cervical ripening and onset of labour, which often take several weeks. Little is understood about these processes. We do know, however, that prostaglandins are important in cervical ripening and that the process of labour is associated with increased sensitivity to oxytocin.

As the process of induction can be associated with problems it is important that there is a clear reason to induce labour. Some of the more common indications include:

• hypertension or pre-eclampsia
• post-maturity
• antepartum haemorrhage
• intra-uterine growth retardation
• diabetes.

Prior to the natural onset of labour (Ch. 1), cervical ripening occurs. This involves progressive softening of the cervix, accompanied by some dilatation and effacement (see Fig. 10, p. 79). The cervix tends to move toward a more anterior position on vaginal assessment and the vertex descends. The extent to which this has already occurred naturally at the time of induction of labour directly affects the chance of success. For this reason the cervix is assessed prior to making the decision to induce, and a Bishop score (see Ch. 1) is assigned.

Induction involves the use of prostaglandins, amniotomy (physical effect + prostaglandin release), and oxytocin. These are used in such a way as to attempt to mimic their natural actions. The natural mechanism of cervical ripening, however, can take weeks to complete. When a decision is made to induce labour it is because one cannot wait weeks for the delivery to occur.

Prostaglandins

Prostaglandins are used to ripen the cervix. They are effective in inducing labour, in reducing the possibility of failed induction, and in reducing the operative delivery rate following an induced labour. The most commonly used is prostaglandin E_2; although others are effective they require higher doses than E_2. Both endocervical and vaginal applications of prostaglandins will induce labour, though the vaginal route is most commonly used now despite the fact that higher doses are required.

The aim of administering prostaglandins is to dilate the cervix and improve the Bishop score. As they can cause the uterus to contract, uterine hypertonus is a possible side-effect, i.e. the uterus can contract excessively and this can impair placental exchange and make the fetus hypoxic and acidotic (hyperstimulation). Other methods of cervical ripening have included oestrogens, oxytocin, physical methods such as Foley catheter insertion, nipple stimulation and sexual intercourse. None of the above methods has proved reliable and prostaglandins are currently the method of choice.

Problems with induction of labour

- Maternal stress
- Maternal pain
- Vaginal discomfort from the use of pessaries
- Hypertonic uterus
- Failed induction leading to caesarean.

Amniotomy and oxytocin

In addition to augmenting slow labour these techniques are useful in the process of induction, provided some cervical ripening has already occurred. As mentioned previously, causing the uterus to contract without ripening the cervix is analogous to driving a car with the brakes on. If some cervical ripening has already occurred, sweeping of the membranes is another useful technique. This increases the likelihood of expediting normal labour without any apparent increase in complication rate. Sweeping involves passing a finger through the cervix and peeling the membranes off the lower segment of the uterus. It is likely that this works through local prostaglandin release.

Amniotomy should generally only be performed once the Bishop score has become favourable (>5) and the cervix dilated, and should be followed by early use of oxytocin infusion. This reduces the time to delivery with no apparent adverse effect.

6.4 Prolonged pregnancy

If a woman has not gone into spontaneous labour beyond her due date, there comes a time when induction of labour should be considered. A policy of induction of labour at 41 weeks + will result in reduced incidence of meconium staining of the liquor and a reduction in perinatal mortality, in comparison with those pregnancies allowed to continue. There is no evidence that maternal or fetal distress are more common or that caesarean rates are increased (see Table 11).

Table 11 The effect of induction of labour in prolonged pregnancy

	At 39–41 weeks	At 41 weeks +
Epidural rate	–	–
Fetal distress	–	–
Meconium staining	↓	↓
Operative delivery rate	?↑	–
Caesarean	–	?↓
Perinatal mortality	?	↓

Because some women feel very strongly against such intervention, pregnancies may be monitored after 41 weeks to look for fetal compromise. Assessment of liquor volume and cardiotocography are most commonly employed for this.

The rate of perinatal death in patients managed conservatively after 41 weeks is 2.4 per thousand.

6.5 Fetal distress

Learning objectives

You should:

- understand the causes of fetal distress
- understand the role of fetal heart monitoring

Fetal hypoxia and acidosis

The two major problems which arise during the course of labour are failure to progress, which has been addressed above, and fetal hypoxia and acidosis. The term 'fetal distress' is used frequently to denote concern that the fetus is not adequately oxygenated, with or without acidosis. This concern may arise as a result of abnormalities detected on intermittent auscultation of the fetal heart, cardiotocograph monitoring or assessment of the liquor.

Hypoxia may be present prior to the onset of labour, an issue addressed in Chapter 2. It also arises in labour, because of the effect of uterine activity which increases resistance to uterine blood flow; impaired intervillous perfusion follows with deterioration in fetal oxygenation. This improves when the uterine contraction ceases. Repeated episodes, however, may result in progressive fetal hypoxia and eventually acidosis. This is more likely to occur if there is compromise of feto-placental oxygen exchange prior to the onset of labour or insufficient recovery time between contractions.

Causes of fetal distress include:

- progressive hypoxia secondary to uterine activity progressing to acidosis
- intra-uterine infection
- acute events
  - cord prolapse
  - placental abruption
  - scar rupture.

It can be seen from the list of causes that fetal conditions can suddenly deteriorate in labour. Management of labour therefore requires vigilance and awareness of these potential complications.

Diagnosis

The diagnosis of fetal hypoxia and acidosis can be difficult and relies on both direct and indirect tests of fetal well-being together with assessment of the progress of the labour.

Assessment of fetal condition in labour involves:

- overall assessment of risk
  — antepartum haemorrhage
  — intra-uterine growth retardation
  — oligohydramnios
- assessment of the liquor
- assessment of the fetal heart.

It must be stressed that the fetal condition must be interpreted in context, i.e. consideration must be given to the progress of the labour and any possible complications.

Abnormalities of the liquor

There may be an abnormality of liquor volume or meconium staining of the liquor. Oligohydramnios may be indicative of fetal compromise prior to labour or prolonged and unrecognised rupture of the membranes. Meconium staining of the liquor may be associated with fetal compromise and is graded as follows:

- grade 1, dilute meconium staining in an otherwise normal liquor volume
- grade 2, moderate meconium staining
- grade 3, thick 'pea soup' meconium staining of a small volume of liquor.

Passage of meconium can be a physiological event and is more common with increasing fetal maturity. Nonetheless, thick meconium staining must be taken very seriously as a sign of possible fetal compromise.

Fetal heart rate monitoring in labour

Fetal heart rate monitoring is the mainstay of detection of fetal hypoxia and acidosis. Cardiotocography has been described in Chapter 2, and the following comments refer to issues specific to labour.

Traditional care in labour involves auscultation to the fetal heart for 1 minute after a contraction at intervals of approximately 15 minutes. If decelerations are noted, action is taken as they can be a sign of fetal compromise. When electronic fetal heart monitors became available it was felt that they would provide better quality information about fetal condition and therefore prevent occasional cases of fetal acidosis which were not detected by intermittent auscultation. This has not been the case, however, and there is substantial concern that continuous electronic monitoring results in increased and unnecessary intervention. In cases deemed at high risk of fetal compromise, there is no concern about the use of such technology. The debate concerning its value has been largely confined to its application in a 'low-risk' setting. In the interim, many midwives and medical staff have lost the skill of intermittent auscultation, and many more have never developed confidence in the use of the technique. Thus electronic monitoring is frequently used despite considerable scepticism about its true role in 'low-risk' women.

If electronic fetal heart rate monitoring is used (in 'low- risk' women) without recourse to fetal blood sampling to confirm suspected fetal acidosis, caesarean rates can be increased 2–3-fold for 'fetal distress'. This term is deliberately used in this context as fetal acidosis has not been confirmed at the time of delivery. Neonatal outcome does not appear to benefit from intervention in this situation.

When electronic fetal monitoring is used in conjunction with fetal blood sampling to confirm acidosis prior to proceeding to caesarean delivery in 'low-risk' women, caesarean section rates are increased by approximately 30%. Operative vaginal delivery rates are also increased by 30%. The benefits of such a policy have never been clear. The rate of neonatal seizures is reduced by 50% but there is no reduction in the incidence of cerebral palsy. It is possible that the lack of demonstrable benefit reflects a failure of midwifery and medical staff to act appropriately when faced with fetal heart rate abnormalities. Such studies must be viewed in context as intrapartum deaths were fewer than one per thousand, i.e. they were performed in units already providing a high level of care.

The role of fetal monitoring is not confined to preventing fetal or neonatal death; it also aims to reduce morbidity. One in a hundred deliveries will have a cord pH <7.05 with a base excess of < -12 mmol/L and this degree of acidosis may lead to significant neonatal morbidity with risk of seizures and ischaemic damage to vital organs. Timely intervention in response to fetal heart rate abnormalities may help prevent such problems.

Interpretation of cardiotographs (CTGs)

If the recording is not clear, the problem may lie in loss of contact. It is then worth considering the use of a fetal scalp electrode. These electrodes penetrate the fetal scalp to ensure good contact and are applied through the cervix. However, they result in fetal scalp trauma and infection in up to 2% of cases and should not be applied without good indication.

In labour, signs of fetal compromise on the CTG include:

- loss of baseline variability
- decelerations
- baseline changes.

Figure 13 demonstrates these changes.

6.6 Analgesia and anaesthesia

Pain relief in labour

Education is an important component of antenatal care. Information regarding contractions and techniques of pain relief will alleviate anxiety in prospective parents when labour begins. Non-pharmacological methods of pain relief such as relaxation techniques, acupuncture and transcutaneous electrical nerve stimulation (TENS) have no good evidence as to their effectiveness but women often prefer to rely on them in the earliest stages of labour.

Nitrous oxide is a form of inhalational anaesthesia normally provided as Entonox, a 50:50 mixture of nitrous oxide and oxygen. It is more effective than pethidine and has a fast onset and limited duration of action. This provides good pain relief, though it is most suitable for short time periods. For this reason it is most commonly used in the second stage or throughout labour in multiparous women with good progress. The use of narcotics such as pethidine provides effective pain relief but is associated

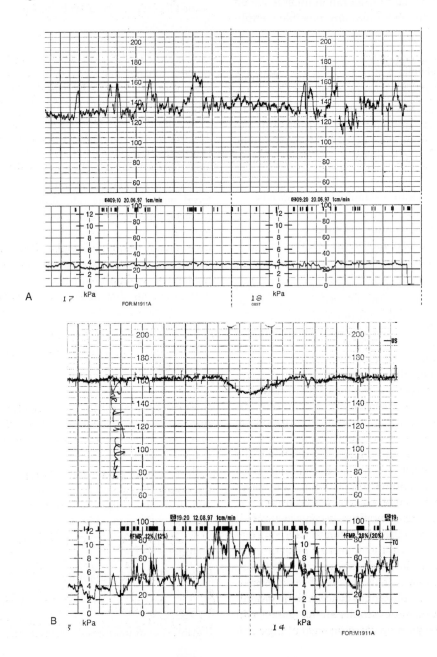

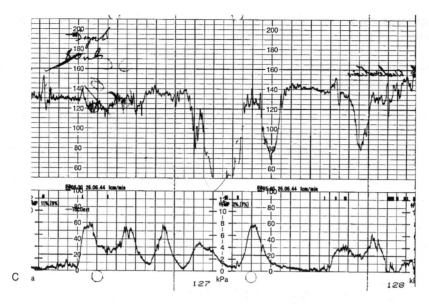

Fig. 13 (**A**) A normal cardiotocograph recording in labour. The baseline is between 150 and 110. The fetal heart has shown two clear accelerations of at least 15 beats per minute. There are no decelerations and the baseline shows beat to beat variation. This is good evidence that there is no fetal compromise. (**B**) This fetus is compromised. The heart rate reveals a tachycardia. There are no reassuring accelerations and no beat to beat variation. The baseline of 165 is flat, reflecting the lack of beat to beat variation, and can be seen to decelerate. From the recording of uterine activity, it can be seen that the deceleration has occurred after the recorded contraction. These are referred to as Type II or late decelerations and indicate a substantial possibility of fetal acidosis. (**C**) The pattern is less clear, as is often the case. There is, however, a normal baseline rate and beat to beat variation, i.e. it is not flat as in (B). There are variable decelerations, which, if persistent, may be associated with fetal acidosis. Fetal blood sampling will help provide reassurance about the fetal condition.

with depressed neonatal Apgar scores. Pethidine may cause maternal nausea, confusion and loss of control. It should therefore be administered with an antiemetic such as metoclopramide. Pethidine also delays gastric emptying, which is of importance if the mother subsequently requires general anaesthesia. It should be avoided in pre-eclampsia as its primary metabolite possesses convulsant properties. Its effect on the neonate is most marked if given to the mother several hours before birth. It can be reversed by administering naloxone 0.2 mg intra-muscularly to the neonate.

Epidural anaesthesia is by far the most effective method of pain relief in labour. Rates of approximately 40% are usual though they will vary depending on availability and the enthusiasm with which it is promoted. Epidural anaesthesia may, however, contribute to delay of up to 2 hours in the length of the second stage, and result in increased use of oxytocin and an increased caesarean section rate. Dural puncture can occur in 0.5% of cases and cause severe headache at a time when the mother is attempting to bond with and commence feeding her newborn baby. Epidural anaesthesia is associated with high rates of instrumental delivery, but this may be due to the fact that instrumental delivery is more likely in labours which are prolonged. There should be appropriate preloading with intravenous

fluids to compensate for the vasodilatation induced by the epidural. Less maternal hypotension occurs with preloading, and less fetal distress.

Strategies with epidurals to prevent operative delivery:

- weaning the block
- different approach to second stage duration (allowing longer time intervals for descent and relocation of the head)
- ? oxytocin.

In the presence of an epidural anaesthetic, oxytocin may reduce the length of the second stage of labour and possibly reduce the need for assisted delivery.

6.7 Primary postpartum haemorrhage

Learning objectives

You must:

- understand the causes of postpartum haemorrhage
- know how to manage postpartum haemorrhage

Primary postpartum haemorrhage is defined as bleeding from the genital tract in excess of 500 ml within 24 hours of delivery. The incidence is 1–2%. In severe cases it can cause maternal shock, possibly emergency hysterectomy, and even death. It occurs most commonly after operative delivery with forceps and ventouse, and also more frequently after twin delivery.

Approximately half the maternal deaths from bleeding are due to postpartum haemorrhage. A major problem is accurate assessment of blood loss. Underestimation by 50% is common. Antenatal care should ensure that the blood group of all women is known so that group compatible uncross-matched blood immediately available if required. Monitoring of full blood counts during antenatal care should ensure that women do not reach term with anaemia due to iron or folate deficiency.

Causes of postpartum haemorrhage (PPH)

Causes of postpartum haemorrhage (PPH) include:

- atonic uterus
- vaginal lacerations
- vulval tears
- cervical tears
- uterine dehiscence
  - previous caesarean
  - previous myomectomy
  - rotational forceps delivery
- broad ligament haematoma.

An atonic uterus is by far the most common cause, though the other causes become more frequent in the most severe haemorrhages. In the acute situation all causes must be considered and the maternal history examined for specific risk factors. Certain specific at-risk groups can be identified:

- multiple pregnancy
- operative delivery (forceps/ventouse)
- antepartum haemorrhage (see Ch. 2)
- placenta praevia
- large fibroids.

Investigations and replacement of the lost intravascular volume must begin immediately. Suspicion of any clotting disorder should prompt the early involvement of a haematologist, and anaesthetic staff should attend to aid in the management of blood loss. Every hospital should have an established protocol for such cases.

Investigation

Investigations are performed at the same time as intravenous lines are inserted to minimise delay:

- full blood count
- clotting screen

- disseminated intravascular coagulation screen
- cross-match 2–6 units, depending on severity
- urea and electrolytes (baseline).

Management

- Deliver the placenta (may already be delivered)
- Ensure the uterus is contracted
- Replace intravascular volume acutely
- Examination under anaesthesia if on-going bleeding after uterus contracts, or if the uterus fails to contract, or if placenta/membranes may not have been completely delivered
- Repair vulval or vaginal lacerations without delay
- Oxytocic drugs:
  - oxytocin 10 IU stat i.v. followed by an oxytocin infusion (40 IU in 0.5 L of saline over 4 hours)
  - ergometrine 0.25 mg i.v.
- 'Rub up' a contraction (may work through local prostaglandin release; also expresses blood clot from the cavity)
- Prostaglandins by direct injection into the uterus.

Emergency hysterectomy is occasionally necessary and is best performed before disseminated intravascular coagulation arises. Indications include:

- primary postpartum haemorrhage
- ruptured uterus
- secondary postpartum haemorrhage.

Placenta accreta

This is a condition in which there is complete adherence of the placenta to the uterine wall, preventing placental detachment. It is more likely to arise in the presence of previous uterine surgery such as caesarean section or myomectomy; if the placenta implants over the scarred area, there may be no plane of cleavage between the placenta and uterus. Treatment options include hysterectomy, or conservative management whereby the placenta is left in place to undergo autolysis under antibiotic cover.

6.8 Infection in labour

Infection represents a significant risk in labour. In Chapter 3 perinatal transmission of maternal infection was reviewed. Ascending infection can also arise during the course of labour, resulting in:

- fetal infection
- chorioamnionitis
- neonatal infection usually manifest as pneumonia
- endometritis and secondary postpartum haemorrhage.

Predisposing factors include prolonged labour, prolonged rupture of the membranes, multiple vaginal examinations, and the use of fetal scalp electrodes. Prevention therefore involves avoiding unnecessary vaginal examination and intervention.

Signs of ascending infection include maternal pyrexia and tachycardia, uterine tenderness, and fetal tachycardia ± meconium staining of the liquor.

The response to any of the above signs involves a thorough assessment of the clinical situation and the possible presence of predisposing factors. If delivery is imminent or the progress in labour rapid, it is reasonable to treat the woman with intravenous broad spectrum antibiotics after collecting all relevant culture specimens including blood cultures and high vaginal swab. If progress is slow and delivery not imminent, immediate caesarean delivery should be considered.

6.9 Amniotic fluid embolism

Amniotic fluid embolism is still a significant cause of maternal mortality, having resulted in 17 deaths in the 3-year period 1994–96 in the latest UK triennial report on maternal mortality. Maternal death may occur despite early recognition and immediate treatment of the condition.

It arises when amniotic fluid gains access to the maternal circulation, resulting in a sudden and massive activation of the clotting cascade leading to disseminated intravascular coagulation. Factors which were believed to predispose to it include the use of oxytocic agents such as oxytocin or prostaglandins, resulting in elevated intrauterine pressure. This was thought to predispose to dissemination of amniotic content into a uterine vein with the systemic sequelae. This association is now less clear and it is also apparent that the condition can arise in nulliparous women as well as multiparous women.

Presentation

- Postpartum haemorrhage of undue severity or without apparent explanation
- Sudden maternal collapse either during or after labour
- Disseminated intravascular coagulation during labour or within hours of delivery
- Respiratory problems such as adult respiratory distress syndrome, haemoptysis, pulmonary oedema and cyanosis
- Convulsions.

It appears to be associated with caesarean delivery but this is not to say that the mode of delivery is causative, though it may be in some instances through leakage of amniotic fluid into uterine veins. The characteristic finding on autopsy examination is fetal squames or hair in the maternal lungs. In cases of collapse which are successfully resuscitated, diagnosis is impossible on these criteria. Therefore the extent to which this condition causes morbidity is unknown. Squames might potentially be detectable in sputum or blood collected from a central line.

Treatment

1. Resuscitative measures to allow time for clearance of the thrombi in the pulmonary vasculature
2. Fresh frozen plasma to correct clotting defects
3. Prevention and/or treatment of postpartum haemorrhage.

6.10 Intrapartum stillbirths

As mentioned in Chapter 9, intrapartum stillbirths have recently been reviewed as part of the Confidential Enquiry into Stillbirths and Deaths in Infancy. Within this enquiry intrapartum related deaths accounted for 4.3% of perinatal deaths. An attempt was made to define suboptimal care that might have contributed to a death.

The median birth weight was 3.39 kg with 40% weighing > 3.5 kg and 14% weighing > 4 kg. This represents considerable loss rates in larger than average babies and emphasises that attention should not be focused solely on babies suffering from impaired fetal growth alone.

Risk factors in the intrapartum period include:

- fetal distress/asphyxia (67%) in the latest CESDI enquiry
- fetal growth retardation
- oligohydramnios
- antepartum haemorrhage
- trauma
  — shoulder dystocia
  — breech delivery
  — delivery of the second twin
  — operative vaginal delivery
  — cord prolapse.

All the above factors serve to emphasise that intrapartum losses are still too common. The enquiry attempted to define the incidence of suboptimal care in this group, and found the following: in 17%, no suboptimal care; in 12%, care suboptimal, but different management unlikely to have altered outcome; in 28%, an avoidable factor was identified, and different management might have made a difference; and in 42%, different management might reasonably have been expected to alter the outcome.

Self-assessment: questions

Multiple choice questions

1. Regarding obstetric haemorrhage:
   a. Women are more likely to die from postpartum haemorrhage than antepartum haemorrhage
   b. O negative blood should be given immediately in the presence of a postpartum haemorrhage of one litre
   c. There is no value in measuring urea and electrolytes in women with postpartum haemorrhage
   d. Disseminated intravascular coagulation should be checked for at the bedside by the attending doctor
   e. Uncross-matched blood should never be transfused in modern obstetric practice

2. Fetal blood sampling is indicated in the presence of delayed decelerations and:
   a. Clinical signs of scar rupture
   b. Slow progress in a nulliparous patient despite oxytocin augmentation for 4 hours
   c. Grade 1 meconium at 7 cm dilatation
   d. Fresh vaginal bleeding suggestive of a possible retroplacental bleed
   e. In an HIV positive patient presenting in labour at 4 cm dilatation

3. One may make a diagnosis of labour:
   a. In a primigravid patient who is 2 cm dilated and experiencing regular contractions
   b. In a multiparous patient with irregular contractions where the cervix is 2 cm dilated as it will admit 1–2 fingers on vaginal examination
   c. In a nulliparous woman who is contracting once every 4 minutes, has ruptured her membranes spontaneously and in whom the cervix is fully effaced though not dilated
   d. In a multiparous patient who is extremely distressed with pains, irregular contractions on the monitor, and who says she lost a show of blood at home
   e. In a woman who is having irregular contractions, is distressed by them and who has had a caesarean delivery in her last pregnancy

4. In current midwifery and obstetric practice:
   a. Liberal use of episiotomy is encouraged
   b. A third degree tear is one which extends to the vaginal fornix
   c. Most episiotomies should be sutured with interrupted polyglycolic acid
   d. Vulval tears may be left unsutured
   e. Swabs must never be put into the vagina unless specifically counted prior to and after the procedure

5. Caesarean delivery is indicated:
   a. In a nulliparous woman at 7 cm who has not progressed over a 4-hour period
   b. In a multiparous woman at 3 cm who is contracting once every 5 minutes with no progress over 6 hours
   c. In a woman who has previously been delivered by caesarean section and is now stuck at 7 cm for 4 hours after labouring spontaneously with good contractions every 2–3 minutes. She is desperate to achieve a normal delivery on this occasion
   d. In an overweight multiparous woman who has laboured spontaneously and reached 8 cm dilatation with strong contractions every 2 minutes. She has not progressed for 4 hours but has not yet had oxytocin; there is marked caput and moulding on vaginal examination and the head is still not engaged
   e. In a multiparous woman who has previously delivered a 4.5 kg baby, and is found to have a footling breech presentation at 5 cm dilatation

6. Induction of labour for postmaturity at term + 10 days:
   a. Results in an increased caesarean section rate
   b. Means the woman is likely to need an epidural anaesthetic
   c. Results in less meconium aspiration
   d. Prevents some late intra-uterine deaths
   e. Is not acceptable to some women

7. Management of a woman who has previously experienced an intra-uterine death due to intrauterine growth retardation at 36 weeks should include
   a. Elective delivery at 34 weeks
   b. Low dose aspirin and heparin from 12 weeks
   c. Delivery by caesarean section
   d. An early dating scan
   e. Hospital-based care

8. With regard to primary postpartum haemorrhage:
   a. It is partly preventable
   b. It should be immediately treated with prostaglandin administration to contract the uterus
   c. It can be helped by rubbing the uterus
   d. Early replacement of lost volume helps prevent coagulation problems
   e. O negative blood must be given immediately

9. Regarding the use of oxytocin and amniotomy:
   a. Oxytocin can cause fetal hypoxia
   b. Abnormalities on a cardiotocograph after amniotomy should prompt vaginal examination
   c. Once amniotomy is performed the process of induction should be regarded as irreversible
   d. Oxytocin must be given in carefully titrated dose depending on the uterine activity
   e. Oxytocin is used more commonly in nulliparous women as they are more sensitive to it

Short notes

1. Write short notes on the mechanism of normal delivery of the fetus.

2. Write short notes outlining your investigation of the cause of a stillbirth.

3. Outline your management of a patient who collapses suddenly in labour, with specific reference to the differential diagnosis.

Self-assessment: answers

Multiple choice answers

1. a. **False.** Deaths from each category are approximately equal.
   b. **False.** O negative blood should only rarely be given in modern practice. The vast majority of women presenting with postpartum haemorrhage will have had their blood group checked in the antenatal period and group compatible uncross-matched blood should therefore be given. Inappropriate use of O negative blood can give rise to anti-C antibodies.
   c. **False.** These measurements need not be performed routinely. In the presence of the most severe haemorrhage, however, it can be useful to know that baseline renal function as assessed by the serum creatinine is normal. Use of large doses of oxytocin (especially with hypotonic solutions) can lead to serious hyponatraemia, and knowledge of serum sodium can be useful in these cases.
   d. **False.** This cannot be performed reliably by most doctors and their time should be spent on the emergency management of the clinical problem, i.e. assessing the patient, correcting the bleeding and ensuring adequate volume replacement.
   e. **False.** See question 2.

2. a. **False.** One should proceed immediately to caesarean delivery. Delay in this situation or in the presence of placental abruption is inappropriate and may result in fetal death.
   b. **False.** There is little point in performing fetal blood sampling as the clinical situation warrants caesarean delivery at any rate due to lack of progress.
   c. **True.**
   d. **False.** See question 1.
   e. **False.** Performance of fetal blood sampling would put the fetus at increased risk of perinatal transmission of the virus.

3. a. **True.**
   b. **False.** Irregular contractions do not support a diagnosis of labour. Many multiparous patients will have a cervix which is 2–3 cm dilated (and 1–2 cm long) in the latter part of pregnancy despite not being in labour; this is often referred to as a 'multips os' and reflects alterations in the cervix secondary to the first delivery.
   c. **True.** Despite the lack of cervical dilatation, spontaneous rupture of the membranes and effacement of the cervix are supportive of the diagnosis of labour.
   d. **False.** This is not sufficient to support a diagnosis of labour. She may subsequently develop more regular contractions, so that the advice to her should be cautious and not dogmatic. More worryingly, her symptoms would be consistent with a retroplacental haemorrhage. Observation on the antenatal ward may be the best option.
   e. **False.** This is not sufficient to support a diagnosis of labour. As with the preceding case, it would be reasonable to observe such a lady on the antenatal ward as it is good practice to monitor any trial of scar in labour and labour is likely to be imminent.

4. a. **False.**
   b. **False.** A third degree tear is one which disrupts the anal sphincter.
   c. **False.** Continuous suturing of the perineal skin is good practice unless there are specific reasons to insert more painful interrupted sutures.
   d. **True.** Vulval tears require suturing only if bleeding as they can be quite painful to repair and heal well without suturing.
   e. **True.** Retained swabs are a cause of infection, foul-smelling discharge and litigation!

5. a. **False.** She should first have a trial of oxytocin administration as inefficient uterine action is common in nulliparous women.
   b. **False.** With this picture, the diagnosis of labour must be reconsidered. If an amniotomy has already been performed she can be induced with the use of an oxytocin infusion.
   c. **True.** This woman should be delivered by repeat caesarean delivery. The use of oxytocin may cause the uterus to rupture. While her wish to avoid caesarean delivery must be considered, she must be advised that rupture of the scar is a possibility with potentially disastrous consequences.
   d. **True.** Fetal macrosomia is associated with increasing maternal weight: the overweight multiparous woman may well have a macrosomic baby and hence the reason for the obstructed labour with the high head. Use of oxytocin in this situation could cause uterine rupture.
   e. **True.** The rationale for caesarean delivery with a footling breech is to avoid cord prolapse and therefore the capacity of the woman's pelvis is not relevant.

6. a. **False.** There is no evidence to support this and the caesarean rate may be decreased by such a policy.
   b. **False.**
   c. **True.**
   d. **True.** Though rare, intra-uterine death may occur at this stage of the pregnancy even in a well-grown baby.
   e. **True.** Some women do not find induction acceptable as they feel it is unnecessarily intrusive and unnatural despite the apparent benefits. Also there is no doubt that induction can fail and the woman can be exposed to a period of stress and discomfort during the process.

7. a. **False.** Her care should involve accurate dating from early in the pregnancy and then serial ultrasound assessment at 2–4-week intervals depending on the level of clinical concern. Any decision to deliver prior to full fetal maturity at 38 weeks would depend on evidence of fetal compromise on ultrasound assessment.
   b. **False**, unless the mother was anticardiolipin positive. Low dose aspirin has been used for this indication in the past and appears not to do any harm, though the benefits have been questioned. Heparin can have serious side-effects and should never be prescribed without a clear indication.
   c. **False**, unless there was significant fetal compromise.
   d. **True.**
   e. **True.**

8. a. **True.** The incidence is reduced by prophylactic administration of oxytocin or ergometrine.
   b. **False.** Oxytocin and ergometrine are used in the first instance. Prostaglandins are normally used only when these have failed and the uterus has been explored under anaesthesia.
   c. **True.** This has never been proven, but it appears to help and may do so by preventing clot accumulating in the cavity and causing some local prostaglandin release within the uterus.
   d. **True.** Allowing the patient to become severely volume depleted appears to increase the possibility of disseminated intravascular coagulation occurring.
   e. **False.** See question 1b. Replacement of intravascular volume with crystalloid and colloid is reasonable in the first instance.

9. a. **True**, if uterine hypertonicity is caused.
   b. **True**, to exclude cord prolapse.
   c. **True**, because there is a risk of ascending infection once the forewaters have been ruptured.
   d. **True**, to minimise the complication of hypertonicity.
   e. **False.** Multiparous women are more sensitive to oxytocin and this is one factor which increases their risk of uterine rupture.

Short notes answers

1. At the onset of labour, the fetal head should be engaged. This will normally be in the occipito-transverse position as the normal gynaecoid pelvis presents the most favourable diameter as the transverse at the pelvic inlet.

   The head will descend in the transverse position through the mid cavity. The oval shape of the inlet, however, is not maintained as the mid cavity is traversed; it becomes more circular in shape and therefore some rotation of the head may occur at this stage. Also as the head descends, flexion is maintained.

   On reaching the level of the levator muscles, however, the head is encouraged to rotate to an occipito-anterior position as a result of the shape of the muscular hammock and the increasing space available in the anterior-posterior diameter as the outlet is approached.

   In parallel with the internal rotation of the head, the fetal body must flex laterally to allow for the concave nature of the sacrum. As the shoulders enter the pelvis they will normally rotate out of the antero-posterior plane as this will provide a more favourable diameter. At delivery the fetal head will externally rotate back to a transverse position (restitution), the shoulders will deliver (anterior first) and the fetal body will follow.

2. Investigation of a stillbirth should be directed towards specific causes.

   1. Postmortem examination of the fetus should be requested. This will determine if there are any underlying congenital abnormalities or evidence of a chromosomal problem such as aneuploidy. Evidence of intra-uterine infection may be found (microcephaly) or of the effects of maternal disease on fetal well-being (macrosomia and cardiomyopathy in infants of diabetic mothers).
   2. If a postmortem is declined, important information can be obtained by an X-ray of the baby (as in dwarf syndromes) or by a specific biopsy such as a trucut liver or renal biopsy. A picture of the baby might provide useful information subsequently for a geneticist reviewing the case.
   3. The baby can be karyotyped from a blood sample obtained by a cardiac stab, or by providing a

sample of tissue such as skin. A placental biopsy can be obtained though there will occasionally be discrepant results due to placental mosaicism.

4. Placental examination is important as evidence of abruption may substantiate the clinical history, or evidence of intra-uterine infection may be seen as in chorioamnionitis.

5. Swabs of the maternal and fetal surfaces may help isolate a particular infectious agent. A biopsy of placental tissue may aid in the culture of infectious agents such as listeria.

6. History taking and physical examination of the mother is important as maternal disease is associated with intra-uterine death. This should include blood pressure and urinalysis.

7. Investigation of the mother should include:

- platelet count, creatinine, clotting   ? pre-eclampsia
- creatinine   ? renal disease
- liver function tests + serum bile acid   ? pre-eclampsia if ? cholestasis
- glucose tolerance   if ? diabetes
- anticardiolipin antibodies + lupus anticoagulant   ?anticardiolipin syndrome
- serum for antibody testing   if ? congenital infection
- screen for alloimmune anti-platelet antibodies   if fetal haemorrhagic complications

Despite all the above investigations the cause of intra-uterine death is often not known. It must be stressed that the most valuable information is gained by a careful review of the maternal history during the course of the pregnancy, and the family history.

3. Sudden collapse in labour is a rare event and the first priority is to summon help. Immediate attention must then be directed towards ensuring:

- the airway is patent
- there is effective respiration
- there is a pulse.

In the absence of any of the above, basic resuscitation should be instituted. The patient should be kept on her left side during the assessment to prevent supine hypotension syndrome. After this, consideration of the cause should dictate the examination and investigation of the patient.

Haemorrhagic complications are common in obstetric practice. Such a complication will normally be indicated by a high pulse rate and low blood pressure. Haemorrhage will either be revealed or concealed. Revealed haemorrhage does not pose a problem for diagnosis, and if severe should be managed by caesarean delivery unless vaginal delivery is imminent (or the baby is dead). Concealed haemorrhage needs to be considered if there is any history of abdominal or pelvic pain, especially in the presence of a uterine scar. Scar rupture would normally manifest with some vaginal bleeding or fetal distress.

Cerebral haemorrhage and eclampsia are predictable risks in patients suffering from pre-eclampsia. Seizure activity should be evident at the time of collapse and neurological signs are likely to be present. In the presence of signs of pre-eclampsia it is reasonable to treat seizures as of eclamptic origin in the first instance. If there is any doubt about the diagnosis, however, a computed tomography (CT) scan should be arranged.

Amniotic fluid embolism may manifest as sudden collapse. Associated features which would support the diagnosis include respiratory distress or cyanosis, or sudden development of a coagulopathy. This diagnosis can only be confidently made by detecting fetal squames or hair in blood taken from a central line, or in the sputum. Management involves resuscitative measures and aggressive treatment of any coagulopathy with fresh frozen plasma.

Pulmonary embolism is a rare event in labour but it would have to be considered in this clinical scenario. It tends to occur with specific risk factors such as prolonged bed rest or thrombophilia, and in the older woman. A history of chest pain or haemoptysis prior to collapse would be supportive, as would cyanosis or respiratory distress. The jugular venous pressure would be raised. An immediate oxygen saturation can be performed on most labour wards and blood gas results should be available within minutes to support or refute the diagnosis. ECG and chest X-ray may help, but a perfusion scan gives the most specific diagnosis. If the embolus is acutely life-threatening, intravenous heparin should be given even though the woman is in labour. Mechanical disruption of the clot may be aided by resuscitative measures if the patient does not have an output, and thrombolytic therapy is useful if the clot is massive.

In the older woman, myocardial infarction must be considered. There would normally have been a history of chest pain or respiratory distress secondary to pulmonary oedema. Other causes that should be considered if there are specific clinical concerns include hypo- and hyperglycaemia, sepsis syndrome, anaphylaxis and intra-abdominal bleeding from a splenic artery aneurysm or hepatic haemorrhage.

7 Malpresentation and operative delivery

Overview

With occipito-posterior, face and brow presentations, there is increased difficulty with delivery as an unfavourable diameter of the fetal head tries to advance through the pelvis. Occipito-posterior positions are the most common and often require operative delivery with a ventouse extractor. Breech presentation often results in caesarean delivery as this seems safest for the baby. This has also resulted in increased use of caesarean section for twin deliveries as the presentation of twin II cannot be determined in advance. Shoulder dystocia is a serious though rare complication of vaginal delivery that can result in serious morbidity for the neonate. Vaginal delivery after caesarean section can be achieved with safety provided certain precautions are adhered to in labour.

7.1 Occipito-posterior, face and brow presentations

Learning objectives

You should:

- be familiar with the causes of malpresentation
- understand the problems associated with malpresentation
- be familiar with the treatment options

Chapter 6 describes normal labour with a well flexed cephalic presentation, eventually delivering a baby in an occipito-anterior position. When the fetus presents in any other way there are increased risks of dysfunctional labour, and difficulty in the second stage.

Causes of malpresentation

- Prematurity
- Multiple pregnancy
- Fetal death
- Congenital abnormalities
- Abnormalities of liquor volume
- Space-occupying lesion in the pelvis
- Small pelvic inlet.

Adverse consequences of malpresentation

- Cord prolapse
- Obstructed labour with risk of:
  — infection
  — ruptured uterus
  — fistula formation if neglected.

Occipito-posterior (OP) positions

Normal labour involves flexion of the fetal head resulting in the occiput being the leading fetal part. The occiput rotates anteriorly when the force of uterine contractions causes it to descend against the gutter of the pelvic floor. In the absence of flexion, the bregma or brow may descend and rotate anteriorly, resulting in the occiput being posterior. Most labours which begin with the occiput in a posterior position result in a delivery of a baby in the occipito-anterior position following successful rotation. In approximately 5% of labours, however, the OP position persists. An android pelvis in which the inlet is a triangular shape and in which there is little room for subsequent rotation predisposes to a persistent OP position.

It is possible to diagnose an OP position prior to labour, though there is little value in doing so as most will rotate. The main feature suggesting an OP position is a flat, almost concave, appearance below the umbilicus. In labour the diagnosis is made by examination of the suture lines and identification of the fontanelles (Fig. 14). It is often associated with a high presenting part.

OP positions are associated with long labour, and this should be considered when analgesia is requested and when determining how best to monitor the fetal condition. Efficient uterine action should be ensured in nulliparous women to maintain flexion of the fetal head. Caesarean section is indicated in the event of failed progress despite ensuring adequate uterine activity. In the second stage of labour, many OP positions will rotate to occipito-anterior. Should the presenting part remain high and in an OP position after pushing, operative delivery should be considered. The options include:

- caesarean section, if the head is two-fifths palpable or more abdominally, or pelvic and abdominal assessment suggest there is disproportion
- ventouse delivery with an occipito-posterior cup
- Kielland's rotational forceps delivery
- manual rotation and delivery
- mid cavity forceps delivery without rotation.

Ventouse delivery is the most favoured method as it results in less maternal trauma. Kielland's forceps have fallen into disrepute in some quarters because of a perception of increased maternal and fetal trauma, but some operators would still prefer them to the ventouse.

Face presentation

If the head is hyperextended, the face presents (Fig. 15A). This occurs in approximately 0.2% of deliveries. Diagnosis is by palpation of the nose, mouth and orbital ridges on vaginal examination.

It may be precipitated by:

- anencephaly
- swelling in the neck region
- any other mechanism causing extension of the fetal head.

The mechanisms of labour will try to achieve anterior rotation of the chin under the symphysis pubis. Successful delivery may occur especially if mento-anterior, but caesarean section will be necessary in a substantial proportion of cases. Fetal scalp electrodes must not be applied with a face presentation and ventouse must not be used. Marked facial oedema may occur with a face presentation and obscure the diagnosis.

Brow presentation

A brow presentation is even less common. The area of the fetal head between the anterior fontanelle and the orbital ridge presents (Fig. 15B). This represents a state between full flexion and extension, which may convert

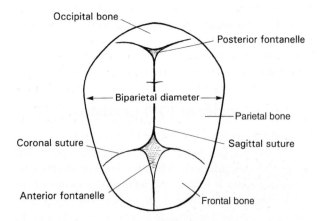

Fig. 14 The suture lines and fontanelles of the fetal skull.

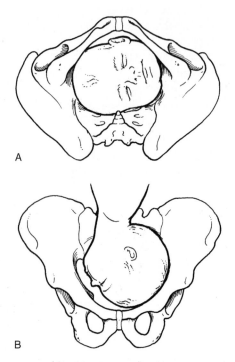

Fig. 15 (**A**) Face presentation. (**B**) Brow presentation.

to either an occiput or face presentation during labour. If the brow presentation persists, vaginal delivery is very unlikely unless there is a large pelvis relative to fetal size.

7.2 Breech presentation and delivery

Learning objectives

You should:

- be familiar with the causes of a breech presentation

- know how to diagnose a breech

- understand the advantages and disadvantages of caesarean and vaginal breech delivery

Breech presentation refers to the unusual situation where the buttocks overlie the pelvis and the head of the fetus is palpable at the uterine fundus. The incidence at term is approximately 3%. Prior to term it is a more common finding as the fetus has not yet settled into a stable position. This is thought to reflect the greater proportion of amniotic fluid (maximal at 32 weeks) creating space for the fetus to continually change position. As term approaches, the relative amount of amniotic fluid diminishes significantly and the fetal lie becomes more stable.

Types of breech presentation

A 'frank breech' presentation whereby the hips are flexed and the legs are extended so that the buttocks lie over the pelvis (Fig. 16A) is the most common type. In a complete breech, the feet and buttocks are alongside each other overlying the pelvis (Fig. 16B). In a footling breech, the feet are below the buttocks and overlie the pelvis (Fig. 16C).

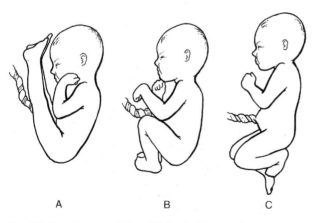

A   B   C

Fig. 16 Breech presentation: (**A**) frank; (**B**) complete; (**C**) footling.

Predisposing factors

- Prematurity
- Polyhydramnios
- Multiple pregnancy
- Factors which displace the presenting part
  — placenta praevia
  — fibroids
- Congenital malformations of the uterus.

As it is not unusual for a fetus to present by the breech prior to term, it only becomes a matter of importance from 34–36 weeks onwards. If a woman goes into labour with a breech presentation prior to 34 weeks it is a matter of individual judgement whether she is delivered by caesarean or not.

Detecting a breech presentation

- Head may be palpable at the fundus
- Fetal heart may be most easily heard above the umbilicus
- The presenting part does not feel as firm
- You may think the head is engaged; think again.

'Beware the well engaged head, for it may not be a head at all.'

If a breech presentation is detected, the options for delivery must be discussed. These include a trial of breech delivery, caesarean section, or external cephalic version.

Vaginal breech delivery

Vaginal delivery with a cephalic presentation is usually uncomplicated because if the head has delivered, the body will automatically follow except in cases of shoulder dystocia (see below). This is because the head is the firmest part of the fetal anatomy and the largest. With a vaginal breech birth, the opposite applies. If the breech is born there is no guarantee that the head will pass through the pelvis without difficulty. Furthermore, the head will have no opportunity to mould as it would with a cephalic presentation. If the breech delivers and the head becomes stuck, the fetus will rapidly become hypoxic as the umbilical cord is compressed in the birth canal. This potentially disastrous complication of a 'trapped aftercoming head' is fortunately rare (0.5%), but is sufficiently alarming to create concern about vaginal breech birth with both prospective parents and professionals. As a result, there has been a trend towards confining vaginal breech birth to situations where there is an extremely high likelihood of success, i.e.:

- proven pelvic capacity
  — previous delivery
  — adequate X-ray pelvimetry
  — adequate clinical pelvimetry
- fetal macrosomia excluded
  — estimated fetal weight on scan < 3.8 kg

— clinical palpation consistent with this
- good progress in spontaneous labour
- exclusion of a hyperextended head.

In a nulliparous woman, the pelvis is untried so caesarean delivery is often preferred. If the woman particularly wants a vaginal delivery, an ultrasound assessment of fetal weight and either a clinical or X-ray assessment of pelvic size are sometimes performed. On X-ray assessment, the following features are sought: good sacral curve, pelvic inlet >11.5 cm, pelvic outlet >11.5 cm. These measurements are not absolute and allow for pelvic soft tissues during delivery and some margin of error. In a multiparous patient, with proven pelvic capacity, the main concern is to exclude fetal macrosomia. Despite these investigations, head entrapment or difficult delivery of the breech remains an unpredictable event.

Caesarean delivery

Caesarean delivery is always an option with a breech presentation because of the concerns outlined above. A recent study suggests unequivocally that it is safest for the baby. One problem with caesarean section is that it increases maternal risk even when performed under optimal circumstances with regional anaesthesia. It also complicates future deliveries in view of the risk of scar dehiscence. An added concern as caesarean rates for breech presentation increase is that medical and midwifery staff become less familiar with vaginal breech birth.

External cephalic version

This refers to the process of manipulating the fetus in an attempt to achieve a cephalic presentation. Analgesia is not generally required but the fetus must be monitored before and after the event. Retroplacental haemorrhage and cord entanglement are very rare complications. Contraindications include a previous caesarean or myomectomy. Anti-D is given to Rhesus negative women.

External cephalic version is contraindicated prior to 37 weeks' gestation because so many fetuses revert to the breech presentation. There is thus no reduction in eventual caesarean section rate. When performed at 37 weeks, however, there is a reduction in both breech births and caesarean sections, but no effect on perinatal mortality.

For the breech presentation at term there is now evidence to suggest that caesarean delivery is best. A policy of routine caesarean section will increase maternal morbidity but reduce perinatal morbidity. It is likely also that where the intention is to deliver vaginally, up to 50% of women will still require caesarean delivery as a result of concerns arising in labour. Attempts at external cephalic version appear to be justified in this context.

7.3 Transverse and oblique lies

The predisposing factors to transverse lie (Fig. 17) are similar to those of a breech presentation, i.e. factors which prevent a presenting part from stabilising within the pelvis or which prevent alterations in fetal position. When faced with such a presentation there is a risk of cord prolapse when the membranes rupture, and a risk of uterine rupture from obstructed labour once uterine activity begins. Caesarean delivery is therefore required.

7.4 Delivery of twins

Learning objective

You should:

- understand the difficulties with twin delivery

Twin pregnancy has been discussed in Chapter 2 and presentation in labour described.

Most of the risk with delivery of twins relates to the delivery of the second twin. After the first twin is delivered the second will enter the cavity. If the second twin is cephalic it should be delivered normally. If transverse, the obstetrician will manipulate the twin to deliver it by the breech, usually by bringing a foot down. The interval between the delivery of each twin is important. During this time the uterus contracts, which can result in shearing of the placenta from the uterine wall with resultant fetal hypoxia. Problems with twin labour and delivery can be summarised as:

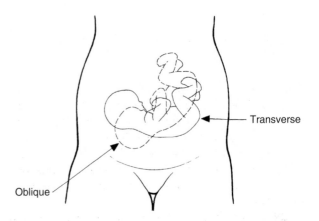

Fig. 17 Transverse and oblique lies.

1. difficulty in monitoring both twins during labour
2. fetal hypoxia arising in the second twin after delivery of the first
3. trauma during attempts at delivering the second twin.

It is generally recommended that the interval between delivery of twins should not exceed 30 minutes. There is no evidence to support a policy of delivering a second twin by caesarean section if not presenting by the vertex, as this exposes the mother to increased risk.

If for any reason there are complications during the course of the pregnancy, or specific concerns about pelvic capacity, elective caesarean may be recommended. If the twins are monoamniotic, elective caesarean section is advisable in view of the risk of cord entanglement and prolapse. Most commonly the leading twin presents by the vertex, and vaginal delivery is appropriate. If the leading twin is transverse, caesarean will be necessary, and if a breech, caesarean is commonly advised. The antenatal presentation of the second twin is not relevant as this often changes once the first twin is delivered.

Outcome

Perinatal mortality rates are significantly higher in all categories with twin pregnancy. Infant mortality rates are also higher once the babies reach home. Furthermore, there is increased morbidity in twins. These problems are often exacerbated by the difficulty in coping with twins under optimal conditions. Multiple pregnancy results in many problems for prospective parents, which emphasises the need for expert care during pregnancy and adequate postnatal support in the home environment.

7.5 Shoulder dystocia

Learning objective

You should:

- be familiar with a management plan for shoulder dystocia

This is an acute obstetric emergency. It occurs when the fetal head is delivered but the anterior shoulder becomes trapped behind the pubic bone preventing delivery of the body. It is more likely to occur in situations where the size of the body is increased relative to the head size, i.e. in some cases of macrosomia (it is more common with diabetes) and other abnormalities.

It is extremely difficult to predict, but becomes more likely with increasing fetal weight. There is a substantial perinatal loss rate associated with this condition. This is a result of:

- trauma due to excessive traction on the baby at delivery – this can cause brachial plexus injury
- asphyxia secondary to hypoxia whilst the baby is stuck.

Management

1. Remain calm and call for senior help
2. Do not apply excessive traction on the head (this is fruitless)
3. Put the patient into McRobert's position, where the patient is in lithotomy with hips hyperflexed and abducted. This increases the effective pelvic diameters and aids delivery.
4. Ensure there is a liberal episiotomy to aid manipulation
5. An assistant should apply gentle but firm supra-pubic pressure to bring the shoulder anteriorly across the fetal chest whilst gentle downward traction is applied to the head
6. The posterior shoulder can be delivered provided there is adequate room in the pelvis for the arm to be reached and brought down.

There are other extreme measures which can be used in desperate situations, but experience in their use is not widespread and they can cause complications for both mother and baby.

7.6 Ventouse delivery

Learning objectives

You should:

- understand when it is safe to use the ventouse and forceps

- be familiar with the advantages and disadvantages of the ventouse and forceps

The ventouse can be used to deliver the fetal head at full dilatation. An alternative is delivery with forceps, which will be described later. Methods to deliver the fetus in the second stage have developed in parallel with increasing safety of caesarean section, and with greater expectation of the parents regarding safety for the fetus. For this reason, attempts at vaginal delivery when the head is high are now no longer acceptable, and vaginal delivery is now only attempted when the obstetrician is confident that delivery can be performed without undue difficulty and with good outcome for mother and baby. The ventouse or vacuum extractor works by the application of suction to the fetal head, following which traction is applied with the aid of maternal effort.

Indications for operative delivery

- Fetal distress (40%)
- Maternal exhaustion or poor maternal effort (50%)
- To avoid maternal effort (e.g. severe hypertension)
- Delivery of a second twin.

It is likely that the proportion of assisted deliveries will vary depending upon the epidural rate. In the presence of an epidural anaesthetic, assisted delivery is more likely to be required, but it is an easier procedure for the obstetrician, and less painful for the mother.

Criteria for ventouse extraction or forceps

- Proper indication
- Maternal analgesia
- Cervix fully dilated
- Position of the fetal head is determined
- Fetal head one-fifth or less palpable abdominally
- Bladder empty
- Membranes ruptured.

Contraindications to the ventouse

- Cephalopelvic disproportion
- Face, brow or breech presentation
- Prematurity (<34 weeks).

Principles of ventouse delivery

The patient is positioned in the lithotomy position. The vulval area is cleansed and draped. Continuous attention to the fetal heart rate is essential. A vaginal examination is repeated to confirm full dilatation, the position of the head and the station. The bladder should be catheterised. Adequate analgesia is important. This is often achieved with local infiltration of the perineum, with or without a pudendal block. An epidural block may be used or may already be in place. Although epidural analgesia represents the best analgesia, it interferes with the urge to push, in a situation where maternal effort is an important component of the delivery. The ventouse should be applied to that area of the fetal head approximately 1–2 cm anterior to the occiput. In this position, if traction is subsequently applied in the direction of the pelvic axis, optimal flexion of the fetal head will be obtained to minimise the presenting diameter. A benefit of ventouse extraction is that if excessive traction is applied the cup will dislodge from the fetal scalp.

Vaginal and cervical tears can arise if the cup is not snugly applied to the fetal skull. This results in vaginal tissue being included in the vacuum and torn (see Box 37). Extreme caution must therefore be taken in applying the cup.

Perinatal mortality rates are sometimes quoted for ventouse or forceps delivery but these are more a reflection of the indication for delivery in the first instance. It is accepted that the vacuum extractor can be applied prior to full dilatation, and traditionally has been used for this purpose. However, delivery prior to full dilatation carries increased risks of failure and of trauma to the mother. If the ventouse is to be applied prior to full dilatation it must be clear that progress is satisfactory, that there is no evidence of disproportion, that the cervix is at least 7 cm dilated and the head no more than one fifth palpable abdominally.

The choice of cup depends upon the initial assessment. Soft cups such as the silc or silastic result in less scalp damage (50% reduction in cephalhaematomata) but metal cups however are less likely to fail with difficult deliveries.

7.7 Forceps delivery

Learning objectives

You should:

- be familiar with the advantages and disadvantages of the ventouse and forceps
- understand when it is safe to use the ventouse and forceps

Forceps are instruments designed to aid delivery through the vagina by exerting traction on the fetal head. They are shaped so that they curve around the fetal head, and also so that their longitudinal curve follows that of the pelvis to allow safe application. Certain criteria must be met to allow safe forceps deliv-

---

Box 37 Ventouse compared with forceps delivery

Advantages of ventouse
- Less analgesia
- Autorotation
- Lies below fetal head, therefore does not use pelvic space
- Less traction required
- Less maternal morbidity

Disadvantages of ventouse
- Vaginal and cervical tears

ery, as outlined above for the ventouse. Only when all these criteria have been met can forceps delivery be performed safely. In modern obstetric practice forceps are seldom applied if the head is at all palpable abdominally though they may be applied after careful assessment if one fifth is palpable abdominally. The indications for forceps delivery are similar to the ventouse. Forceps are very effective instruments in safe hands and allow rapid delivery of the fetus in the presence of fetal heart rate abnormalities.

Following application of the blades, traction is applied as the mother pushes with a contraction. An episiotomy is normally made just as the head crowns. Delivery should occur with between one and three pulls on the forceps without excessive force being used. Despite all the above precautions, complications can arise (see Box 38).

Shoulder dystocia is more common and postpartum blood loss tends to be increased after forceps delivery.

Ventouse or forceps?

The choice of ventouse or forceps for an assisted delivery will reflect local practices, an individual's training and specific concerns about the delivery to be performed. Current evidence appears to favour the ventouse because it involves less maternal injury, is less painful, and causes less facial injury. Ventouse, however, may fail where forceps may have succeeded in effecting delivery, and it is more likely that cephalhaematomata will develop with ventouse.

7.8 Caesarean section

Learning objectives

You should:

- understand when caesarean delivery is recommended
- understand why it poses problems in future pregnancies
- be familiar with the protocol to be followed with subsequent labours

The decision to perform a caesarean section is a serious one, with implications for neonatal well-being and the future reproductive career of the mother. However, the maternal mortality from this operation is substantially less than it was 25 years ago.

Indications for elective caesarean section include:

- placenta praevia
- two previous caesarean sections

Box 38 Complications of forceps delivery

• Fetal	Forceps marks on the face (not serious, transient)
	Neonatal seventh nerve palsy (rare)
• Maternal	Vulval and vaginal tears
	Third degree tears
	Cervical tears
	Problems with bladder emptying in the puerperium

- some breech and twin pregnancies
- serious fetal compromise
- transverse or unstable lie.

Emergency caesareans are generally performed for failure to progress in labour or fetal distress in labour. Other rare emergency circumstances include placental abruption, placenta praevia and cord prolapse.

An elective caesarean is safer than an emergency procedure.

Efforts to improve safety of the operation

1. Thromboprophylaxis in selected cases and awareness of the benefits of mobilisation in all cases. There is no evidence that the use of subcutaneous heparin preoperatively increases blood loss at caesarean section.
2. Sodium citrate or H_2 antagonists such as cimetidine given within 60 minutes of caesarean section help to increase gastric pH. These measures may reduce complications in cases at high risk of requiring caesarean section.
3. Spinal versus epidural anaesthesia has the advantage of speed of onset, but has the potential to cause spinal headache. Epidural anaesthesia carries the benefit of less hypotension, and greater duration of block post-operatively. There appears to be no difference in neonatal condition with either form of blockade. Currently combined spinal-epidural anaesthetics are being evaluated, as are alterations in the drugs used including opiates.
4. The operation should be performed with the patient tilted approximately 15° to the left to minimise aorto-caval compression.
5. Prophylactic antibiotics prior to caesarean section reduce the risk of infectious morbidity, including wound infection and endometritis.

Cephalosporins, broad spectrum penicillins and metronidazole have all been shown to be effective in this context.

7.9 Trial of scar

Learning objectives

You should:

- understand when caesarean delivery is recommended

- understand why it poses problems in future pregnancies

- be familiar with the protocol to be followed with subsequent labours

Following delivery by caesarean section, a decision must be made as to the route of delivery in any subsequent pregnancy. An attempt at vaginal delivery following a previous caesarean section is termed a 'trial of scar'. This term reflects the concern about possible scar rupture. As a general rule repeat caesarean is advised only if the obstetrician feels there is very little chance of a successful vaginal delivery. The decision to allow a trial of scar will have a major impact on overall caesarean rates.

Complications of a trial of scar include:

- need for an emergency caesarean section
- scar rupture (rare)
  — with maternal shock (occasional death), possibly requiring a hysterectomy
  — with serious fetal compromise, possibly death.

Although the risks of a trial of scar are low, some women will prefer an elective caesarean. The majority of women undergoing a trial of scar have a vaginal delivery. The incidence of scar rupture is significantly less than 1%, though it should still be discussed as part of the procedure of informed consent. Women undergoing a trial of scar should have:

- continuous monitoring of fetal heart, and maternal observations throughout labour
- a large bore I/V cannula in place
- a haemoglobin estimation, and serum saved in labour
- continuous medical supervision in labour.

Signs of possible scar rupture in labour include:

- fetal heart rate abnormalities
- slowing or cessation of contractions
- blood loss vaginally
- tenderness overlying the scar
- signs of intraperitoneal bleeding
- superficially palpable fetal parts.

Care during labour therefore should include close monitoring by medical and midwifery staff for the warning signs as outlined above.

Self-assessment: questions

Multiple choice questions

1. Regarding occipito-posterior positions:

   a. They are detected by finding the anterior fontanelle in the posterior aspect of the pelvis
   b. A minority will rotate prior to full dilatation
   c. They are sometimes delivered by caesarean even though full dilatation has been reached
   d. The incidence is increased where the presenting part is very low in the pelvis
   e. They may be delivered by ventouse

2. In face and brow presentations:

   a. A face presentation may be confused with a breech
   b. Fetal distress is more common with a face presentation and therefore a fetal scalp electrode should always be applied
   c. A caesarean should be performed once a face presentation is diagnosed
   d. A caesarean should be performed if a brow presentation is associated with no progress
   e. Both are rare and often only diagnosed in labour

3. Forceps:

   a. In skilled hands do not require analgesia
   b. Can be safely applied in a multiparous patient at 8–9 cm dilatation
   c. Cause shoulder dystocia
   d. Can lead to urinary retention in the puerperium
   e. Allow vaginal delivery in all cases once full dilatation has occurred

4. Ventouse delivery:

   a. Is more painful than forceps because of the suction used
   b. Is better than forceps because the head does not have to be engaged
   c. Is less likely to result in a third degree tear than forceps
   d. Is suitable for delivery of a second twin
   e. Is just as successful as forceps even in the presence of marked caput and moulding

5. Regarding previous caesarean delivery:

   a. It is reasonable to repeat the caesarean section if there is a persistent breech presentation in the second pregnancy
   b. A sudden and marked deterioration in the fetal heart rate in a subsequent labour should prompt a fetal blood sample
   c. Two caesarean deliveries prevent any further attempt at vaginal delivery
   d. Women should have no more than three caesareans
   e. Long labours can be tolerated after a previous caesarean if it was performed for reasons other than cephalopelvic disproportion

6. With regard to breech presentation

   a. All associated fetal morbidity will be prevented by caesarean delivery
   b. It occurs in about 10% of all deliveries
   c. It occurs more often with premature labour
   d. It should be diagnosed during antenatal care
   e. Entrapment of the aftercoming head can always be predicted by the use of ultrasound and pelvimetry

7. With regard to shoulder dystocia

   a. It is more common with larger babies
   b. It is more common with babies of diabetic mothers
   c. Strong traction should be applied immediately because of the risk of imminent asphyxia
   d. Episiotomy is not necessary as the problem is not at the pelvic outlet
   e. Erb's palsy is a complication

True/false questions

Are the following statements true or false?

1. Caesarean delivery has been shown to be safest for the fetus/neonate with a breech presentation.
2. Caesarean delivery for the breech baby ensures an easy and atraumatic delivery.
3. External cephalic version poses no risk to the fetus.
4. A history of previous caesarean section with twins is sufficient to warrant a repeat section.
5. Abdominal pain in a woman with a previous caesarean should provoke concern about the integrity of the scar.

Case history

A primiparous lady progresses well in labour until she reaches 9 cm dilatation. She then fails to achieve any progress over the ensuing 2 hours and oxytocin is prescribed. She is diagnosed fully dilated 2 hours later and commences pushing. After 1 hour of pushing it is clear that the vertex is not advancing and an operative delivery is recommended. Forceps are applied and the baby is delivered face-to-pubes. There is a brisk bleed following delivery and a tear has to be sutured in the right vaginal fornix. She has difficulty passing urine some hours later and requires a urinary catheter.

1. Is it reasonable to prescribe oxytocin in this situation?
2. Might caesarean not be a better option?
3. Should a ventouse delivery have been performed?
4. Should a urinary catheter have been inserted immediately after delivery?

Self-assessment: answers

Multiple choice answers

1. a. **False.** In an occipito-posterior position, the occiput and hence the posterior fontanelle will be posterior, and the anterior fontanelle will be found anteriorly.
   b. **False.** At least 80% will rotate prior to full dilatation.
   c. **True**, as the head is often high and this may be the least traumatic method of delivery.
   d. **False.**
   e. **True.** This is the optimal instrumental method of delivery.

2. a. **True.** The mouth may be mistaken for the anus.
   b. **False.** Fetal scalp electrodes should never be applied unless the anatomy has been identified and a face presentation excluded.
   c. **False.** Many proceed to vaginal delivery.
   d. **True.**
   e. **True.**

3. a. **False.** Adequate analgesia should always be provided (normally epidural, spinal or pudendal block).
   b. **False.** Forceps should not be used prior to full dilatation.
   c. **False.** Shoulder dystocia occurs more commonly where forceps have been applied but they are not the cause.
   d. **True.** Women who have had a particularly difficult forceps delivery or who had bladder emptying problems in the past may warrant urinary catheterisation after delivery.
   e. **False.** This is absolutely not the case. At full dilatation the safest method of delivery may still be by caesarean section, though it is normally by forceps or ventouse.

4. a. **False.** It is generally less painful than forceps.
   b. **False.** No matter which technique is used the same degree of caution is required and an unengaged head is not suitable for assisted vaginal delivery.
   c. **True.**
   d. **True.**
   e. **False.**

5. a. **True.** In the presence of complications the balance will often favour repeating the caesarean electively.
   b. **False.** Such a sudden change suggests a possible scar rupture and emergency caesarean is indicated.

   c. **True**, though in some countries selective cases would be allowed a trial in labour.
   d. **False.** There is no absolute number which represents the limit, but the surgery gets progressively more difficult. The risk of adhesions and bladder injury become greater as the number increases.
   e. **False.** Long labours should always be avoided with a trial of scar.

6. a. **False.** Much of the morbidity associated with breech presentation is due to associated congenital abnormalities, effects of premature delivery and events occurring during the antenatal period. Only those specific problems caused by the delivery process will be prevented by caesarean delivery.
   b. **False.** 3%
   c. **True.**
   d. **True.** This allows discussion with the parents of all the options in relation to management of breech presentation, and the performance of external cephalic version. When diagnosed in labour, such a discussion cannot occur, external cephalic version will not be possible and ultrasound assessment of fetal weight may not be possible.
   e. **False.** It can still occur.

7. a. **True**, but it can arise with average size babies also.
   b. **True.** These babies tend to be bigger than average and can also have substantial soft tissue swelling due to hyperglycaemia.
   c. **False.** Strong traction only causes harm, as the shoulder is impacted on the pubic bone and brachial plexus injury will result (Erb's palsy).
   d. **False.** Although the problem is at the level of the pelvic inlet, room must be created within the pelvis to allow access to correct the problem.
   e. **True.** See answer to c above.

True/false answers

1. **True.** This has been demonstrated. This does not mean however that all attempts at vaginal breech birth should be abandoned. It may well be that for women planning a large family that maternal considerations should sway one to vaginal breech birth. In practice, experience in conducting vaginal breech birth is likely to diminish and caesarean will be increasingly favoured in the developed world.

2. **False.** Caesarean delivery can be difficult and fetal/neonatal trauma has been documented. This is especially the case at premature gestations when the lower segment may not be well developed.

3. **False.** Large series of cases suggest this technique is generally safe. However there is significant anecdotal experience suggesting occasional intra-uterine death or retroplacental bleeding in association with the technique. For this reason most units insist on monitoring the fetus after the procedure has been completed.

4. **True.** Most obstetricians would view the combined risks of scar rupture and the problems with twin delivery as sufficient justification for caesarean section. Furthermore intra-uterine manipulation is sometimes required for the delivery of twin II and this would pose a specific risk of scar rupture.

5. **True.** Such pain should always provoke concern about scar integrity. This is best tested in the first instance with fetal monitoring as the fetus will often demonstrate fetal distress and this has to be acted on immediately.

Case history answer

1. It is reasonable to prescribe oxytocin. Sometimes progress slows because of inefficient uterine action and sometimes because of an occipito-posterior position. Oxytocin directly addresses the question of inefficient uterine action and can help the occiput to rotate. Oxytocin can do harm in two ways. It can cause the uterus to contract strongly even though the labour is obstructed. This could result in a ruptured uterus but in practice this is hardly ever seen in primiparous patients. The other way in which oxytocin could do harm relates to overstimulation of the uterus. This is monitored continuously in conventional practice and oxytocin is stopped immediately if fetal distress occurs with any suspicion of hyperstimulation.

2. A caesarean could be considered but a significant proportion of women will achieve vaginal delivery if oxytocin is commenced. A caesarean in this situation is emergency and high risk as the patient is nearing full dilatation. Risks of bladder trauma and excessive haemorrhage are increased at and near full dilatation. Furthermore a caesarean would compromise the next pregnancy, i.e. a repeat caesarean would be required or labour with a risk of scar rupture.

3. Both ventouse and forceps depend on knowing the correct position of the baby's head for their safe application. If an occipito-posterior position was diagnosed ventouse would be the preferred mode of delivery for most operators. It is felt that forceps carry greater risks of maternal trauma, especially anal sphincter damage.

4. If there was any prior history of voiding problems, a urinary catheter would have been advisable. In the absence of such a history, it is reasonable to avoid catheterisation but to watch the patient very carefully and intervene at the earliest sign of a voiding problem.

8

The puerperium and its disorders

Overview

The puerperium refers to that period of time when the pelvic organs return to normal and the physiological adaptations to pregnancy are reversed. Much of the systemic physiological change is reversed within 2 weeks of delivery but it takes 6 weeks minimum for complete resolution. Secondary post-partum haemorrhage may occur and often coexists with some intra-uterine infection requiring antibiotic treatment. Thromboembolic disease is sometimes a problem especially in those with risk factors or following operative delivery. Postnatal depression is a cause for concern mainly among general practitioners and practice nurses as it commonly presents after discharge from hospital services.

8.1 The normal puerperium

Learning objectives

You should understand:

• how the uterus involutes

• how genital tract bleeding resolves following delivery

The puerperium is the term used to describe the time when the pelvic organs return to the pre-pregnant state; this takes approximately 6 weeks and is accom-

panied by a reversal of physiological adaptations to pregnancy, and by the establishment of lactation. This occurs as a result of the withdrawal of placental hormones. During this time the mother will be predominantly under the care of her midwife, though the obstetrician and family doctor may be involved if there are problems. Physiotherapists also play a role through advice on pelvic floor exercises to ensure restoration of muscle tone. Circulatory and other changes have usually reversed by approximately 6 weeks post partum.

Pelvic organs

Uterine involution is the term given to the return of the pregnant uterus to its pre-pregnant size. By approximately 10 days post partum the uterus will no longer be palpable abdominally. This occurs as a result of the withdrawal of influences originating in the fetoplacental unit, and is aided by oxytocin produced in response to breast feeding. The process of involution is usually checked by palpation as delay may be a sign of retained products of conception, with or without infection. The external os of the cervix may remain open or patulous, but the internal os should have closed by the second week post partum.

Lochia

Involution of the uterus is accompanied by passage vaginally of the lochia, comprised of decidua and blood constituents. While initially it resembles a dark red blood loss, it gradually becomes clearer over the second week and clears completely at around 4–6 weeks post partum. There is considerable variation in the timing of cessation of lochial flow and bleeding. The timing of the first menstrual period will depend on breast feeding. It usually occurs at approximately 6 weeks post partum in those not breast feeding. It is important for women to understand that they may ovulate and therefore conceive before their first menstrual period.

Engorged breasts

Management includes firm support, analgesia and avoidance of expression of breast milk.

Episiotomies

Episiotomies and tears usually heal well within 2–3 weeks of delivery if properly sutured and kept clean.

8.2 Medical care on the postnatal ward

Learning objectives

You should:

- be familiar with the clinical issues in the immediate puerperium
- know how to perform a clinical examination in the puerperium

The examination involved in the postnatal check is outlined in Table 12. While checking that the uterus is involuted is routine, breast and vaginal examinations should only be performed for specific symptoms.

Other issues which must be considered during this period include smear tests, anti-D prophylaxis and Rhesus status.

It is important that those women who are found not to be immune to rubella at antenatal screening are immunised in the immediate postpartum period. This achieves immunity in the majority of patients. It is advisable that such vaccination is performed when the patient is not pregnant, hence the advisability of puerperal vaccination. Nonetheless, no adverse effect of rubella vaccination during pregnancy has been noted in cases where this has occurred accidentally.

Anti-D immunoglobulin should be given to those women who are Rhesus negative who deliver a Rhesus positive baby. This is normally done by intramuscular injection of anti-D immunoglobulin 500 IU and will substantially reduce the risk of anti-D sensitisation in the postpartum period. The overall risk of sensitisation with such a protocol is approximately 1–2% and will be further reduced by the use of antenatal prophylaxis. A Kleihauer test may be performed to ensure that an appropriate dose of anti-D is administered. A 30 ml fetomaternal bleed will require at least 500 IU of anti-D prophylaxis. Only 0.6% of deliveries will have a fetomaternal bleed of this magnitude.

The length of hospital stay depends upon a number of factors, including:

- level of help and support at home
- mode of delivery (longer if lower segment caesarean section)
- presence or absence of any neonatal problems
- presence of any medical complications such as pre-eclampsia.

The duration of hospital stay is much shorter than previously despite higher levels of intervention. It is now common for women to be discharged home within 24–48 hours of delivery in the absence of complications. The most common reasons for longer stays are difficulty in establishing breast feeding or recovery from caesarean section. Some women choose to be discharged home 6 hours following delivery, though this most often applies to women with good home circumstances and no complications.

8.3 Secondary postpartum haemorrhage

Learning objectives

You should:

- know how to assess bleeding in the puerperium
- know how to manage a secondary haemorrhage

Secondary postpartum haemorrhage (PPH) is defined as haemorrhage from the genital tract 24 or more hours after delivery, but within 6 weeks. It usually occurs in association with retained pieces of placenta, membrane or blood clot within the uterus. This typically presents within 1–2 weeks of delivery and initially with fresh red bleeding against the background lochia. The patient may be shocked if blood loss is heavy.

Symptoms and signs of secondary PPH

- Heavy vaginal bleeding
- Lower abdominal pain
- Shock, if substantial blood loss

Table 12 The postnatal check

Examination	Rationale
Blood pressure	? pre-eclampsia ? hypotension
Temperature	? puerperal pyrexia
Breast examination if indicated	? breast abscess
Abdominal examination	re uterine involution. If tender, ? endometritis. Check bladder emptying
Inspect vulval region	? episiotomies healing
Vaginal examination	only if specifically indicated
Legs	watch for thromboses

- Larger than expected uterus
- Associated signs of uterine infection (pyrexia, uterine tenderness).

Management

- Resuscitation
- Oxytocin or ergometrine
- Removal of any products of conception from the cervical os *if it is easy to do so*
- Antibiotics
- ± evacuation of retained products.

The decision to perform an evacuation of the uterus in a postpartum patient is a very delicate one in view of the increased risk of uterine perforation. It should be considered, however:

1. if the placenta or membranes were thought to be incomplete
2. if there is good ultrasound evidence of retained products or
3. if bleeding is persistent following a course of antibiotics.

Ultrasound examination has a useful role to play in diagnosis of retained products of conception. However, within 10 days of delivery there is often some retained blood clot in the uterus, confusing the ultrasound interpretation, and the clinical picture should determine management at this time.

Following a caesarean section, the diagnosis is usually one of endometritis and should be treated with antibiotics. In this situation uterine exploration may cause scar rupture which might lead to hysterectomy and therefore should be avoided.

When there is persistent bleeding in the postpartum period trophoblastic disease should be considered and HCG assayed.

8.4 Puerperal sepsis

Learning objectives

You should understand:

- the risk factors for puerperal sepsis
- the differential diagnosis
- how to treat genital tract sepsis in the puerperium

Maternal death in the puerperium from sepsis is now very rare. There were 11 cases of death from puerperal sepsis in the last triennial report of the Confidential Enquiry into Maternal Deaths in the UK. Most pyrexias in the puerperium are due to pelvic infection. Puerperal pyrexia is defined as a temperature of 38°C or greater in the 2 weeks following delivery.

Factors contributing to an increased incidence of pelvic infection include:

- caesarean section
- multiple vaginal examinations or internal monitoring
- prolonged rupture of the membranes
- prolonged labour
- bacterial vaginosis
- chorioamnionitis preceding delivery
- intra-uterine manipulation
- retained placental or membranous tissue.

Prophylactic antibiotics at caesarean delivery reduce the incidence of wound infection from 7 to 2%, and also the incidence of endometritis. Serious sepsis may be difficult to diagnose and become fulminating over a short time period. The differential diagnosis of puerperal sepsis includes:

- endometritis, with or without retained products
- salpingitis, which may be associated with endometritis
- urinary tract infection
- wound infection
- breast infection, abscess
- venous thromboembolic disease
- incidental causes such as respiratory infection
- meningitis post spinal anaesthesia (very rare).

The investigation of a puerperal infection will depend on the presence of predisposing factors and mode of delivery. Pelvic infection usually involves the uterus only (endometritis) but occasionally involves the parametrial tissues also.

Clinical features of postpartum pelvic infection

1. Lower abdominal pain
2. Foul-smelling lochia
3. Pyrexia, rigors, tachycardia
4. Uterine and lower abdominal tenderness
5. Delayed uterine involution
6. Non-specific flu-like symptoms.

Investigations

- High vaginal swab
- MSU
- Blood culture
- White cell count
- Wound swabs if appropriate.

The above investigations are not always helpful, so antibiotics are indicated on clinical grounds even when all investigations are negative.

Treatment

Treatment is with intravenous antibiotics. Cephalosporins, amoxycillin alone or with metronidazole, or clavulinic acid with amoxycillin may be used. In general if there is any suspicion of endometritis it is best to treat early with broad spectrum antibiotics to prevent any associated salpingitis. This will on occasion result in over-treatment.

Respiratory causes of febrile morbidity are almost always related to general anaesthesia for caesarean delivery. Causes include:

1. aspiration pneumonia
2. atelectasis
3. bacterial pneumonia.

The possibility of underlying thromboembolism must be considered in any pregnant patient with respiratory symptoms.

Pyelonephritis may arise in the puerperium. Predisposing factors include:

1. residual urinary stasis of pregnancy
2. catheterisation in labour
3. retention of urine related to instrumental delivery
4. renal tract trauma during caesarean delivery (rare).

Breast abscess and engorgement may also contribute to puerperal pyrexia, as may deep vein thrombosis.

8.5 Venous thromboembolic disease

Thromboembolism can be a major postpartum problem. This topic is covered in Chapter 3. Prevention with early mobilisation, use of compression stockings and appropriate use of heparin prophylaxis are important components of postpartum care.

8.6 Psychological and psychiatric problems

Learning objectives

You must:

- understand that depression is an important cause of morbidity
- know that psychosis can occur

The arrival of a newborn baby represents a joyous occasion to most families, but may on occasion be a source of stress. This may occur as a result of financial pressures or fears of inability to cope with feeding and other needs of the child.

Psychological problems may therefore arise and vary from expected anxieties to 'fourth day blues' to major psychiatric emergencies. It is not known to what extent the major hormonal changes which arise in the puerperium contribute to these problems. It is possible, at least in a proportion of patients, that the puerperium unmasks a patient's long-term tendency to psychiatric disorder.

Staff involved with the care of mothers must be vigilant for signs of psychological instability such as antisocial behaviour or problems with bonding with the newborn child. Early recourse to help from a psychiatrist is advised. If during the antenatal period there is concern about the possible stability of the mother in the puerperium, referral to a psychiatrist should occur at that time. Should a mother require inpatient management, then this should occur in a designated 'mother and baby' unit.

'Fourth day blues'

This is experienced by up to half of all women in the puerperium and is evidenced in tearfulness and mild depression. It is difficult to know whether this reflects an underlying endocrine change, but no specific abnormality has been identified. It normally resolves over a period of days without specific medical intervention.

Postnatal depression

This term refers to episodes of moderate depression which most commonly arise within 2–3 months of delivery. It affects up to 10% of women. Predisposing factors include adverse social circumstances, past psychiatric history and earlier concerns regarding desirability of the pregnancy. However, depression can also arise without any apparent adverse factors. Anti-depressant medications may be indicated.

Puerperal psychosis

This is a most serious psychiatric complication, affecting up to 1 in every 500 mothers. It may be manifest by irrational behaviour and an abnormal pattern of bonding with the baby, usually within weeks of delivery. There is a 10% risk of recurrence in subsequent pregnancies and this often raises considerable anxiety about planning further children.

8.7 Advice and counselling

While in the postnatal ward, midwifery staff are available to advise women on the benefits of breast feeding and to help them develop confidence in this method. Advice on contraception is also offered, as is guidance on positioning and handling of the baby to minimise subsequent problems such as cot death.

Women who have a caesarean delivery or a complicated vaginal delivery should have an explanation of the course of events and advice on management in subsequent pregnancies. More specific counselling is offered to women who may have suffered a poor outcome to the pregnancy and appropriate arrangements are made for out-patient follow-up.

Self-assessment: questions

Multiple choice questions

1. The following statements apply to pre-eclampsia in the postpartum period:
   a. Abdominal pain and vomiting are never due to pre-eclampsia once the fetus has been delivered
   b. Fits in the postpartum period should only be diagnosed as eclampsia after thorough neurological investigation
   c. Controlling the blood pressure is not a serious problem once the fetus is delivered
   d. Pre-eclampsia prior to delivery increases the risk of thromboembolism post partum
   e. If the hypertension or proteinuria persist, alternative diagnoses should be considered

2. Care on the postnatal wards includes:
   a. Administration of anti-D to all rhesus-D negative women who have given birth to rhesus-D negative babies
   b. Arranging rubella immunisation where appropriate for 3 months post partum
   c. Discussion of contraceptive needs
   d. Regular checks to ensure bladder emptying for 24–48 hours following delivery
   e. Women delivered by caesarean should be counselled regarding mode of delivery in future pregnancies

3. After delivery:
   a. Monitoring uterine fundal height is not necessary after caesarean delivery
   b. Women delivered by caesarean require strict bed rest for 24 hours to allow the uterine incision time to heal
   c. Women may go home 6 hours after delivery if they wish
   d. Blood transfusion should be recommended if the haemoglobin is less than 10 grams post partum
   e. Non-steroidal anti-inflammatories should never be used for analgesia in the postpartum period

True / false questions

Are the following statements true or false?

1. Vaginal bleeding has always completely stopped by 6 weeks postnatal.
2. Headaches are common in the postpartum period and do not require investigation.
3. Leg swelling is common in the first 10 days after delivery and does not require investigation unless particularly severe or localising signs are present.
4. Ovarian cyst accidents are more common in the first 2 weeks of the puerperium.
5. Appropriate treatment of endometritis depends on bacteriology results and should not be commenced until such results are available.

Short notes

1. Describe the purpose of the 6-week postnatal check.

2. Describe the causes and management of sudden postpartum collapse.

Self-assessment: answers

Multiple choice answers

1. a. **False.** These symptoms should always prompt consideration of underlying pre-eclampsia and this still applies for at least 48 hours post partum. Pre-eclampsia often presents with such symptoms.

   b. **False.** Eclamptic fits often arise in the postpartum period for the first time. This still represents the most likely cause of fitting within 48 hours of delivery. Alternative diagnoses are most likely in the absence of hypertension or proteinuria and with increasing interval from delivery.

   c. **False.** Controlling the blood pressure to prevent cerebral complications is extremely important in the postpartum period. Parenteral anti-hypertensive medications are often required in serious cases for 24–48 hours following delivery. Blood pressure can rise during the first week after delivery and therefore must be watched carefully during this period, though oral treatment is normally sufficient at this time. Methyldopa should be stopped in the postpartum period and another anti-hypertensive substituted. This is because the side-effect profile is particularly unsuited to nursing mothers and the arguments for methyldopa in terms of fetal safety no longer apply.

   d. **True.** This is likely to be due to the underlying vascular damage in pre-eclampsia, the increased risk of operative delivery in these women, greater likelihood of in-hospital bed rest, increased maternal age and coexistent medical problems such as diabetes and SLE.

   e. **True.** Pre-eclampsia is cured by delivery of the fetus and placenta. It may take up to 48 hours in serious cases for sustained recovery to begin, and improved blood pressure control and a diuresis are normally evident by then. The longer the interval from delivery that hypertension and/or proteinuria persist, the more alternative diagnoses must be considered, though hypertension due to pre-eclampsia may take some weeks to resolve.

2. a. **False.** Anti-D will only be necessary when the baby is Rhesus-D positive, raising the possibility of sensitisation.

   b. **False.** Rubella immunisation should be performed immediately to prevent any possibility of conception prior to administration. This will apply to those women who have been shown on antenatal testing to be non-immune or to have low levels of immunity.

   c. **True.** This issue should always be discussed prior to discharge home, and every effort made to ensure the mother understands that she may conceive before having a period.

   d. **True.** Problems with micturition often arise in the immediate postpartum period. This may be as a result of painful vulval tears, or operative delivery resulting in tissue oedema around the bladder base.

   e. **True.** This is important as not all women attend for postnatal checks. Information should include the type of scar which is present on the uterus and the rationale for the caesarean delivery.

3. a. **False.** The uterus can fill with blood after caesarean delivery and cause haemorrhagic shock. This may only be detected by monitoring the fundal height after the delivery.

   b. **False.** On the contrary, they must be mobilised as soon as possible because of the risk of thrombosis.

   c. **True.** Few complications occur after this time that cannot be detected by the district midwife. Discharge home at this time depends on adequate social support and the confidence of the mother.

   d. **False.** There is no absolute cut-off after which transfusion is required. Any decision should be made by the patient with reference to the symptoms she is experiencing. Below 8 grams, transfusion will normally be advised as the patient is often symptomatic.

   e. **False.** They provide excellent analgesia.

True/false answers

1. **False.** It has normally stopped at 6 weeks post partum but not always.
2. **False.** There is always a risk of coincidental pathology. Diagnoses that must be specifically considered in the puerperium include cerebrovascular accidents, meningitis and cerebral sinus thrombosis.
3. **True.** Significant leg oedema is common in the first 10 days after delivery and emphasises that the physiological changes of pregnancy are resolving slowly over that 2 week period.
4. **True.** As the uterus involutes the ovary may twist on its pedicle as it returns to the pelvis. This is most likely to happen if there is an undiagnosed dermoid cyst.

5. **False.** Once a clinical diagnosis is made antibiotics must be commenced immediately rather than waiting for culture results.

Short notes answers

1. Women are traditionally asked to have a postnatal visit at 6 weeks post partum. This may be with the family doctor if the pregnancy has been free of complications, or with the hospital specialist if complications have arisen or are anticipated with a future pregnancy.

   This visit allows the clinician to ensure that any medical problems such as hypertension, proteinuria or anaemia have resolved. The mother may be questioned regarding any new symptoms such as incontinence, or problems with breast feeding. Examination need not routinely include a vaginal examination. There are occasions, however, when it is sensible to perform such an examination, i.e. if there are concerns following vaginal tears. Cervical smears may be taken as necessary and contraception discussed.

   This visit also allows the woman to discuss any issues she considers important, either concerning her care during the pregnancy or regarding future pregnancies. It is an ideal opportunity to discuss any complications that may arise in future pregnancies. While many aspects of pre-conceptual care may be covered by the obstetrician, this may represent an ideal time to request referral to a geneticist or paediatrician. Women who have lost a baby will require a detailed explanation of the events and postmortem and other findings.

2. The differential diagnosis of postpartum collapse is dependent upon the timing and the clinical circumstances in which it arises. Collapse occurring within 6 hours of delivery is usually due to postpartum haemorrhage or eclampsia. Postpartum haemorrhage is the most common cause and only represents a diagnostic problem if the bleeding is not revealed, such as with a broad ligament haematoma or bleeding concealed within the uterus. Eclampsia may occur in a woman who has had no previous problem with hypertension or proteinuria. Cerebral haemorrhage and sepsis must also be considered.

Anaesthetic problems can include failure to reverse the agents causing respiratory depression, and toxicity of local anaesthetics. Toxicity from agents used in regional blocks arises as a result of accidental intravascular injection, or use of excessive doses. Side-effects include confusion, respiratory compromise, myocardial depression and apnoea.

Cardiac arrhythmias or infarction may also present in this manner. Myocardial infarction is rare in pregnancy, occurring in approximately 1 in 10 000 deliveries. Management in the puerperium is similar to that in the non-pregnant state except that fibrinolytic agents must be used with caution in view of the possibility of genital tract haemorrhage.

Amniotic fluid embolism is a rare cause of postpartum collapse. It was responsible for 17 maternal deaths in the last triennial report of the UK Confidential Enquiry into Maternal Deaths. The spread of amniotic fluid into the maternal circulation results in pulmonary vasoconstriction and left ventricular failure. Disseminated intravascular coagulation (DIC) rapidly ensues. It is associated with uterine trauma, placental abruption, use of oxytocic agents and caesarean section. The diagnosis may be made by the finding of fetal squames and other components of amniotic fluid in blood taken via a central line, or by the presence of fetal squames in the maternal lungs on postmortem. Management includes ventilation if pulmonary problems predominate, maintenance of intravascular fluid volume via a central line, and consideration of dopamine. DIC should be managed by infusion of fresh frozen plasma, cryoprecipitate, platelet transfusion if necessary, and replacement of blood loss.

Pulmonary embolism in the puerperium will normally present with sub-acute symptoms and signs. It may, however, present with collapse of the patient if massive, or with sudden onset of chest pain, dyspnoea, cyanosis and tachycardia. Investigations will include examination of blood gases for hypoxaemia, ECG for right axis deviation, a chest X-ray for atelectasis, pleural effusion or an elevated hemidiaphragm. Management of massive pulmonary embolus includes maintenance of ventilation and oxygenation, and anticoagulation with intravenous heparin.

9 Measures of outcome in pregnancy

Overview

Obstetrics has a strong history of audit of clinical outcome. Audit of maternal mortality over 3 year cycles takes place in the UK and provides valuable data on pregnancy outcome and major contributors to maternal morbidity and mortality. Perinatal mortality and morbidity is audited on a departmental basis as is the level of intervention within the departments concerned. Both maternal and perinatal mortality have fallen progressively over the last 30 years.

Introduction

The field of obstetrics lends itself to accurate measurement of outcome such as maternal or perinatal mortality. Traditionally these aspects of care have been kept under rigorous review, though the rates of mortality, both maternal and perinatal, are now relatively low. As a result of this, emphasis is now being placed on methods of assessing morbidity following pregnancy, and also on the level of satisfaction of parents with the service being provided.

9.1 Definitions

Learning objective

You need:

- to understand the information available on fertility, abortion and on-going pregnancy rates

In determining rates of mortality or morbidity in relation to pregnancy, it is imperative that accurate information is available concerning the number of pregnancies occurring each year, and the proportion progressing beyond the first trimester. Some definitions are therefore important for the interpretation of figures to be referred to later.

Fertility rates refer to births per thousand women per year aged 15–44 years. Fertility increased in the 1950s, peaked in 1964, and then declined until 1974. It has fluctuated a little since and the current fertility rate is approximately 61 per thousand women aged 15–44 years. The average age at childbirth is currently increasing, as is the number of multiple pregnancies. In 1994–1996, 2% of births were to women aged 40 years or more.

The number of conceptions per year in the UK is calculated from the combined total number of maternities, legal abortions and the number of hospital admissions for spontaneous abortions and ectopic pregnancies. This will underestimate the total number of conceptions, as some miscarriages will occur very early at home and not be recorded in the above statistics.

The outcome following conception based on the above statistics is as follows:

- 75% live or stillbirth
- 18% legally terminated
- 7% spontaneous abortion or ectopic.

Approximately 14 abortions per 1000 women aged 15–44 years are performed annually in the UK and there was a steady upward trend until 1990, and a slight fall since. The Abortion Act 1967 obliges operating practitioners to notify abortions. Since 1970 there has been a steady decline in the maternal mortality rate from illegal abortion, such that in the more recent reports no mortalities from this cause have been recorded.

A maternity is any pregnancy which results in the birth of one or more live or stillborn children. There are approximately 700 000 maternities in the UK per year. A birth may be either a live birth or stillbirth. A live birth is defined as the complete expulsion or extraction of a product of conception from the mother, irrespective of the duration of pregnancy, which shows any sign of life. Fetal death is death prior to complete expulsion or extraction irrespective of the duration of pregnancy. Signs of life include a heart rate, breathing, umbilical cord pulsation or movement. Abortion is therefore defined as the complete expulsion of a fetus showing no signs of life from a woman prior to 24 weeks' gestation.

9.2 Maternal mortality

Learning objectives

You should:

- be familiar with the conduct of the maternal mortality enquiry
- understand the trends in the different categories of maternal mortality

There are currently 500 000 maternal deaths per year worldwide. The vast majority of these occur in developing countries, and maternal mortality rates vary greatly depending upon underlying socioeconomic conditions. Improvements in socioeconomic conditions reduce the number of maternal mortalities through a variety of mechanisms including access to appropriate antibiotic treatment, improved blood transfusion services and greater availability of contraception.

Historical perspective

Maternal mortality has declined to currently low levels from earlier this century when one in 250 women died in pregnancy. A clear fall has occurred since 1935, and mortality rates in developed countries have converged. The leading causes of maternal death prior to 1935 included puerperal infection with β haemolytic streptococcus, septic abortion, hypertensive disorders of pregnancy, eclampsia, and haemorrhage. Factors that have contributed to the rapid decline in maternal mortality since then include availability of antibiotics, safer anaesthesia and caesarean delivery, availability of ergometrine, development of blood transfusion services and general improvement in health services.

Given the huge effect these developments have had, it is clear that marginal improvements in the provision of care to developing countries could have a huge impact on worldwide maternal mortality. The challenge in developed countries such as the UK is clearly different in that further improvements in care are likely to have only a minor impact on maternal mortality rates without further advances in research into the underlying causes.

The Triennial Report

The Triennial Report on Confidential Enquiries into Maternal Deaths in the United Kingdom is the mainstay of audit in relation to maternal mortality in Great Britain. This report focuses on the worst possible outcome to pregnancy, namely maternal death. On the basis of this enquiry recommendations are made concerning the delivery of care in the UK, aiming to minimise maternal mortality in future years. Between 1952 and 1984, maternal mortality halved every 10 years. The latest report concerns the triennium 1994–1996 and the maternal mortality is currently approximately 12 per 100 000 maternities. This translates into 268 maternal mortalities over the 3-year period, or approximately 89 women per year. This figure represented no change in mortality rate since the last report, and as before, substandard care was reported in up to half the cases.

The Triennial Report reviews maternal deaths in England, Wales, Scotland and Northern Ireland. The report is confidential to ensure privacy for the patients concerned and to ensure ongoing cooperation from obstetric and other medical staff contributing to the enquiry. Completion of the case reports is not a statutory requirement. In order to maintain confidentiality, the identity of the patient is erased from all relevant documents, and just prior to publication all such documents are destroyed. Deaths are identified through inspection of death certificates, but only about 50% are detected in this way. The enquiry therefore also relies on the relevant health service staff to notify deaths on their own initiative.

Maternal deaths are classified as outlined in Box 39.

Only direct and indirect deaths are counted for statistical purposes. There are generally twice as many direct as indirect deaths. Late deaths refer to deaths occurring between 6 weeks and 1 year after the pregnancy. Some maternal deaths may occur outside the limits of the enquiry as a result of life support measures while others will be of no relevance to the pregnancy. Currently they are included in the report if they occur up to 12 months after delivery.

While maternal mortality represented 1.1% of all deaths in females aged 15–44 years in 1973, this has now fallen to 0.7%. Maternal mortality is expressed as deaths per number of maternities. Approximately one third

Box 39 Maternal deaths: classification in Triennial Report	
• Direct	Those deaths resulting from obstetric complications of pregnancy
• Indirect	Those resulting from previous existing disease, or disease that developed during pregnancy and which was not due to direct obstetric causes, but which was aggravated by the physiologic effects of pregnancy
• Fortuitous	Those deaths from other incidental causes which happen to occur during pregnancy or the puerperium

Box 40 Maternal mortality by causes (% of direct deaths for the UK, 1991–1993)

• Hypertensive disease	15.5
• Pulmonary embolus	27.1
• Haemorrhage	11.6
• Amniotic fluid embolus	7.8
• Early pregnancy	14.0
• Sepsis, excluding abortion	7.0
• Anaesthesia	6.2

occur prior to 28 weeks. The most common causes of maternal mortality are thromboembolism, hypertension in pregnancy and haemorrhage. Maternal deaths generally increase with increasing maternal age and parity (see Box 40).

The maternal mortality report provides continuous audit for obstetricians in the UK. It also serves as an unpleasant reminder of the possible consequences of substandard care. There are undoubtedly aspects of care which are not covered by this report and which will serve as subjects for investigation and audit under the heading of maternal morbidity. These are likely to include immediate postpartum morbidity including transfusion requirement, renal failure, postpartum pain, and more long-term effects such as urinary or faecal incontinence. There is little or no data at present on long-term morbidity following pregnancy.

9.3 Perinatal mortality

Learning objectives

You should:

• know the definitions of the components of perinatal mortality

• understand the level of fetal and neonatal loss

• be familiar with the causes of perinatal loss

Perinatal mortality is thought to reflect the quality of care of pregnant women within society and is therefore the most studied and quoted statistic in obstetric practice. The Office of Population Censuses and Surveys (OPCS) publishes a review of perinatal and infant deaths annually for England and Wales. The Department of Health now also publishes the Confidential Enquiry into Stillbirths and Deaths in Infancy (CESDI) Annual Report. This report was established to identify ways by which perinatal and infant deaths may be reduced. Scottish statistics are published in the Stillbirth and Infant Death Report by the Information and Statistics Division of the NHS Scotland.

Some definitions

It is a legal requirement in England and Wales that all births are notified to the Directors of Public Health within 36 hours of occurrence, and in Scotland within 24 hours. This does not apply to deliveries before 24 completed weeks of pregnancy showing no signs of life. Births after 24 weeks must also be legally notified to the Registrar for Births and Deaths. The time limit for registration is 42 days in England and Wales, 21 days in Scotland.

A fetal death is defined as death prior to the complete expulsion or extraction from its mother of products of conception without signs of life, irrespective of the duration of pregnancy.

Stillbirths are defined as delivery of an infant after 24 weeks of pregnancy which shows no sign of life. The rate quoted is per thousand live and stillbirths, currently 5 per thousand. It appears to be reaching a plateau at this level, having fallen consistently in the 70s and early 80s. Antepartum stillbirth is death of a baby before the onset of labour. Intrapartum death is death occurring during labour.

Perinatal deaths include those deaths occurring in the first week of life and stillbirths, per thousand total births. The perinatal mortality rate is currently 7.9 per 1000 births. Comparable statistics are collected for Scotland by the Information and Statistics Division, NHS Scotland.

Neonatal deaths are deaths during the first 28 days of life per 1000 live births and is currently 3.8 per thousand. This is subdivided into early (within the first week) and late (7–27 days). Post-neonatal deaths are deaths of babies aged 28 days and over, but less than 1 year of age, per thousand live births. This fell to 1.8 in 1998.

Infant deaths refer to all deaths in the first year of life, per thousand live births. This rate has shown a steady decline to present levels of approximately 5 per thousand live births. This fall has been due mostly to a steady fall in neonatal mortality, and a less steep fall in post-neonatal mortality.

Birthweight is the first recorded weight of fetus or newborn after birth. It is optimal that this measurement is performed within the first hour of life. Low birthweight is defined as less than 2.5 kg. It may be caused by babies being born prematurely (<37 weeks) or being growth retarded. Both categories are at increased risk of perinatal death.

There are approximately 3300 stillbirths in the UK each year. Births outside marriage, have slightly higher stillbirth rates than births within marriage, the difference reflecting altered socioeconomic conditions. There are also differences with age, the rate being lowest for the age group 25–29 years, and highest for mothers aged 35 years and over. Parity also influences stillbirth rates, being lowest for women who have had one previous child.

Perinatal mortality rates reflect similar influences, being lowest in those women who have had one previous child, are married, and are aged 25–29 years. In total there are approximately 5300 perinatal deaths in the UK each year.

There are approximately 2500 neonatal deaths in the UK annually. The neonatal death rate is lowest for those mothers aged 25–29 years, who have had one child previously and who are married.

As mentioned above, there is a confidential enquiry system into perinatal care, similar to the maternal mortality enquiry. The CESDI inquiry (Confidential Enquiry into Stillbirths and Deaths in Infancy) is published annually. Causes of perinatal loss are outlined in Box 41.

Perinatal mortality is influenced by many factors. Because deaths due to congenital abnormalities are not thought to be a reflection of the quality of care, perinatal mortality rates are often corrected for these. Other factors which will influence interpretation of such statistics include gestational age. Table 13 is a guide to neonatal survival rates. They will vary markedly depending on the level of local service being provided.

Table 13 Neonatal survival

Gestational age		Neonatal mortality rates/ 1000 live births
Postmature (42 weeks +)		1
Term	(37–41 weeks)	1–2
Pre-term	32–36 weeks	12
	28–31 weeks	110
	26–27 weeks	300
	<26 weeks	800

Approximately 50% of babies born weighing between 500 and 1000 g will be alive 1 year later, based on national figures for 1983–1991. Fetuses which weigh 500 g or more are generally considered viable. Only a small proportion weighing <500 g will survive.

Perinatal mortality rates have fallen due to significant improvements in survival of premature infants. There has, however, been little improvement in the stillbirths rate in normally formed infants. Current methods of antenatal surveillance and fetal assessment do not appear to be sufficient to prevent such deaths. There then remains that proportion of deaths due to problems in labour including asphyxia and birth trauma. While the incidence of these problems declines with improved intrapartum care, there will always be some deaths which at present must be considered unpreventable.

Congenital malformations

Approximately 7000 reports of congenital malformations are received annually. A congenital malformation is defined as any physical malformation, including a biochemical abnormality, which is present at birth.

The Office of Population Censuses and Surveys (OPCS) publishes an annual review of congenital malformations in England and Wales; Scottish statistics are recorded separately. OPCS has monitored the incidence of notification of congenital malformations since 1964 as a result of the thalidomide epidemic. Notification is voluntary and only covers malformations noted up to 10 days after birth. It includes multiple malformations associated with chromosomal abnormalities, but not diseases such as Rhesus disease.

As a result of the fall in infant deaths from other causes such as infection, congenital malformations constitute an increasing proportion of infant mortality. In 1991 approximately 5000 infants died aged under 1 year. 25% of these had a major condition or underlying cause of congenital malformation resulting in death. Approximately 6% of all stillbirths now are due to a congenital malformation. Current trends include a long-term decrease in central nervous system (CNS) malformations, the decrease being greatest in those CNS malformations which may be detected by ultrasound or

Box 41 CESDI enquiry findings 1993

• Unexplained antepartum stillbirth	35%
• Immaturity	18%
• Lethal or severe congenital malformation (50% were neonatal deaths)	15%
• Intrapartum related death	9%
• Infection	6%
• Other specific causes	9%
• Sudden unexpected infant death	5%
• Unclassifiable	2%
• Accident or non-intrapartum trauma	0.7%

AFP screening. The incidence is decreasing even allowing for those terminated in early pregnancy. Some notifications are gender specific, for example hypospadias. The incidence of congenital dislocation of the hip is higher in females.

There are thus many problems in the interpretation of perinatal mortality statistics. For comparative purposes they must be corrected for the incidence of congenital malformation, and specific gestational age ranges must be compared. Nonetheless, such statistics provide a valuable method of on-going audit of the provision of obstetric care.

9.4 Perinatal morbidity

Learning objective

You should:

- understand the causes of perinatal morbidity

Attention is now increasingly focused on ways of reducing perinatal morbidity, as perinatal mortality rates have fallen. While the main focus has been on the incidence of cerebral palsy as described below, the quality of obstetric care affects morbidity in many other ways. Premature neonates may suffer in the long term as a result of chronic lung disease of prematurity, necrotising enterocolitis and infectious morbidity. Term infants may suffer from meconium-related morbidity and the consequences of perinatally acquired infection.

9.5 Cerebral palsy

Learning objectives

You should:

- be familiar with the potential causes of cerebral palsy

- and therefore understand how obstetric practice might influence the incidence of cerebral palsy

The incidence of cerebral palsy has changed little over recent decades (2–2.5 per thousand live births), and until recent years this was thought to be a reflection of intrapartum asphyxia. The list of causes is outlined in Box 42, though the vast majority are of unknown aetiology possibly due to problems during the antenatal period.

Box 42 Cerebral palsy: aetiology

- Cause unknown
- Complications of prematurity
- Peripartum asphyxia (< 15%)
- Postnatal (encephalitis, accidents)
- Perinatal infection (CMV, rubella)
- Associated with multiple pregnancy (especially with co-twin death)
- Chromosomal anomalies
- Other congenital abnormalities
- Toxicity (rare)
- Trauma (rare)

As most cases of cerebral palsy are of unknown origin it remains very difficult to know how to prevent them. Cerebral palsy is strongly associated with low birth weight and there is now concern that the prevalence may be increasing due to increased survival of brain-damaged pre-term infants. It has been suggested in the past that close monitoring of the fetus in labour may help prevent cerebral palsy, but with the increasing recognition that the origin is likely to be much earlier in pregnancy this has been discredited other than for exceptional cases. There is to date no evidence that monitoring of the fetus in labour by currently available methods reduces the incidence of cerebral palsy.

9.6 Maternal satisfaction and rates of operative delivery

In attempting to achieve optimal perinatal outcome it is imperative that no excessive cost is incurred in maternal mortality or morbidity. This may be the case if inappropriate operative vaginal delivery is attempted or an unnecessary caesarean section performed. For this reason rates of operative delivery are closely monitored.

Current rates of caesarean delivery vary in the UK between 7% and 20%. While much of the variation results from higher risk populations attending some hospitals, and some is patient-led, most arise from different opinions of obstetricians regarding risk and benefits of caesarean delivery. Rates of caesarean delivery have increased over the past 2 decades, without very clear evidence of improved perinatal outcome as a result. It is likely that only very small gains in perinatal survival result from substantial increases in the caesarean section rate. Nonetheless, even a small risk of perinatal death and handicap are unacceptable within society today, and therefore it is often not clear at exactly which threshold a caesarean delivery should be performed. In parallel with these changes, elective caesarean section has become much safer, with the maternal risk now approaching that of a vaginal delivery. There is, however, unequivocal evidence that emergency caesarean section carries a higher risk. This raises the dilemma for the clinician as to whether in the presence of a significant chance of caesarean delivery during labour, an elective caesarean is not the best option.

Morbidity from operative vaginal delivery is an equally important issue. The increased incidence of third degree tears and trauma associated with operative deliveries has long-term implications with regard to prolapse and incontinence in later life.

9.7 Information availability and meta-analysis in obstetrics

Learning objective

You should:

- understand the rationale behind metaanalysis

As a result of the dilemmas outlined above it is important for the obstetrician and the patient that good quality information is available to guide decision-making. Given the now very low incidence of adverse perinatal outcome, it is difficult for studies to address these questions other than by way of surrogate markers. For this reason, meta-analysis of trials is being increasingly used as a guide to best clinical practice. Faced with an ever increasing volume of literature on obstetrics and gynaecology, it is increasingly difficult for obstetricians to read all the individual studies. This provides further reason for the use of meta-analysis of studies. Such meta-analyses for the UK are currently coordinated by the Cochrane Centre in Oxford which acts in parallel with the National Perinatal Epidemiology Unit.

The National Perinatal Epidemiology Unit in Oxford is a Department of Health funded research unit, responsible for both conducting and facilitating research. Its work includes facilitating randomisation in multicentre studies, and synthesising and disseminating results of research. The unit monitors data collected from government sources and elsewhere to determine trends in relation to childbirth, and publishes an annual report summarising its work.

9.8 Audit

Learning objective

You should:

- understand the audit cycle

All forms of medical intervention should be subjected to regular audit to ensure that appropriate care is being delivered in a cost-effective way. Standards must be set so that performance can be compared. This involves formally recording outcomes of procedures, reviewing the results, implementing any necessary changes and then assessing whether the changes have had the desired effect. Information must be gathered systematically and the evidence interpreted objectively. Comparison of performance with peers is then carried out and deficiencies identified, together with the action required to remedy them. Following change of practice, the effects of such change are then monitored, closing the audit loop. This function is served by the processes of perinatal and maternal review as outlined above, and is currently being extended to include many routine procedures within obstetrical and gynaecological practice.

Self-assessment: questions

Multiple choice questions

1. In relation to maternal mortality:
   a. Ectopic pregnancy accounts for more maternal deaths than thromboembolism
   b. Sepsis is no longer a concern since antibiotics became available
   c. Regional anaesthesia is safer than general anaesthesia
   d. Deaths from amniotic fluid embolism are declining
   e. Caesarean delivery is now as safe as vaginal delivery provided a regional anaesthetic is used

2. With regard to perinatal mortality:
   a. It is increasing
   b. Improvements reflect better prevention of preterm labour
   c. Intrapartum loss rates can be reduced further by more widespread availability of CTG monitoring
   d. Neonatal deaths are independent of obstetric care
   e. The incidence of cerebral palsy is decreasing, reflecting improved management of the fetus in labour

Short notes

1. Discuss methods of improving perinatal mortality.

Self-assessment: answers

Multiple choice answers

1. a. **False.** Thromboembolic disease is now the greatest cause of maternal death, resulting in 27% of direct maternal deaths.
   b. **False.** There are still maternal deaths due to sepsis. To some extent this reflects the lack of effectiveness of antibiotics in treating intra-uterine sepsis prior to delivery of the fetus or the placenta. Diagnosis and management of incidental causes of sepsis such as pneumonia are also complicated by pregnancy.
   c. **True.** Regional anaesthesia should always be used when possible.
   d. **False.** The lack of success in this area reflects our inability to predict when it may occur and also our poor understanding of the pathophysiology, reflected in limited treatment options.
   e. **False.** While caesarean delivery is now safer than in previous decades, it cannot be regarded as equal in safety to vaginal delivery. Mothers should always be fully informed of the potential risks if elective caesarean is planned.

2. a. **False.** Perinatal mortality is falling. This reflects improvements in antenatal care in preventing intra-uterine death, and neonatal care in preventing early neonatal death. Further improvements in the stillbirth rate are likely to depend on improved understanding of pathophysiological mechanisms.
   b. **False.** Efforts at preventing pre-term labour have not met with success to date. This is another area where improved understanding of the underlying pathophysiology should be beneficial.
   c. **False.** CTG monitoring is not likely to confer much benefit as CTGs are of limited use and are already used for most high risk pregnancies.
   d. **False.** Obstetric care can influence the well-being of the neonate substantially. This is why early neonatal deaths are included as 'perinatal', such that the overall statistic reflects quality of obstetric care. Good management will allow prompt treatment of perinatal infection, prevention of asphyxia, optimal timing of delivery of the premature fetus, and a coordinated approach to care of the infant with a congenital abnormality.
   e. **False.** The incidence of cerebral palsy is not decreasing. Only a small proportions of all cerebral palsy is thought to arise from events during labour. This means that any attempt at reducing the incidence will have to concentrate on understanding the potential causes in utero.

Short notes answer

To reduce perinatal mortality significantly it is likely that a major advance in the management of one of the major causes would be required. Stillbirths comprise the major cause of mortality and there has been little improvement in the prevention of this problem in the past decade. Many antepartum stillbirths occur without any clear cause on postmortem examination, and prevention of these is impossible until such time as the aetiology is understood. The other major subgroup of stillbirths occurs where there is suboptimal growth in utero. Improvements here will depend on improved detection of intra-uterine growth retardation, improved surveillance of such fetuses, including appropriate use of Doppler ultrasound in their management, and extending the use of steroids where such fetuses have to be delivered prior to lung maturity. None of the above measures will make a major impact, however, and it is likely that major improvements will only be made when an improved screening method for IUGR becomes available or a better understanding of the pathophysiology leads to preventative measures. Of the stillbirths which occur in the absence of IUGR, a small proportion may be prevented by improved care of diabetic women, and greater awareness of cholestasis in pregnancy. Stillbirths also arise in association with placental abruption. In these situations maternal well-being is the major concern and there is no screening or therapeutic measure which is likely to prevent such stillbirths in the near future. As with many causes already mentioned, research leading to a better understanding of the underlying pathophysiology represents the best hope of long-term improvement.

The next largest cause of perinatal mortality is that associated with prematurity. Substantial improvements have been made in the provision of neonatal care, resulting in improved survival of pre-term babies. It is possible that further significant improvements may come about through greater use of steroids in women threatening to deliver pre-term, and further research into other therapeutic measures to improve fetal lung maturity. The treatment of pre-term labour is more difficult, and to date no major improvement in perinatal outcome has been shown with tocolytic drugs. It is possible that improved rationale for the use of tocolysis to allow in-utero transfer or administration of steroids will help. Newer tocolytic agents currently being researched may prove to be more effective. These drugs include oxytocin receptor antagonists and selective cyclo-oxygenase inhibitors.

Congenital abnormalities are also a major cause of perinatal mortality. Most of these are not preventable, but it is very important when specific preventative measures are available, such as the administration of folic acid to prevent neural tube defects, that these are used across the whole population. The vast majority of congenital abnormalities are not preventable, and improvements in their care can only arise through improved diagnosis and management in utero, and effective communication between obstetricians and the neonatal and paediatric surgical staff.

Intrapartum losses contribute less to perinatal mortality than all of the above causes. Nonetheless, intrapartum loss causes considerable stress and is the subject of much litigation. It is perceived by parents that once they are admitted to a delivery suite with a normally formed baby and under continuous care, problems should not arise. Some intrapartum losses may not be preventable (some placental abruptions or cases of shoulder dystocia) though others are preventable provided ideal care is delivered. Errors will of course arise for human and organisational reasons. The rate of intrapartum death is considered a measure of quality of care within a unit. While the absolute number of intrapartum deaths that are preventable is small, it is likely that some reduction may be achieved through appropriate training and supervision of labour ward staff, rehearsed management of emergencies, and appropriate recourse to caesarean delivery in the presence of fetal distress.

In summary, some improvements in perinatal mortality are achievable by ensuring that the current best standards of care are provided universally for all patients. Major improvements, however, are only likely to be achieved by breakthroughs in the field of perinatal research leading to improved understanding of the pathophysiology of these conditions.

2

10 Disorders of childhood and puberty

Overview

Disorders of childhood and puberty comprise a small yet important part of gynaecological practice. Normal gender development requires a normal chromosome complement, normal hormone production, end organ sensitivity, and normal anatomy. The ovaries play no part in the development of the genital tract, in that the presence of testes cause male genital organs to develop and in their absence female genital organs will develop. When normal mechanisms fail, there may be ambiguous genitalia present at birth. When this occurs, a decision has to be made about gender assignment.

10.1 Determination of sex

Learning objectives

You should know:

- the chromosomal difference between male and female
- the different ways in which the sex of an individual can be defined

The sex of an individual can be defined at phenotypic, chromosomal, gonadal, or behavioural level. Most cases are easily classified as either male or female by the appearance of the external genitalia at birth. The normal female has two X chromosomes, making a complement of 46XX. The normal male has a 46XY chromosome complement. When development is abnormal, sex determination can be difficult. Such individuals may have the phenotype of one sex but the gonads or chromosomes of the other.

10.2 Normal development

Learning objective

You should understand:

- how the presence of the Y chromosome affects sexual development

The sex of the fetal gonads can be determined from 6 weeks' gestation. Prior to this, the fetal gonad is undifferentiated. The internal genitalia are represented by two systems of ducts, the Wolffian system with potential for male development, and the Müllerian system with potential for female development. The external genitalia are common to both sexes up to 8 weeks' gestation, consisting of a midline genital tubercle, a urogenital groove, and labio-scrotal swellings. In the female, the absence of a Y chromosome allows the Müllerian system to develop. The paired Müllerian tracts fuse in the midline to form the fallopian tubes, uterus and vagina. In the male the presence of the Y sex chromosome causes development of testes. The testes produce testosterone and Müllerian inhibiting factor (MIF). Testosterone causes development of the male external genitalia and formation of the vas deferens and epididymis from the Wolffian duct. Müllerian inhibiting factor prevents the development of the female upper genital tract.

10.3 Anatomical malformations of the female genital tract

Isolated anatomical abnormalities of the female tract may occur in the presence of entirely normal chromosomal and gonadal configuration. The common forms are described below.

Vaginal atresia

This is described under delayed menarche.

Incomplete fusion of the Müllerian ducts

Incomplete fusion of the Müllerian ducts results in varying degrees of duplication of the uterus and vagina (Fig. 18). These are associated with anomalies of the urinary tract such as double ureter and pelvic kidney.

Septate vagina

The vagina may be separated into two distinct passages by an anteroposterior septum (Fig. 18D). This may occur in isolation or be accompanied by duplication of the uterus. There is rarely any problem with intercourse, but a septum may occasionally need to be divided to allow a normal vaginal delivery.

Uterine duplications

There are several varieties. In complete lack of Müllerian duct fusion there is a double uterus and double vagina (Fig. 18A). In bicornuate uterus the two uterine horns may be of unequal size, and have completely separate cavities (Fig. 18B). A rudimentary horn (Fig. 18E) may have no patent connection with the lower genital tract. A septate uterus has a normal external appearance but the cavity is partly divided by a septum (Fig. 18C). These abnormalities may interfere with placentation, leading to miscarriage, and with fetal lie in late pregnancy, leading to malpresentations. A rudimentary uterine horn should be excised because of the risk of rupture if pregnancy occurs within it.

Wolffian duct remnants

Remnants of the Wolffian duct are occasionally seen as cysts, found in the broad ligament, the outer end of the fallopian tube or the lateral wall of the vagina.

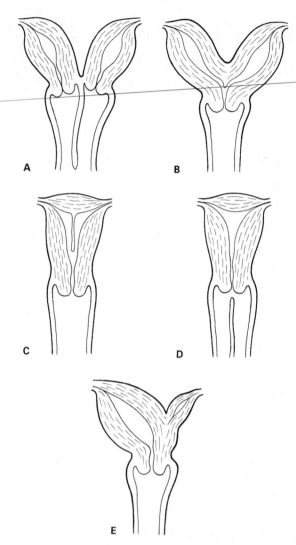

Fig. 18 Common anomalies of the uterus and vagina: (**A**) complete lack of Müllerian duct fusion: double uterus and double vagina; (**B**) bicornuate uterus; (**C**) septate uterus; (**D**) septate vagina: (**E**) rudimentary uterine horn.

10.4 Intersex

The term intersex is used in cases where there is difficulty or contradiction in deciding the appropriate sex designation. It is extremely rare. If the ascribed gender is at odds with chromosomal or gonadal sex, this may only become apparent at a later stage in life. Then it is rarely either necessary or desirable to reassign gender and the situation must be handled with extreme care and sensitivity to avoid immense psychological upset. The chromosomal complement will usually determine the sex of the gonads.

Types of intersex

- Chromosomal
- Gonadal
- Partial masculinisation of chromosomal and gonadal females
- Incomplete masculinisation of chromosomal and gonadal males.

Chromosomal intersex

There are many varieties of chromosomal intersex. The majority of chromosomally abnormal embryos spontaneously abort. The more common ones are described below.

Turner's syndrome

This has an incidence of 1 in 2500 live births. The chromosome abnormality is 45,X0 with deletion of the Y sex chromosome. Rarely there is a chromosomal mosaic appearance with 2 different cell lines such as 46,X0/46,XX. The ovaries are present as rudimentary streaks due to developmental failure at around 20 weeks' gestation. The absence of the Y chromosome means that normal female internal organs develop with a uterus and vagina, but menstruation and ovulation are absent because of ovarian failure. Individuals are of short stature, with poorly developed secondary sex characteristics. Other features include a webbed neck, increased carrying angle, wide spaced nipples, low hair line and shortening of the fourth metacarpal.

Klinefelter's syndrome

This has an incidence of 1 in 1000 live births. The chromosome abnormality is 47,XXY. The presence of a Y chromosome allows development of testes and a male phenotype, despite the abnormal chromosome complement. Individuals are phenotypic males, many of whom enjoy normal active sex lives. Clinical features include small testes, gynaecomastia, diminished body hair and marginally low intelligence. Many individuals are azoospermic, and have degeneration of the seminiferous tubules on testicular biopsy. Sometimes the condition is diagnosed when karyotyping is performed as part of investigations into male infertility. Delicate handling of the situation is then needed. Sterility is not absolute because of the occasional small 46,XY cell line.

Gonadal intersex

Ovotesticular states

The presence of both ovarian and testicular tissue is termed hermaphroditism. It is extremely rare. Most cases are 46,XX rather than 46,XX/46,XY. It is characterised by mixed development of internal and external genitalia. Most individuals are reared as males.

Pure gonadal dysgenesis

In this condition the female phenotype develops regardless of chromosomal sex which may be 46,XX or 46,XY. In contrast to Turner's syndrome there are no other features apart from absent secondary sex characteristics.

Partial masculinisation of chromosomal and gonadal females

Congenital adrenal hyperplasia

There are several types, all consisting of abnormalities in steroid synthesis. The common form is 21-hydroxylase deficiency, which is an autosomal recessive disorder. There is an inability to produce cortisol in normal quantities, leading to an increase in adrenocorticotrophic hormone (ACTH), and increased production of cortisol precursors which are converted to androgens. The build-up of androgens causes masculinisation of a female child and thus ambiguity of genitalia at birth. The infant may become systemically ill with disordered blood biochemistry. Early diagnosis is important because treatment with cortisol allows normal development. Diagnosis is made by finding increased urinary pregnanetriol and serum 17 hydroxy-progesterone levels. The late onset variety presents at puberty with hirsutism and clitoral enlargement.

Masculinisation of a female fetus

This can occur from exogenous steroid administration during pregnancy.

Incomplete masculinisation of chromosomal and gonadal males

Androgen insensitivity syndrome

This was previously called testicular feminisation. A defect of androgen receptors prevents masculinisation of a 46,XY karyotype. Individuals are phenotypically female, and are often happily married. Breast development occurs at puberty. A blind ending vagina is present, which permits coitus, but the uterus is absent. Testosterone levels are elevated but produce no clinical effects due to end organ insensitivity. Testes are found in the lower abdomen or occasionally in hernial sacs, but the woman need not be burdened with this information, or informed of her male karyotype. They should be advised that they have abnormal gonads which need to be removed because of a 30% risk of malignancy.

5 alpha-reductase deficiency

This is an autosomal recessive condition characterised by a failure to convert testosterone into the active dihydrotestosterone, due to an enzyme deficiency. Testosterone is present but ineffective, so the external genitalia have a female appearance. The uterus is absent.

Management of intersex

Early and correct assignment of gender is important in cases where there is ambiguity of the external genitalia at birth. This may require an examination under anaesthetic, imaging of the internal genital organs and a karyotype. Once an individual has adjusted to a particular sex there can be serious psychological problems in trying to change it later. With the exception of the adrenogenital syndrome, fertility is rarely possible, but sexual intercourse often is. As mentioned above, intra-abdominal gonads should be surgically removed in the androgen insensitivity syndrome because of a 30% risk of malignancy.

10.5 Puberty

Learning objectives

You should know:

- the five stages of puberty and when they usually occur
- the hormonal changes involved at puberty

Puberty is a time of profound physical and psychological development linking childhood to adulthood. The most obvious change is the appearance of the secondary sex characteristics. These begin to appear at a mean age of 10.5 years, but there is great individual variation.

The stages of puberty

Five morphological changes are seen:

- breast growth
- pubic hair growth
- axillary hair growth
- growth spurt
- menstruation.

Breast growth is the first sign of puberty, and is called thelarche. It begins with budding below the areola. Full development takes 5 years. Breast growth may initially be asymmetrical but this is usually transitory. Pubic hair begins to appear shortly after breast budding, and is followed by development of the labia. Axillary hair appears slightly later than pubic hair, at around 13 years of age. The adolescent growth spurt takes place between 10 and 14 years and coincides with sexual development. Peak growth reaches 11 cm per year. Most girls reach their maximum height by 14 years when the bony epiphyses fuse. Menstruation occurs by the age of 13 in 95% of girls, but the range is 10–16 years. During the growth spurt there is a 120% increase in body fat, from about 5 to 11 kg. In contrast, lean body weight increases by under half this amount. Body fat is a significant source of extragonadal oestrogen production. Body weight and fat have a significant effect on both menstruation and reproductive function in later life. Too little or too much fat are associated with infertility, due to disturbance of the hypothalamic–pituitary–ovarian (HPO) axis (see p. 139). Both anorexia nervosa and intensive athletic training can delay the onset of puberty because of the low percentage of body fat.

These physical changes occur in response to a maturation of the hypothalamus, and an alteration in the secretion of gonadotrophin-releasing hormone (GnRH). The precise trigger for this is unknown, but GnRH secretion is influenced by several brain neurotransmitters and by impulses from the amygdala and hippocampus. During childhood, the hypothalamus is extremely sensitive to the negative feedback effect of small amounts of circulating oestrogen and testosterone, so only small amounts of GnRH are released. As puberty approaches, hypothalamic sensitivity decreases and there is a progressive increase in the amplitude and frequency of pulsatile GnRH secretion. This initially occurs only during sleep, but gradually extends to waking hours. GnRH reaches the anterior pituitary via the hypothalamic–

hypophyseal portal circulation, where it stimulates increased synthesis and release of the pituitary gonadotrophins lateinising hormone (LH) and follicle-stimulating hormone (FSH). The ovarian granulosa cells respond to the increased FSH by producing oestradiol, and ovarian follicular development commences. Oestradiol is the primary sex steroid and it induces development of the secondary sex characteristics. It also has a positive feedback effect on LH production. When a dominant ovarian follicle develops, increasing oestrogen levels induce a surge of LH which in turn causes ovulation.

The secretion of adrenal androgens takes place as early as 6–7 years of age and is called the adrenarche. Androgen levels continue to rise throughout puberty and this instigates both the prepubertal growth spurt and the appearance of axillary and pubic hair.

Abnormalities of puberty

The onset of puberty varies within a wide age range, and is dependent on the integrity of the HPO axis. Abnormalities of puberty include:

- delayed puberty
- delayed menarche
- precocious puberty
- pseudo-precocious puberty.

10.6 Delayed puberty

Learning objective

You should:

- know the definition and causes of delayed puberty

This means failure of the development of secondary sex characteristics by 14 years of age.

Causes

- Constitutional
- Primary hypogonadism
- Secondary hypogonadism
- Trauma.

Constitutional

There is an idiopathic delay in the maturation and activation of the HPO axis. There is often a family history of the same. It is self-limiting and no treatment is required apart from reassurance.

Primary hypogonadism

The defect here is due to ovarian failure. Inability of the ovary to secrete adequate amounts of oestrogen results in a lack of negative feedback on the hypothalamus and pituitary, so gonadotrophin levels are increased. It is thus also known as hypergonadotrophic hypogonadism. The most common cause is Turner's syndrome. Other causes include chemotherapy, radiotherapy or autoimmune disease.

Secondary hypogonadism

This is a rare cause of delayed sexual development, resulting from a lack of endogenous gonadotrophin secretion, gonadotrophin levels are low so it is known as hypogonadotrophic hypogonadism. Causes of gonadotrophin deficiency include a chromophobe adenoma of the pituitary, craniopharyngioma, the Laurence–Moon–Biedl syndrome and the Prader–Willi syndrome.

Trauma

Cerebral trauma and hydrocephalus causing hypothalamic damage are rare causes of delayed puberty.

10.7 Delayed menarche

Learning objective

You should:

- know the definition and causes of delayed menarche

If menstruation has not started by 16 years of age in the presence of otherwise normal sexual development it is considered delayed and required investigation.

Causes of delayed menarche

Vaginal atresia

Atresia of the vagina caues retention of the normal menses. This is called cryptomenorrhoea. The atresia is usually in the form of a thin membrane just above the hymen. Menstrual blood is unable to escape and the vagina becomes distened with blood to form a haematocolpos. This may be accompanied by cyclical pain. Examination reveals a bulging membrane at the introitus, and an abdominal mass may be present if the uterus has been pushed above the symphysis pubis. Treatment is by simple incision of the membrane. Complete vaginal atresia presents in a similar way but requires more extensive reconstructive surgery to correct the anatomy.

Defective cycle initiation

This is a common cause of delayed menarche, an is due to immaturity of the HPO axis. Endocrine investigations are usually normal. Such women occasionally experience lifelong irregular ovulation and reduced fertility, but this is usually responsive to treatement with clomiphene.

Androgen insensitivity syndrome

An end organ androgen receptor defect prevents masculinisation of a 46,XY karyotype. Patients are thus phenotypically female, and are reared as such. The uterus is absent and testosterone levels are elevated.

10.8 Precocious puberty

Learning objective

You should:

- know the definition and causes of precocious puberty

True precocious puberty is the appearance of secondary sex characteristics before the age of 8 years. It is due to early activation of the HPO axis. In contrast, pseudo-precocious puberty is the result of sex steroid stimulation which is independent of the HPO axis. The only long-term stigma is short stature, which results from early epiphyseal closure. The accelerated physical growth and development makes these children look older than they are. This can lead to difficulties because emotional and intellectual development remain normal for chronological age.

The pattern of early sexual development follows the same sequence as that of normal puberty, and is always in accordance with phenotypic sex. No cause is found in 80% of females, but in males a space-occupying lesion is found in 50%.

Aetiology of precocious puberty

- Idiopathic
- Cerebral tumour
- Hydrocephalus
- Head injury, seizure, central nervous system (CNS) infection
- von Recklinghausen syndrome
- McCune Albright syndrome.

Incomplete precocious puberty

Isolated early features of puberty such as breast development, pubic hair growth or onset of menstruation are occasionally seen. These are called premature thelarche, adrenarche and menarche respectively.

Managemnt of precocious puberty

All causes need hormonal and radiological investigation in order to identify causal factors such as tumours. In the more common idiopathic variety treatment aims to arrest the development of secodnary sex characteristics and delay the progress of bone maturation. Luteinising hormone releasing hormone (LHRH) agonists are used to produce a reversible down-regulation of the pituitary.

10.9 Pseudo-precocious puberty

Learning objective

You should:

- understand the difference between precocious and pseudo-precocious puberty

The clinical picture is similar to true precocious puberty. There is early development of the secondary sex characteristics, but without activation of the HPO axis. The most common cause is an oestrogen-secreting ovarian tumour. Oestrogen levels will be high but in contrast to true precocious puberty gonadotrophin levels will be suppressed.

10.10 Eating disorders

Learning objectives

You should appreciate that:

- dieting to lose weight in adolescent girls may become obsessional, leading to anorexia
- anorexia may be a response to the psychosexual pressures of adolescence

The eating disorders anorexia nervosa and bulimia nervosa are becoming increasingly common, especially among ballet dancers and models. Presentation is frequently around the time of puberty or during the teenage years, often with a gynaecological problem, such as amenorrhoea, infertility or symtpoms of oestrogen deficiency. The fundamental problem is that extreme fears about weight gain or fatness lead to rigid dieting, vomiting or laxative abuse. In bulimia, dieting is interspersed by episodes of massive overeating. The hormonal profile in anorexia resembles that of a pre-pubertal girl. There is diminished pulsatile LH release, hypothalamic dysfunction, and impaired oestrogen secretion. This results in amenorrhoea, a failure to ovulate, reduced sex drive and infertility. The bone loss which also occurs is thought to result from a primary osteoblast dysfunction, related to poor nutrition.

Treatment of eating disorder

Treatment focuses on nutritional recovery, which may be combined with psychological and self-help measures, to encourage a more normal adaptation to adulthood. If the treatment is successful, weight gain is accompanied by the establishment of normal menstruation and fertility.

Follow-up studies have shown that treatment is not always successful in the long term, especially where there are poor child–parent relationships or associated psychiatric problems, when mortality approaches 20%.

Box 43 Features of anorexia nervosa		
Symptoms	**Signs**	**Sequelae**
Lack of periods	Emaciation	Amenorrhoea
Poor sleep	Bradycardia	Infertility
Cold intolerance	Anaemia	Psychosexual
Constipation	Increased body hair	dysfunction
Loss of head hair		Osteoporosis

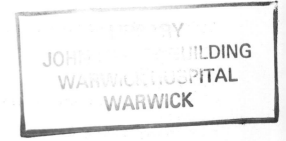

Self-assessment: questions

Multiple choice questions

1. Which of the following are true?
   a. In the absence of a Y chromosome, fetal development is female
   b. The Wolffian ducts develop into the male reproductive collecting system
   c. Development of male external characteristics is controlled by androgens
   d. The sex of the fetal gonad cannot be determined prior to 6 weeks' gestation
   e. Development of the Müllerian ducts is dependent upon the presence of ovaries

2. Precocious puberty:
   a. Results in tall stature
   b. Can be distinguished from pseudo-precocious puberty by measurement of LH levels
   c. Breast buds are the first sign
   d. Has no causative factor in 80% of girls
   e. Is difficult to define precisely because of the marked variation in the age of normal puberty
   f. Causes psychosocial difficulties

3. Concerning normal puberty:
   a. The first event is thought to be nocturnal release of gonadotrophins
   b. Once initiated, occurs at the same speed in both sexes
   c. The average age of onset is falling
   d. Initial cycles are often anovulatory
   e. Growth stops after the menarche

4. Concerning Turner's syndrome (45,X0):
   a. Gonadotrophin levels are usually elevated
   b. Streak gonads should be removed because of the risk of malignancy
   c. Withdrawal bleeding can be induced with hormone replacement therapy
   d. There is an increased incidence of congenital cardiac lesions
   e. Individuals are usually under 147 cm

Short notes

1. An 18-year-old girl has not yet started her periods. What are the possible causes and how could you differentiate between them?

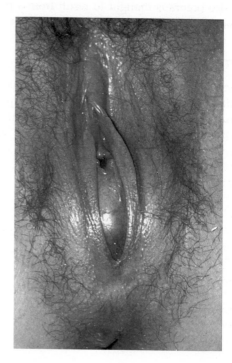

Fig. 19

Picture question

Figure 19 shows the clinical appearance of the vulva of a 16-year-old girl who complains of monthly episodes of pelvic pain. She says her periods have not started yet. On examination, there was a tender suprapubic mass.

1. What clinical abnormality do you see?
2. What is the likely nature of the abdominal mass?
3. What is the appropriate treatment?
4. What would be the most likely karyotype?

Self-assessment: answers

Multiple choice answers

1. a. **True.**
   b. **True.**
   c. **True.**
   d. **True.**
   e. **False.** The Müllerian duct always develops unless Müllerian inhibiting factor is produced by the testes.

2. a. **False.** Precocious puberty results in short stature due to premature epiphyseal closure.
   b. **True.**
   c. **True.**
   d. **True.** Most cases are constitutional.
   e. **True.**
   f. **True.** Precocious sexual activity and behavioural problems are common in affected girls.

3. a. **False.** The first event of puberty is the nocturnal release of GnRH which stimulates gonadotrophin release.
   b. **False.** Puberty begins on average 9 months earlier in girls, and once started is usually complete within 3 years, compared to 5 years in boys.
   c. **True.** The average age of puberty has shown a gradual decrease over the last 4 decades. This is thought to be due to improved nutrition and less physical work.
   d. **True.** Postmenarchal cycles are often anovulatory, and dysfunctional uterine bleeding is common. The frequency of ovulatory cycles gradually increases as the reproductive system continues to mature.
   e. **False.** Growth slows but does not stop after the menarche.

4. a. **True.**
   b. **False.** It is only phenotypically female individuals with XY karyotypes who require gonadal excision because of the increased risk of malignancy.
   c. **True.** The uterus is intact so withdrawal bleeds can be induced by giving hormone replacement therapy. Hormone replacement therapy (HRT) will also allow development of secondary sex characteristics.
   d. **True.**
   e. **True.** Short stature is typical of Turner's syndrome.

Short notes answer

1. This is a difficult question to answer, which requires a thorough understanding of the physiological mechanisms and embryological development necessary for normal menstruation. The possibilities include:

- idiopathic delay in an otherwise normal female
- physiological reason such as pregnancy
- anatomical disorder in an otherwise normal female, such as imperforate hymen
- chromosomal disorder such as Turner's syndrome (45,X0)
- androgen insensitivity syndrome in a 46,XY karyotype
- cerebral lesion such as a craniopharyngioma
- primary gonadal failure, either 46,XX or 46,XY (gonadal dysgenesis).

The history and clinical examination will point to the cause in the majority of cases. The relevant points are:

1. Has there been normal development of female secondary sex characteristics?
2. Has a local anatomical abnormality in the genital tract been excluded?
3. Has pregnancy been excluded?
4. Is the patient of short stature (below 147 cm)?

If the answer to 1, 2 and 3 is yes, spontaneous onset of menstruation can be expected with time, or alternatively withdrawal bleeds can be induced by administration of oestrogen and progestogen.

An anatomical abnormality such as vaginal atresia may be an isolated finding in an otherwise normal female with normal sex characteristics. A blind ending vagina and absent uterus on examination is suggestive of androgen insensitivity syndrome. Karyotyping will show 46,XY.

If the woman is of short stature, there may be features of Turner's syndrome such as a wide carrying angle or widely spaced nipples, together with an absence of female secondary sex characteristics. Karyotyping will confirm the diagnosis. If the karyotype is 46,XX then rare causes such as craniopharyngioma should be excluded by CT scan. A diagnosis of panhypopituitarism is equally rare and will usually have been made earlier.

If normal female secondary sex characteristics are absent and the stature is normal, gonadal dysgenesis is a possibility. Karyotyping is essential in these cases. In 46,XX individuals there will be elevation of LH and FSH levels secondary to the ovarian failure. If gonadotrophin levels are normal or low, the diagnosis is hypogonadotrophic hypogonadism.

Those individuals with 46,XY will require excision of the gonads due to the 30% risk of malignancy.

Picture answer

1. The tense bulging membrane visible is an imperforate hymen. It results from distension of the vagina by the retained menstrual fluid haematocolpos.

2. Haematometra – a uterus distended with fluid. It is displaced upwards by the haematocolpos.
3. Incision of the hymen, under general anaesthetic, which allows the retained menses to drain, and normal menstruation to commence.
4. As this is an isolated anatomical problem, the karyotype should be 46XX.

11 Disorders of menstruation

Overview

The menstrual cycle is under the control of the hypothalamic–pituitary–ovarian endocrine axis. Menstruation occurs as a result of falling progesterone levels. Many different factors can affect the menstrual cycle, and disorders of menstruation are common. There are now a wide variety of different treatment options for heavy periods. Abnormal vaginal bleeding, especially after the menopause, may be the presenting symptom of gynaecological cancer, although in the majority of cases a less serious cause for the bleeding will be found.

Introduction

The monthly vaginal bleeding which occurs due to the shedding of secretory endometrium is called menstruation. It occurs in response to falling levels of the steroid hormone progesterone. Typically the bleeding lasts 4–5 days. It is heaviest on the first 2 days and then gradually diminishes as the endometrium begins to regenerate. The average monthly menstrual loss is 30 ml but there is great individual variation. Menstruation is usually accompanied by some lower abdominal cramping pains, caused by myometrial contractions. The first menstruation is called the menarche. This occurs at an average age of 13 years. Menstruation ceases at the menopause, which occurs at an average age of 51 years. Disorders of menstruation are extremely common and can result from a wide variety of causes. In order to understand these it is necessary to consider the mechanism of normal menstruation in more detail.

11.1 The menstrual cycle

Learning objectives

You should:

- understand the changes which occur throughout the menstrual cycle
- understand what controls the menstrual cycle

The menstrual cycle has an average duration of 28 days with a range of 21–35 days. It consists of proliferative and secretory phases that correspond with the follicular and luteal phases of the ovarian cycle (Fig. 20). It is the result of complex interactions between the hypothalamic–pituitary–ovarian (HPO) endocrine axis. During the proliferative phase of the cycle, oestrogen causes growth of endometrial glands and stroma. The glands elongate and the endometrium becomes thicker. This renders conditions favourable for implantation of a blastocyst, should fertilisation occur. After ovulation, progesterone is produced by the corpus luteum. Progesterone causes secretory change in the endometrium. The glands become distended and the stroma loose and oedematous. This is termed decidualisation. When progesterone levels fall with the demise of the corpus luteum, vasoactive substances such as prostaglandins, histamine and bradykinin are produced by the endometrium. Prostaglandins cause spasm of the spiral arterioles which results in ischaemic necrosis and shedding of all but the basal layer of the endometrium. The spiral arterioles then relax, allowing blood to pass into the distal part of the endometrium, resulting in menstruation. Clotting does not normally occur because of the

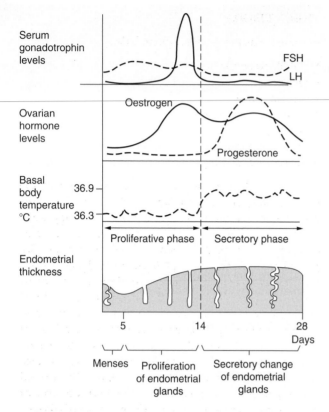

Serum gonadotrophin levels

FSH

LH

Ovarian hormone levels

Oestrogen

Progesterone

Basal body temperature °C

36.9

36.3

Proliferative phase   Secretory phase

Endometrial thickness

5   14   28
Days

Menses   Proliferation of endometrial glands   Secretory change of endometrial glands

Fig. 20 The hormonal and endometrial events in the menstrual cycle.

enhanced fibrinolytic activity and reduced clotting factors in menstrual blood. Clots only occur if the amount of menstrual loss exceeds the capacity of the local fibrinolytic system. The endometrium begins to regenerate within 48 hours of the onset of bleeding and is complete by the fifth day.

Regulation of menstrual blood loss (MBL) is thus controlled by 3 factors:

- vasodilation of spiral arterioles
- fibrinolytic activity of menstrual blood
- endometrial regeneration.

Menstrual disorders (see Box 44) are extremely common amongst women of reproductive age, and are capable of causing significant disruption to both work and family life. Menstrual disorders account for:

Box 44 Abnormalities of menstruation

• Menorrhagia	menstrual blood loss exceeding 80 ml
• Oligomenorrhoea	infrequent periods
• Amenorrhoea	absent periods
• Hypomenorrhoea	reduced menstrual blood loss

- 3% of all female consultations in general practice
- one third of all referrals to gynaecologists
- 60 000 hysterectomies per annum in the UK.

There are a wide variety of different medical and surgical treatment options for menorrhagia. Medical treatment with drugs is the usual first line treatment. Minimally invasive treatments offering a reduction or cessation of menstrual bleeding include the progestogen releasing intra-uterine device, hysteroscopically guided endometrial destruction, and thermal destruction via a water-filled balloon. Hysterectomy, which can be achieved via the abdominal, vaginal or laparoscopic route, offers guaranteed permanent relief from menstruation.

11.2 Menorrhagia

Learning objectives

You should:

- know how to define menorrhagia

- be aware of the different causes

Excessive menstrual bleeding is defined as menstrual blood loss exceeding 80 ml per cycle. It is estimated to affect between 9 and 14% of the female Western population, and it is a common cause of iron deficiency anaemia. However, there are no easily available facilities to measure actual menstrual blood loss in menorrhagic women, and studies attempting to estimate this from collected sanitary pads have found that it is frequently below 80 ml. This underlines the subjectivity of the complaint, and the unreliability of the diagnosis from the history. Some women are undoubtedly inconvenienced by and receive treatment for a physiologically normal menstrual blood loss. The complaint of menorrhagia appears to be increasing, which may reflect the changing role of women in society, whereby for example increasing work commitments cause menstruation to be a problem. In addition, the combined tendencies towards an earlier menarche, a later menopause and a smaller family size mean that women nowadays are likely to experience many more periods than previously.

Aetiology of menorrhagia

Menorrhagia may result from both local and systemic diseases (see Box 45), but in 50% of cases there is no obvious cause, when the term dysfunctional uterine bleeding (DUB) is used. Organic pathology may be discovered on clinical examination, and the use of

Box 45 Causes of menorrhagia

Systemic
- Thyroid dysfunction
- Coagulation disorder

Local
- Fibroids
- Endometriosis
- Endometrial polyps
- Endometrial hyperplasia/neoplasia/infection
- Pelvic inflammatory disease
- Intra-uterine contraceptive device

Dysfunctional
- Ovulatory
- Anovulatory

hysteroscopy to visualise the genital tract will further identify a percentage with a local cause such as endometrial polyps or submucous fibroids. DUB may be associated with anovulation, which commonly occurs at the extremes of reproductive life, but may also occur in otherwise normal ovulatory cycles as a result of an increase in either endometrial prostaglandins or fibrinolytic activity.

11.3 Investigation of menorrhagia

Learning objective

You should:

- understand how to assess and investigate a patient with menorrhagia

The history should seek details regarding the quantity, rhythm and duration of bleeding, method of contraception and desire for future pregnancy. Additional symptoms such as dysmenorrhoea, premenstrual syndrome, prolapse or urinary incontinence should be sought. Breathlessness or palpitations suggest anaemia, whilst excessive bruising suggests a coagulation disorder. Examination should include inspection for any signs of endocrine disease. The vulva, vagina and cervix should be visualised to exclude an extra-uterine source of bleeding, and a cervical smear should be taken if due. Uterine size and mobility, adnexal enlargement and any local tenderness are assessed by pelvic examination. A precise and quick assessment is required to identify the minority of patients needing further investigation.

Investigations

Investigations in menorrhagia include:

- full blood count
- ferritin
- cervical smear
- thyroid function tests
- clotting screen
- hysteroscopy
- pelvic ultrasound.

In women below the age of 40 years, further investigation is usually only undertaken if first line medical treatment fails or if there are symptoms and signs suggestive of pathology. Endometrial biopsy can be performed as an outpatient procedure using a small plastic sampler passed through the cervix. Alternatively, hysteroscopy can be undertaken, either under local or general anaesthetic. This provides more information as it gives direct visualisation of the endocervical canal and uterine cavity. Endometrial polyps and submucous fibroids are often found, although their precise causal relationship to menorrhagia is difficult to determine as they are also commonly found in asymptomatic women. Ultrasound and laparoscopy are useful in the investigation of coexisting pain or a pelvic mass. Over the age of 40 years hysteroscopy is more readily undertaken, in order to exclude both endometrial carcinoma and atypical hyperplasia, which may present with menorrhagia or irregular bleeding in the perimenopausal age group.

Indications for hysteroscopy include:

- failed medical therapy
- intermenstrual or post-coital bleeding
- irregular heavy menstrual blood loss
- suspected uterine pathology.

11.4 Treatment of menorrhagia

Learning objectives

You should:

- be able to discuss the different treatment options for menorrhagia

- be aware of the relative merits and disadvantages of the different treatments

General

Sometimes all that is required is explanation and reassurance that nothing sinister is present. For example, women stopping the oral contraceptive pill or having an intra-uterine device fitted should be advised that a small increase in menstrual blood loss is to be expected. Women with a high body mass index should be advised that weight loss often results in a return to ovulatory cycles and lighter periods. If thyroid disease has been discovered, treatment may improve menstrual blood loss and regularity. Iron deficiency anaemia should be treated with iron supplementation. Finally, the ability to cope with the inconvenience and discomfort of menstruation may be reduced by any existing anxiety or depressive illness. Such patients may derive most benefit by measures to relieve these symptoms rather than by treatment directed at reducing menstrual blood loss.

Medical

Medical therapy has an important role to play in the treatment of menorrhagia, particularly in the younger woman. Although no single drug offers a permanent solution, and all have potential side-effects, many women have no wish to undergo surgery for a self-limiting condition, particularly if childbearing is incomplete (see Box 46).

Prostaglandin synthetase inhibitors

Prostaglandin synthetase inhibitors such as mefenamic acid are a popular first line therapy. They are cheap, effective and need only be taken immediately before and during menstruation. The analgesic properties make them especially suitable for women with coexisting dysmenorrhoea.

- Mode of action: inhibit the synthesis of endometrial prostaglandins
- Effectiveness: reduce MBL by 30%
- Side-effects: nausea, dizziness and headache.

Combined oestrogen–progestogen formulations

The combined oral contraceptive pill is suitable for women who also require contraception or cycle regulation. Smoking, obesity and a history of cardiovascular disease are relative contraindications (see p. 184).

- Mode of action: induce regular shedding of a thinner endometrium
- Effectiveness: up to 50% reduction in MBL
- Side-effects: headache, weight gain, breast tenderness.

Antifibrinolytic agents

The antifibrinolytic agent tranexamic acid has been shown in randomised controlled trials to effectively reduce MBL. It is given only during menstruation.

- Mode of action: reduces endometrial fibrinolytic activity
- Effectiveness: 50% reduction in MBL
- Side-effects: nausea, dizziness, tinnitus, rashes, abdominal cramps.

Progestogens

Progestogens such as norethisterone and medroxyprogesterone acetate are widely prescribed for menorrhagia although there are few studies to validate them as a first line choice. They are a more logical choice when cycle regulation is required, when they are given for 3 out of 4 weeks. Menstruation should then occur during the pill-free week.

- Mode of action: induce secretory change in the oestrogen-primed endometrium
- Effectiveness: little objective evidence in ovulatory cycles
- Side-effects: mild androgenic effects, weight gain.

Danazol

This drug is a synthetic derivative of ethinyl testosterone. It is given in a daily dose of 200–600 mg. It is relatively expensive and sometimes poorly tolerated due to androgenic side-effects such as acne and hirsutism. It appears to have the benefit of a carry-over effect for up to 6 months after cessation of treatment.

Ethamsylate

Ethamsylate is a haemostatic agent, which is given immediately prior to and throughout menstruation. It

---

Box 46 Drugs used in treatment of menorrhagia

First line drugs	Second line drugs
• Prostaglandin synthetase inhibitors	• Danazol
• Combined oestrogen-progestogen formulations	• Ethamsylate
• Antifibrinolytics	• luteinising hormone releasing hormone (LHRH) agonists
• Progestogens	• Progestogen-releasing intra-uterine (contraceptive) device (IUD)

acts by increasing capillary stability. Side-effects include headaches, rashes and nausea.

Luteinising hormone releasing hormone (LHRH) agonists

LHRH agonists are potent synthetic derivatives of the endogenous decapeptide LHRH. They induce down-regulation of the HPO axis which results in hypo-oestro-genisation and amenorrhoea. Administration is usually by monthly depot subcutaneous injection. High cost and side-effects limit their long-term use. The hypo-oestrogenic state produces symptoms of hot flushes and vaginal dryness. Long-term use carries a risk of osteo-porosis resulting from loss of bone calcium. Their main use is in thinning down the endometrium prior to endometrial resection.

Progestogen-releasing intra-uterine (contraceptive) device (IUD)

The levonorgestrel-releasing IUD is inserted into the uterine cavity where it continually releases a small locally-acting dose of progestogen. This results in endometrial atrophy and a marked reduction in men-strual blood loss. It also provides reliable contraception. It is proving to be extremely effective, with many women having complete amenorrhoea after 3 months. The main side-effect is irregular bleeding within the first 3 months of insertion.

Surgery

One in five women in the UK currently undergo hys-terectomy, with menstrual problems being the most common indication. Unlike medical therapy it offers a permanent solution, and has an accordingly high satis-faction rate. However, it is generally only recommended when medical treatment or less invasive procedures have proved unsatisfactory, or as first line treatment for large uterine fibroids. A tender or fixed uterus, chronic dysmenorrhoea and severe chronic anaemia are all relative indications for hysterectomy.

Minimally invasive surgical treatments for menor-rhagia, such as endometrial ablation, are of great benefit in selected women. The outcome is less certain in terms of therapeutic benefit, but it is a less invasive procedure than hysterectomy with a correspondingly quicker recovery. Patient preference will greatly influence the final choice of treatment. Some women, for example, may prefer to opt for surgery, in full knowledge of the various medical alternatives, rather than trying or persisting with drug treatments.

Hysterectomy

Vaginal hysterectomy is usually preferred to abdominal hysterectomy for treatment of menorrhagia because it avoids the need for an abdominal incision. This allows a shorter hospital stay and quicker convalescence. As a rough guide, patients can return to normal activities after 6 weeks following a vaginal hysterectomy and after 12 weeks following an abdominal hysterectomy, but there is great individual variation. The abdominal route is often preferred if there is significant uterine enlargement or fixation, if there is other suspected pathology or if the ovaries are to be removed. Laparoscopically-assisted vaginal hysterectomy is an alternative to abdominal hysterectomy. This combines the advantages of vaginal hysterectomy with an improved view of the abdomen and pelvis, and allows easy removal of the ovaries without the need for a laparotomy. It requires particular surgical skills and can be a more time-consuming operation, but the recovery is as quick as with vaginal hysterectomy. Subtotal hys-terectomy, whereby the cervix is conserved, is gaining popularity in the UK. It is reported to be associated with less impairment of sexual and bladder function, although this remains unclear. Complications of hysterectomy are listed in Box 47.

Endometrial destructive techniques

Endometrial destructive techniques aim to stop or greatly reduce menstrual blood loss by producing endometrial fibrosis and obliteration. The most com-monly used techniques employ either laser or electro-cautery to destroy the endometrium down to and including the basal layer (see Box 48). This is done under direct vision using a hysteroscope. Operating time is approximately 30 minutes, with return to normal activi-ties within 2 weeks. Hysterectomy can thus be avoided, which is both a considerable attraction to patients and a cost saving to the community. Prolonged follow-up is required to assess the long-term benefit. A perforation of

---

Box 47 Complications of hysterectomy

Early	Late
● Infection	● Vaginal vault prolapse
— wound	● Bladder problems
— pelvic	● Ovarian adhesions
— urinary	
● Haemorrhage	
● Bladder injury	
● Ureteric injury	
● Thromboembolism	

Box 48   Surgical treatment choices for menorrhagia

Endometrial destruction	Hysterectomy
• Resection/ablation	• Abdominal
• Laser ablation	• Vaginal
• Radiofrequency radiation	• Laparoscopically assisted
• Thermal balloon ablation	• Subtotal

the uterus may rarely be sustained during endometrial resection (see Fig. 21). Approximately one in five women undergoing endometrial resection still eventually come to hysterectomy, usually because of persistent troublesome menstruation or pain (see Box 49). A rela-

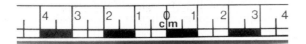

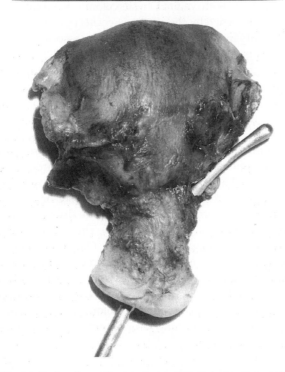

Fig. 21 Perforation of the uterus sustained during endometrial resection, necessitating hysterectomy. The perforation has occurred through an old caesarean section scar.

Box 49   Complications of endometrial resection

Early	Late
• Uterine perforation	• Haematometra
• Haemorrhage	• Pain
• Absorption of irrigating fluid	

tive disadvantage of endometrial resection as compared to hysterectomy is the continued need for both contraception and cervical screening.

Outcome after endometrial resection:

- 30% have amenorrhoea
- 50% have reduced MBL
- 20% have no change.

Fibroid embolisation

Uterine artery embolisation is a recently introduced alternative to hysterectomy for the treatment of symptomatic uterine fibroids. A success rate of 81% has been reported, as defined by an improvement in menorrhagia, pain and pressure symptoms. The technique involves introducing a catheter, via the femoral artery, into the uterine artery, which is then used to inject the embolising material. It can also be used as a method of controlling pelvic bleeding, when the internal iliac artery is embolised.

11.5 Oligomenorrhoea

Learning objective

You should:

- understand the mechanisms which may give rise to oligomenorrhoea

Oligomenorrhoea means infrequent menstrual periods. It may reflect an unusually long follicular phase in an otherwise normal ovulatory cycle, but it is more commonly due to disorder of the HPO axis causing anovulation. The resulting absence of a corpus luteum and therefore progesterone leads to unopposed oestrogen stimulation of the endometrium. This causes cystic hyperplasia, whereby the endometrium becomes thickened and polypoid. Periods may occur anywhere between every 6 weeks and 6 months, and are frequently heavy.

The causes of oligomenorrhoea overlap with those of amenorrhoea (see p. 146). Oligomenorrhoea due to anovulatory cycles is commonly seen in the years immediately following the menarche and preceding the menopause, and in women with an abnormal body mass index.

It is important to exclude treatable causes of oligomenorrhoea such as prolactinoma, androgenic tumour and thyroid disorders (see Box 50). These are further discussed under amenorrhoea.

11.6 Polycystic ovary syndrome

Clinical features

Polycystic ovary syndrome (PCOS) is a common but heterogeneous endocrine disorder with a poorly understood aetiology. It is characterised by ovarian hypersecretion of androgens, and an increase in the pulsatile secretion of luteinising hormone (LH). Common clinical features include menstrual irregularity, hirsutism and infertility. 25% of patients are obese. Persistently increased LH secretion results in ovarian theca cell hyperplasia. The ovaries then become typically enlarged with a thickened 'icing sugar' capsule. The characteristic appearance on ultrasound examination is of multiple small peripherally-placed follicles.

Androgen hypersecretion increases the sensitivity of the pituitary to GnRH. This results in increased pulsatile LH secretion and elevated serum LH levels. LH causes further androgen secretion from ovarian theca cells. A vicious circle is thus established. Hypersecretion of LH is associated with both anovulation and an increased risk of miscarriage.

A raised fasting insulin and increased insulin responses to oral glucose are seen in many individuals with polycystic ovary syndrome. Thus it may be that hyperinsulinaemia is the key to the pathogenesis of PCOS, as insulin stimulates androgen secretion by the ovarian stroma and appears to affect the normal development of ovarian follicles.

Biochemical features

Biochemical features include:

- increased LH:FSH ratio
- raised serum androgen index
- decreased sex hormone binding globulin (SHBG)
- increased prolactin
- increased serum insulin

Differential diagnosis

- Anovulatory cycles
- Late onset congenital adrenal hyperplasia
- Androgen-secreting tumour
- Cushing's syndrome.

Treatment

Weight loss is the cornerstone of management in obese women. This is usually associated with improvement in both menstrual irregularity and acne, together with a normalisation of the hormone profile. In women of normal weight the combined low dose oral contraceptive pill is useful for cycle control. It is important to avoid preparations containing androgenic progestogens, such as norethisterone, as these may aggravate hirsutism. The most appropriate contraceptive formulation is one containing a combination of 35 µg of ethinyl oestradiol with the anti-androgen cyproterone acetate. Menstrual irregularity can alternatively be treated with cyclical progestogen therapy for 10 days a month. If infertility is the presenting feature, ovulation can be induced with clomiphene. 20% of such women will not ovulate in response to clomiphene alone, and will require more potent ovarian stimulation using gonadotrophins. For clomiphene resistant cases, laparoscopic ovarian surgery is a useful measure which can bring about a reduction in serum LH concentrations, and thereby restore regular ovulation. The surgery consists of partial ovarian destruction, using laser or diathermy.

Long-term effects

There is an increased risk of endometrial hyperplasia and endometrial carcinoma due to the long-term effect of unopposed oestrogen stimulation. The metabolic consequences of long-term hyperinsulinism may increase the incidence of both coronary heart disease, due to a lowering of high-density lipoprotein, and non-insulin-dependent diabetes.

11.7 Hyperprolactinaemia

Learning objectives

You should:

- understand how prolactin secretion is controlled
- be able to recognise the symptoms of hyperprolactinaemia
- understand the principals of management of hyperprolactinaemia

Prolactin is secreted from the anterior pituitary gland. It is under negative control from hypothalamic dopamine. Any disease process in the hypothalamus or pituitary stalk can result in hyperprolactinaemia due to a reduction in dopamine secretion. A pituitary adenoma accounts for 50% of pathological cases. These are benign tumours but are potentially serious because of their proximity to the optic chiasma. Even slight enlargement may cause chiasmal compression and threaten eyesight.

Hyperprolactinaemia is a physiological event during breast feeding. Elevated prolactin blocks the effects of gonadotrophins on the ovary. This results in anovulation and low oestrogen levels. The common symptoms are menstrual irregularity, infertility and galactorrhoea.

Symptoms associated with hyperprolactinaemia

- Oligomenorrhoea
- Galactorrhoea
- Headache
- Visual field defects
- Hot flushes.

Pathological causes of hyperprolactinaemia

- Pituitary tumours: prolactinoma, non-prolactin secreting pituitary tumours.
- Hypothalamic tumours: craniopharyngioma, meningioma, glioma.
- Drugs: phenothiazines, haloperidol, tricyclic antidepressants, benzodiazepines, metoclopramide.
- Others: idiopathic hyperprolactinaemia, polycystic ovary syndrome, primary hypothyroidism.

Investigation of hyperprolactinaemia

Very high serum levels of prolactin are almost always due to a prolactinoma. Detection requires neuroradiological investigation of the pituitary fossa by computed tomography (CT) or magnetic resonance imaging (MRI) scan. Plain tomography of the pituitary fossa may show erosion of the floor, but may not detect a small microadenoma. Hypothyroidism should be excluded, as an elevated thyroid stimulating hormone (TSH) level can cause secondary hyperprolactinaemia.

Treatment of hyperprolactinaemia

Troublesome symptoms require lowering of prolactin levels, but minor degrees of hyperprolactinaemia can often be ignored. Treatment with dopaminergic drugs such as bromocriptine and cabergoline is highly effective in correcting both infertility and menstrual disorders. Bromocriptine treatment is usually continued for at least 1 year. Side-effects of nausea and headache are a problem which lead to discontinuation of treatment in up to 5% of patients. The daily dose is up to 7.5 mg, given in small divided doses with food. Cabergoline is a longer-acting and more tolerable dopaminergic agent. It is given only once a week. Surgery is reserved for large macroadenomas and non-secreting pituitary tumours, and is usually performed via a trans-sphenoidal approach. Radiotherapy is occasionally used as an adjunct to surgery and for parasellar tumours. During pregnancy there is a small risk of tumour enlargement from the effect of oestrogen.

11.8 Amenorrhoea

Learning objectives

You should:

- understand the different mechanisms resulting in amenorrhoea
- be able to use investigations to determine the likely cause
- understand when and why treatment may be indicated

Amenorrhoea is the absence of menstruation in a woman of reproductive age. There are a wide variety of causes, and these may be pathological or physiological. Pathological causes are nearly always endocrine in origin. Anatomical causes are rare but important. It is a physiological occurrence during pregnancy and breast feeding. Amenorrhoea is often subdivided into primary and secondary amenorrhoea. Primary amenorrhoea is defined as a failure to menstruate by the age of 16 years, whilst secondary amenorrhoea is the absence of menstruation for 6 months or more. This distinction is of little practical significance since many of the causes overlap.

Endocrine causes of amenorrhoea

Endocrine causes include:

- polycystic ovary syndrome
- stress and exercise
- weight-related
- hyperprolactinaemia
- psychological disorders
- systemic illness, e.g. renal failure
- drugs
- premature ovarian failure
- ischaemic necrosis of the pituitary
- primary HPO axis failure.

Excessive loss of body fat results in a reversible hypothalamic dysfunction due to loss of the normal gonadotrophin-releasing hormone (GnRH) release. The eating disorder anorexia nervosa accounts for 15% of all cases of amenorrhoea. The other features include severe weight loss, bradycardia, dry skin and altered hair distribution. Athletes are frequently amenorrhoeic, even when weight is in the normal range, because of a high muscle to fat ratio.

Any severe illness can cause amenorrhoea by upsetting the balance of the HPO axis. Exercise and stress cause amenorrhoea due to a modification of hypothalamic catecholamines and endogenous opioids. Polycystic ovary syndrome has already been discussed (p. 145).

Drugs such as phenothiazines may cause amenorrhoea because they raise serum prolactin levels. Continued suppression of the HPO axis may go on for up to 6 months after stopping the combined oral contraceptive pill. This is called post-pill amenorrhoea, and is always short-lived. By contrast irreversible HPO failure occurs due to ischaemic necrosis of the pituitary gland following profound postpartum haemorrhage. This is known as Sheehan's syndrome. There is failure of secretion of all the anterior pituitary hormones, including TSH and adrenocorticotrophic hormone (ACTH). It is very rare.

Primary HPO axis failure is extremely rare. In Kallmann's syndrome there is a primary failure of GnRH production, accompanied by anosmia.

Anatomical causes of amenorrhoea

Congenital

- Intersex – e.g. 46, XY female phenotype with androgen insensitivity syndrome
- Turner's syndrome
- Imperforate hymen
- Vaginal atresia or horizontal septum
- Congenital absence of the uterus.

Acquired

- Endometrial fibrosis (Asherman's syndrome)
- Cervical stenosis
- Hysterectomy.

Endometrial fibrosis results in obliteration of the uterine cavity. This may occur following traumatic uterine curettage, and is the therapeutic aim of endometrial resection. Cervical stenosis is a rare complication which occurs as a result of post-operative scarring following a cone biopsy or a Manchester repair. Menstrual fluid is unable to escape because of the obliterated endocervical canal, causing the uterus to distend with blood to form a haematometra.

Investigation of amenorrhoea

A well-directed history often points to the cause. Symptoms of breast tenderness or nausea would be suggestive of early pregnancy. Headache or breast discharge suggest hyperprolactinaemia. The date of the last menstrual period and the age of the menarche are important. Any recent weight change should be sought and a full contraceptive and drug history taken. Symptoms such as cold intolerance or constipation would suggest a thyroid disorder. Cyclical pain with a history of previous cone biopsy and amenorrhoea suggests cervical stenosis. Secondary amenorrhoea accompanied by symptoms of oestrogen deficiency indicate a premature menopause.

Examination should include a full assessment to look for any generalised medical or endocrine disorder. The presence of secondary sex characteristics should be documented. Pelvic examination may reveal congenital malformation or signs of oestrogen deficiency.

The need for any biochemical or radiological investigations will be directed by the above findings, and may include:

- pregnancy test
- follicle-stimulating hormone (FSH), LH, prolactin, oestrogen, androgen index
- thyroid function tests
- CT scan of pituitary fossa
- pelvic ultrasound
- karyotype
- autoantibody screen.

Treatment of amenorrhoea

Treatment is directed at the cause, and by any desire by the patient for contraception, cycle restoration or fertility. Treatment of a prolactinoma will restore menstruation and ovulation. Ovulation induction using clomiphene or gonadotrophins can be used in other instances of HPO dysfunction (see p. 201), and is further discussed in the chapter on infertility. Secondary amenorrhoea may spontaneously resolve following weight correction or a reduction in the intensity of athletic training. Patients with oestrogen deficiency from premature ovarian failure or gonadal dysgenesis should be given balanced hormone replacement therapy both for symptomatic relief and to offset the increased risks of both osteoporosis and cardiovascular disease. Patients with adequate oestrogen levels and long-standing amenorrhoea should be given cyclical progestogens for 10 days every month to allow regular endometrial shedding and prevent the development of endometrial hyperplasia.

11.9 Hirsutism

Learning objectives

You should:

- understand the principles of normal androgen metabolism

- be able to use investigations to detect abnormalities of androgen metabolism

- understand the principles of treatment of hirsutism

Hirsutism is defined as the presence of excess coarse hair which is socially unacceptable to the patient. The areas usually involved are the face, chest, lower abdomen and thighs. It may be accompanied by both menstrual irregularity and acne, and is aggravated by obesity. It is especially common among Mediterranean women. Virilism by contrast is much rarer, and is usually caused by adrenal hyperplasia or tumour. The features in addition to hirsutism are clitoromegaly, deepening of the voice, muscular prominence and temporal balding. Hirsutism is often associated with a moderate increase in circulating androgen levels, whereas in virilism there is a marked increase.

Androgen metabolism

Androgens are produced by the ovaries, the adrenal glands and peripheral fat. The main varieties are testosterone, androstenedione and dehydroepiandrosterone sulphate (DHEAS). Testosterone (T) circulates in the serum tightly bound to sex hormone binding globulin (SHBG). Only a small fraction circulates unbound, and this is the biologically active part. Low SHBG levels permit more T to circulate in the free form, whereas high levels of SHBG do the reverse. The hepatic production of SHBG is inhibited by androgens and stimulated by oestrogens. The availability of biologically active T is

therefore increased by androgens and decreased by oestrogen. In obesity, androgen production in peripheral fat is increased. Hyperinsulinism may be associated with obesity, which increases the pituitary secretion of LH, thus further stimulating androgen production by the ovarian theca cells.

Causes of androgen excess

Ovarian

- Polycystic ovary syndrome – common
- Androgen-secreting tumours – rare.

Adrenal

- Late onset congenital adrenal hyperplasia – rare
- Cushing's syndrome – rare
- Androgen-secreting tumours – rare.

Drugs

- Danazol
- Phenytoin
- Androgenic progestogens.

Diagnosis

Cases of mild hirsutism with regular menses do not require further investigation. In more severe cases accompanied by menstrual disturbance, investigation of the serum endocrine profile in the follicular phase of the cycle is indicated. Measurement of plasma levels of androgens, gonadotrophins, 17 hydroxyprogesterone, thyroid function and SHBG may all be useful. Very high T levels in the presence of virilism are suggestive of an androgen-secreting tumour. These are often small tumours, requiring CT scanning and vaginal ultrasound to locate. Cushing's syndrome is diagnosed by the finding of an elevated 24-hour urinary free cortisol. Congenital adrenal hyperplasia is usually diagnosed in the neonatal period. The late onset variety is characterised by an elevated plasma 17 hydroxyprogesterone. It is treated with glucocorticoid therapy. An elevated LH:FSH ratio, slightly elevated T and reduced SHBG level is the typical hormonal profile seen in the polycystic ovary syndrome. Elevated DHEAS levels are suggestive of adrenal overproduction of androgen.

Treatment of hirsutism

Treatment is directed at the cause. Androgen-secreting tumours require excision. Cortisol is given for congenital adrenal hyperplasia. In most cases there is only a minor abnormality of androgen metabolism, and the following measures are useful:

- weight loss
- removal of unwanted hair
- anti-androgen therapy.

Weight loss is frequently associated with a return to menstruation and a normalisation of the hormonal profile. The aim should be a body mass index (BMI) of ≤ 21 kg/m². Cosmetic removal of unwanted hair is best achieved by waxing or electrolysis. If anti-androgen therapy is used, this needs to be continued for at least a year to be effective. The best regimen is a combination of cyproterone acetate and ethinyl oestradiol. Cyproterone acetate acts by blocking the androgen receptor and inhibiting gonadotrophin secretion, whilst ethinyl oestradiol increases the production of SHBG, so reducing the amount of free circulating I. Ethinyl oestradiol is given in a dose of 30–50 µg for 21 days out of 28, with 50–100 mg of cyproterone for the first 10 days. The above regimen will inhibit ovulation and therefore provide contraceptive cover. Cyproterone is contraindicated during pregnancy as it is both teratogenic and capable of causing feminisation of a male fetus. In less severe cases a combined oral contraceptive pill consisting of 35 µg of ethinyl oestradiol and 2 mg of cyproterone can be tried. Hirsutism accompanied by elevated DHEAS levels suggests an adrenal source of excess androgen. This is best treated with low-dose dexamethasone.

11.10 Intermenstrual and post-coital bleeding

Learning objectives

You should:

- understand the potential significance of abnormal vaginal bleeding

- understand the different pathophysiological mechanisms which may cause abnormal vaginal bleeding

- know how to investigate abnormal vaginal bleeding

Bleeding occurring in between periods is called intermenstrual bleeding (see Table 14). It is a common symptom. Bleeding after sexual intercourse is called post-coital bleeding. Although rarely serious, both these abnormal bleeding patterns require investigation in order to exclude neoplasia of the genital tract, and in particular carcinoma of the cervix. Bleeding from a complication of an unsuspected pregnancy should also be remembered.

Intermenstrual and post-coital bleeding may originate from the delicate epithelium of the endocervix, in the absence of any serious pathology. This is especially common in women taking the combined oral contraceptive pill, as this causes prominence of the endocervical epithelium, giving rise to a characteristic vascular appearance to the cervix called ectopy. This is easily traumatised by sexual intercourse or contact with a tampon, giving rise to bleeding. Cervicitis due to infection with Chlamydia will also result in a cervix which bleeds early. Intermenstrual bleeding may also originate from the endometrium. This is a thin, inherently unstable epithelium, the growth and maintenance of which is under hormonal control. Irregular secretion of oestrogen and progesterone, as seen in anovulatory states, or a thin endometrium as seen with the combined low dose oral contraceptive pill, commonly give rise to intermenstrual bleeding. Investigation is frequently thus unrewarding, but only then can serious disease be excluded.

Management of intermenstrual and post-coital bleeding

A speculum examination of the vagina and cervix is indicated to look for a causative lesion. A bimanual pelvic examination is needed to feel the consistency of the cervix, which may feel indurated in the presence of a carcinoma, and to detect any pelvic masses. A cervical smear should always be taken. If the woman is taking contraceptive hormones, and both clinical examination and a smear are normal, consideration should be given to increasing the dose of progestogen in order to try to stabilise the endometrium and prevent breakthrough bleeding which commonly occurs due to low serum hormone levels. If genital tract infection is suspected, swabs should be taken and appropriate antimicrobial

Table 14 Causes of intermenstrual and post-coital bleeding

Cervix	Uterus	Vagina	Ovary	Fallopian tube
Ectopy	Pregnancy complication	Atrophic vaginitis	Oestrogen-secreting tumour	Carcinoma
Cervicitis	Endometritis	Infective vaginitis	Irregular ovulation	
Polyps	Endometrial polyps	Vaginal carcinoma		
Carcinoma	Endometrial hyperplasia			
	Endometrial carcinoma			
	Oral contraceptive pill or HRT			

treatment started. Colposcopic examination of the cervix and hysteroscopic examination of both endocervical canal and uterine cavity are required to exclude a lesion higher up in the genital tract if symptoms persist for more than a few weeks or are unresponsive to the above simple measures.

11.11 Post-menopausal bleeding

Learning objective

You should:

- be aware that post-menopausal bleeding may be caused by gynaecological cancer

Post-menopausal bleeding is defined as genital tract bleeding which occurs 6 months or more after the menopause. It always requires investigation. Endometrial carcinoma is found in 10% of cases. This is discussed further in the chapter on gynaecological neoplasia.

Self-assessment: questions

Multiple choice questions

1. Regarding the normal menstrual cycle:
   a. FSH promotes follicular development
   b. Oestrogen is produced mainly by theca cells
   c. Progesterone peaks in the follicular phase
   d. Prostaglandins stimulate myometrial contractions
   e. The basal layer of the endometrium is not shed

2. Which of the following are true?
   a. Pulsatile secretion of GnRH controls the synthesis of FSH and LH
   b. Secretion of prolactin from the anterior pituitary is needed to maintain a regular cycle
   c. Prostaglandin-induced constriction of the spiral arterioles causes endometrial ischaemia
   d. Growth of ovarian follicles occurs in the luteal phase of the cycle
   e. Progesterone causes decidualisation of the endometrium

3. Which of the following drugs are useful in the treatment of menorrhagia?
   a. Tranexamic acid
   b. Cabergoline
   c. Oil of evening primrose
   d. Diazoxide
   e. Naproxen

4. Regarding the polycystic ovary syndrome:
   a. SHBG levels are increased
   b. Androgens are increased
   c. LH secretion is decreased
   d. Galactorrhoea is a feature
   e. Menstrual irregularity is a common feature

5. Regarding hirsutism:
   a. It is more common in Chinese than in Greek women
   b. SHBG is usually decreased
   c. It may be successfully treated with the combined oral contraceptive pill
   d. It may be caused by diazepam
   e. In the presence of a regular menstrual cycle it is usually idiopathic

Short notes

1. What are the indications for treatment of menorrhagia by hysterectomy? Under which circumstances is the abdominal route preferred to the vaginal route for this operation?

2. Why are normal ovaries frequently removed at the time of hysterectomy in women over the age of 45 years?
3. Describe the management of a 14-year-old girl with menorrhagia and iron deficiency anaemia.
4. What is post-pill amenorrhoea?

Case histories

Case history 1

A 24-year-old woman with a previously regular menstrual cycle presents with oligomenorrhoea. Investigations show her serum prolactin level is markedly elevated.

What are the likely causes, and how would you differentiate between them?

Case history 2

A 45-year-old multiparous woman presents with a 2-year history of heavy, irregular periods and increasing tiredness. On examination she appears pale. The uterus is enlarged to 12 weeks in size. The cervix and adnexae are unremarkable.

Describe, giving reasons, how you would manage the case.

OSCE questions

OSCE 1

You have been asked to design a patient information leaflet on menorrhagia:

1. List what you consider to be the essential information for this leaflet, under separate headings.
2. List four different possible medical therapies for menorrhagia.
3. List four different possible operations for menorrhagia.
4. List the disadvantages of endometrial resection as compared with a total hysterectomy (when the cervix is removed).

OSCE 2

A 22-year-old woman has been started on the oestrogen/progesterone combination called Dianette. Each tablet contains 35 mg ethinyloestradiol and 2 mg cyproterone acetate. She has been instructed to take this for 3 out of every 4 weeks, and advised that this will improve her complaint of acne and hirsutism. She asks you the following questions:

1. Will this provide her with safe contraception?
2. How does Dianette work in acne and hirsutism?
3. How long should Dianette be taken in order to improve her symptoms?

Self-assessment: answers

Multiple choice answers

1. a. **True.**
   b. **False.** Oestrogen is produced by the granulosa cells.
   c. **False.** Progesterone peaks in the mid-luteal phase of the cycle, 8 days following the LH surge.
   d. **True.**
   e. **True.**

2. a. **True.**
   b. **False.** Prolactin secretion is not required for regulation of the menstrual cycle, although excessive secretion may disrupt it.
   c. **True.**
   d. **False.** Ovarian follicular growth occurs in the proliferative phase of the cycle.
   e. **True.**

3. a. **True.** Tranexamic acid produces a specific effect by inhibiting endometrial fibrinolysis.
   b. **False.**
   c. **False.**
   d. **False.**
   e. **True.** Naproxen is a prostaglandin synthetase inhibitor which reduces menstrual blood loss via effects on endometrial prostaglandin synthesis.

4. a. **False.** SHBG levels are suppressed by the excess testosterone.
   b. **True.** There is excess androgen secretion which causes hirsutism and interferes with ovulation.
   c. **False.** Pulsatile LH secretion is increased.
   d. **False.**
   e. **True.** Menstrual irregularity is common and reflects disordered ovarian function.

5. a. **False.** Hirsutism shows great variation between different races, and is more common in Mediterranean women.
   b. **True.**
   c. **True.**
   d. **False.** It may be caused by drugs such as diazoxide, danazol and phenytoin, but not diazepam.
   e. **True.**

Short notes answers

1. Large uterine fibroids causing troublesome menorrhagia rarely respond to medical therapy and are best treated by hysterectomy, provided that childbearing is complete. Symptoms of severe dysmenorrhoea and menorrhagia with the clinical findings of a tender enlarged uterus are suggestive of adenomyosis. Such patients usually benefit considerably from hysterectomy. Coexisting but unrelated symptoms may suggest other surgically amenable conditions which could with benefit be treated at the same time as hysterectomy. Examples include uterovaginal prolapse which could be treated by vaginal hysterectomy and pelvic floor repair, or genuine stress incontinence of urine due to urethral sphincter incompetence, which could be treated by colposuspension at the time of hysterectomy.

   In the absence of uterine pathology, hysterectomy as a treatment for menorrhagia is greatly influenced by patient preference. Failure or dissatisfaction with medical treatment, and the desire for permanent relief from the inconvenience of heavy periods are the usual indications. An informed decision regarding hysterectomy can only be made by a woman after a full explanation of the likely benefits and risks of surgery.

   The vaginal route is generally preferred for uncomplicated hysterectomy, because of the advantage of avoiding an abdominal incision. The abdominal route is reserved for cases when the uterus is grossly enlarged or fixed, when adnexal disease is suspected, or when vaginal access is limited.

2. Bilateral oophorectomy is usually offered to women over the age of 45 years who are undergoing hysterectomy. The benefits are protection against ovarian cancer, which affects 1 in 100 women by the age of 70 years, and prevention of residual pain and cyst formation due to entrapment of the ovaries in post-operative scar tissue. Subsequent surgery to remove painful cystic ovaries involves a risk of trauma to the ureter, as it often lies just beneath the ovary on the pelvic side wall. Lastly, hysterectomy appears to advance the age of the menopause by up to 4 years, probably because of interference with the ovarian blood supply. This limits the remaining useful function of conserved ovaries in a woman undergoing hysterectomy beyond the age of 45 years.

   The disadvantage of prophylactic oophorectomy is a premature menopause. Oestrogen replacement therapy is therefore advisable in order to prevent the increased risk of osteoporosis and cardiovascular disease which result from a premature menopause.

3. A history and general examination are indicated to identify endocrine disorders. Vaginal examination is preferably avoided in this age group as it is unlikely to be rewarding and is traumatic for the patient. Pelvic assessment may be done by rectal examination or transabdominal ultrasound, looking for significant uterine enlargement. Blood should be screened for coagulation and thyroid disorders. Examination of a blood film will exclude other causes of anaemia. The majority of cases of menorrhagia in this age group are due to dysfunctional uterine bleeding due to anovulatory cycles. This will be aggravated by obesity. Uterine fibroids are a rare cause of menorrhagia in this age group.

Diagnostic curettage is not necessary. Reassurance should be given that spontaneous improvement usually occurs with age, and with normalisation of any weight problem. Treatment with the combined oral contraceptive pill can produce an effective reduction in menstrual blood loss in this situation. Iron supplementation should also be given.

4. Post-pill amenorrhoea is the absence of normal menses following discontinuation of the combined oral contraceptive pill. It results from continued suppression of the HPO axis, and this may last up to 6 months. Use of the combined oral contraceptive pill is not associated with any increase in the incidence of long-term infertility or amenorrhoea.

Case history answers

Case history 1

The most important diagnosis to exclude is a pituitary tumour, which accounts for the majority of cases where prolactin levels are markedly elevated. This can be done by CT or MRI scan of the pituitary fossa. A hypothalamic tumour such as a craniopharyngioma is a less common cause of hyperprolactinaemia which may also be demonstrated by neuroradiology. The other causes of a raised prolactin are hypothyroidism, pregnancy and drugs such as phenothiazines. These should be sought by thyroid function and pregnancy tests, and by a drug history.

Case history 2

Her tiredness and pallor are suggestive of anaemia, which should be confirmed with a full blood count and film. If iron deficiency anaemia is confirmed it should be treated with oral iron supplementation. The cervix should be inspected to exclude a carcinoma, and a cervical smear should be taken to look for neoplastic cells, as irregular bleeding may be the presenting symptom of cervical carcinoma. Endometrial sampling should be performed in order to exclude significant pathology such as endometrial hyperplasia, polyps, fibroids, and the rare occurrence of endometrial carcinoma in this age group. This is best achieved by hysteroscopy, which provides a direct visualisation of the endometrial cavity and endocervical canal. If a likely causative lesion is found, such as a submucous fibroid or endometrial polyps, hysteroscopic excisional biopsy may bring about relief of symptoms. If all the investigations are normal the most likely diagnosis is dysfunctional uterine bleeding secondary to unopposed oestrogen stimulation of the endometrium. A therapeutic trial of a progestogen such as norethisterone 5 mg 8-hourly from day 7–28 of the next three cycles could then reasonably be offered, both to reduce the amount of bleeding and to regulate the cycle. If unsuccessful, a second choice would be the antifibrinolytic agent tranexamic acid. A third possibility would be to fit the levonorgestrel-releasing IUCD.

If medical therapy fails or is unacceptable to the woman, surgery should be offered. The choice rests between the less invasive destructive endometrial techniques and hysterectomy. An informed choice should be made by the woman after a full discussion of the relative merits and disadvantages of each method. Endometrial ablation may help by either stopping menstruation completely or by reducing the amount of loss to acceptable levels, and has the advantage of a rapid recovery. Hysterectomy has a more certain outcome but is a bigger procedure with a longer recovery time. Morbidity is minimised with the vaginal route.

OSCE answers

OSCE 1

1. This leaflet could be designed in a variety of ways, but the essential information headings are as follows:
   a. Definition of menorrhagia. It is the subjective complaint of excessive menstrual bleeding.
   b. Reassurance. It is a common problem among women, is rarely life-threatening, and there are a wide variety of different treatment options.
   c. Explanation of common symptoms. Tiredness from anaemia, inconvenience and embarrassment, interference with family and work committments if problems such as flooding are encountered.
   d. Explanation of likely causes. No cause is found in many women. Fibroids, coexisting use of intra-uterine contraceptive device, thyroid disorder, coagulation disorder, are all examples of potential causes.
   e. What to expect when the GP is consulted. Expect to be asked questions about periods: amount of blood loss, regularity of cycle, how it affects day to day activities, etc. Pelvic examination. Possible blood tests or ultrasound scan if anaemia or fibroids are suspected. May be referred to gynaecologist.
   f. Treatment options. Simple measures such as reassurance, or removal of the coil. Medical treatments. Surgical treatments. Women need to know that menorrhagia is frequently a chronic condition, so treatment may need to be long term. Any discussion of medical treatments needs therefore to include likely side-effects, and the expected reduction in menstrual blood flow. Medical therapies are usually the first line treatment, but some women will prefer, in the full knowledge of the alternatives, to opt for surgery rather than trying or persisting with drug treatment. The nature of each surgical procedure should be outlined, together with their suitability, likelihood of cure, associated risks, and how they compare with drug treatments. For example, endometrial resection allows preservation of the uterus, a shorter operating time, a smaller risk of complications, a shorter hospital stay and a sooner return to full activities as compared with hysterectomy. However, in a few women, the operation will not result in less bleeding and therefore some will still go on to have a hysterectomy.

2. Tranexamic acid, mefenamic acid, oral contraceptive pill, danazol.

3. Endometrial resection, thermal balloon ablation, laser ablation, hysterectomy.

4. Continued need for contraception and cervical smears. Risk of cervical cancer and endometrial cancer remain. Occasional need for emergency hysterectomy if uterine perforation occurs during the procedure. The operation sometimes does not result in less menstrual blood loss.

OSCE 2

1. The contraceptive efficacy of Dianette is similar to that of any orthodox combined oral contraceptive, and will therefore provide safe contraception.

2. Acne and hirsutism are androgen-dependent conditions. Androgens cause over activity of the sebaceous glands, leading to acne, and stimulate the growth of a typically male distribution of hair. Dianette works in several ways. The cyproterone acetate acts as an antiandrogen by displacing androgens at the receptor, thereby blocking androgen at the target organ. In addition, both cyproterone acetate and ethinyloestradiol have antigonadotrophic properties which cause suppression of ovarian androgen production. Ethinyloestradiol also reduces free circulating androgens by increasing plasma levels of sex hormone binding globulin. By these mechanisms, the drug reduces sebum production and decreases hair growth.

3. With regard to acne, an improvement is usually seen by 3 months, but treatment may be needed for up to a year. Treatment of hirsutism generally takes longer before any significant improvement is seen, with a period of a year or longer being necessary.

Gynaecological infections

Overview

During the reproductive years, the healthy vagina is colonised by the lactobacillus. This bacteria metabolises glycogen to lactic acid, thus creating an acidic environment in the vagina. This provides protection against infection and, together with cervical mucus, maintains the sterility of the upper genital tract. When organisms such as *Chlamydia* do gain access to the upper genital tract, the result may be pelvic inflammatory disease. The potential sequelae of pelvic inflammatory disease, namely chronic pelvic pain, infertility and ectopic pregnancy, are a major cause of gynaecological morbidity.

Introduction

The upper genital tract is normally sterile, whereas both the vulva and vagina harbour commensal organisms.

12.1 Vulval infections

Learning objectives

You should know:

- how to recognise and treat genital warts
- the pathophysiology of Bartholin's swellings

Learning objectives *(continued)*

- the implications of painless vulval ulceration
- the implications of a genital herpes simplex infection

Infections of the vulva may present as swellings, ulceration or infestations (see Box 52).

Vulval swellings

Genital warts

Genital warts are caused by infection with the human papillomavirus (HPV). HPV types 16 and 18 are associated with an increased risk of preinvasive and invasive neoplasia of the cervix. Genital warts are usually transmitted by sexual contact, and have an incubation period of up to 8 months. The warm moist skin folds of the vulva are ideal conditions for the virus. The clinical appearance is of multiple small papillary excrescences which are most common on the vulval and perineal skin. Warty lesions may also be found in the vagina and on the cervix. Warts are generally painless, but they may cause skin irritation and are usually a cosmetic concern to the patient. The particular strains of papillomavirus responsible for genital warts differ from those causing common skin warts.

Box 52 Presentations of vulval infections

Vulval swellings

Infective	Non-infective
- Warts	- Tumour
- Vulval abscess	- Sebaceous cyst
- Bartholin's abscess	- Lipoma
- *Molluscum contagiosum*	- Hernia

Vulval ulcers

Infective	Non-infective
- Herpes simplex	- Vulval carcinoma
- Primary or secondary syphilis carcinoma	- Basal cell
- Chancroid	
- Granuloma inguinale	- Trauma
- *Lymphogranuloma venereum*	

Vulval infestations

- Lice
- Scabies

Women with genital warts should be offered a cervical smear and colposcopic examination of the cervix because of the association with cervical intraepithelial neoplasia. Screening should be undertaken for other sexually transmitted diseases (STDs) such as gonorrhoea, trichomonas and *Chlamydia*. During pregnancy genital warts often enlarge markedly. There is a small risk of neonatal infection at delivery which may result in laryngeal papillomas.

Treatment

Treatment is best carried out at a genitourinary clinic which has facilities for STD screening and contact tracing. Caustic agents such as podophyllin or trichloracetic acid are applied twice weekly to the lesions, taking care to avoid contact with the surrounding skin. Excision, diathermy or laser is reserved for large or resistant warts.

Treatment of warts does not lead to eradication of the virus from the genital tract, and characteristic warty cytological changes may persist on cervical smears. Genital warts may recur, particularly in the immuno-compromised patient.

Vulval abscess

The vulval skin is prone to cellulitis and abscess formation. This commonly starts with a staphylococcal infection at the base of a hair follicle or in a sebaceous gland. The clinical course is of increasing pain and swelling followed by a discharge of pus. Early treatment with antibiotics may avert this but once a fluctuant swelling has developed incision and drainage is required.

Bartholin's cyst and abscess

The duct of the Bartholin's gland which opens out on the posteromedial aspect of the labium majus is prone to obstruction. Secretions then build up and dilate the duct to form a Bartholin's cyst, which may reach the size of an egg. These are usually painless but if the cyst becomes infected an extremely painful abscess develops. This will require drainage, and pus should be sent for culture and sensitivity. Bartholin's cysts are treated by marsupialisation, which involves eversion and suturing of the cyst wall, so allowing it to drain.

Molluscum contagiosum

Molluscum contagiosum is a contagious virus which causes small pearly white skin papules, which may occur on the vulval and perineal skin. Treatment is by piercing the lesions with phenol on the end of an orange stick.

Vulval ulceration

Vulval ulceration is commonly due to infection and rarely due to malignancy. Acutely painful ulcers are usually due to genital herpes, whereas the syphilitic chancre is painless.

Herpes simplex

Genital herpes simplex virus infection (herpes simplex virus (HSV) type 1 or 2) is a common STD. The primary attack occurs following sexual contact with an infected person, after an incubation period of 7 days. Acutely painful vulval ulceration, occasionally preceded by prodromal tingling, is the most prominent feature. Systemic symptoms such as headache and photophobia are not uncommon. The vesicles progress over 14 days to weeping infectious ulcers, which then crust over and finally heal like a cold sore. The cervix is usually infected and may be covered in vesicles. The inguinal lymph nodes may be enlarged and tender. The diagnosis is confirmed by culture of vesicle fluid. After a primary infection the herpes virus is carried for life in the dorsal root ganglia. Recurrent attacks of genital herpes often follow, which may be triggered by stress, illness or sexual intercourse. These attacks are rarely as severe as the primary attack, and may even pass unnoticed, which allows infection to be easily transmitted to other sexual partners. Recurrent attacks of painful ulceration together with the knowledge that the virus is carried for life frequently leads to long-term psychosexual difficulties amongst sufferers.

Complications

- Urinary retention
- Secondary bacterial infection
- Neonatal infection.

Treatment

Cure is not possible as the viral genome becomes integrated into the host neuronal cell deoxyribonucleic acid (DNA), and antiviral agents can only act when the virus is replicating. During acute attacks, pain relief is by simple analgesics and warm salt bathing. Aciclovir is given orally 200 mg five times daily for 5 days in conjunction with aciclovir ointment, which speeds healing of the ulcers and reduces the duration of infectivity. Famciclovir and valaciclovir are newer antiviral agents having improved bioavailability and longer half-lives, thus allowing less frequent administration.

Long-term antiviral therapy can be used to reduce the frequency of acute attacks in those patients suffering from recurrent infections.

Syphilis

The primary chancre of syphilis is painless, and this may present as a highly infectious vulval ulcer. The incubation period is 9–90 days, by which time the spirochaete has disseminated throughout the body. The characteristic lesions of secondary syphilis are condylomata lata, which appear as moist flat infective erosions on the vulva, vagina or cervix. Treatment is a 10-day course of procaine penicillin. All patients should be referred to a genitourinary clinic for full STD screening, treatment, contact tracing and follow-up.

Serological testing for syphilis is part of routine antenatal screening, because of the risk of transmission to the fetus. This practice has enabled the virtual elimination of congenital syphilis.

Vulval infestations

Lice

A particular type of louse called *Pediculosis pubis* may be found clinging to pubic hairs, using its three sets of legs. Clinical features are intense pruritus and sky blue spots at the bite sites. Both sexual partners should be treated with 1% gamma benzene hexachloride powder.

Scabies

Scabies is caused by a small slow-moving mite called *Sarcoptes scabei* which is transmitted by prolonged close physical contact. The female burrows under the skin and lays eggs, which causes unbearable itching. A favourite site is in the finger clefts. Diagnosis is made by deroofing the burrow and extracting the mite for identification under a microscope. Treatment is with 25% benzyl benzoate solution.

12.2 Vaginal infections

Learning objectives

You should:

- understand how the vagina maintains an acidic environment
- know how to manage the common symptom of vaginal discharge
- be aware that chlamydia infection may be asymptomatic
- understand how alterations in vaginal pH may occur

The healthy vagina is colonised by the Lactobacillus, which prevents infection by other micro-organisms. The Lactobacillus metabolises glycogen, which is produced by the squamous epithelial cells under the influence of oestrogen, to lactic acid. This maintains a vaginal pH of 4.5. Any conditions which reduce the vaginal acidity or eradicate the Lactobacillus will predispose to infection.

Vaginal discharge

The healthy vagina produces a variable amount of physiological vaginal discharge. This is called leucorrhoea. It is yellowish/white in colour and does not cause any irritation or offensive smell. It contains a mixture of secretions from endometrial and cervical glands, exfoliated vaginal cells, bacterial flora and white blood cells. It has a cyclical variation in common with cervical mucus, so women may notice their discharge increases at mid-cycle or prior to menstruation. Vaginal discharge may increase in pregnancy and in women who are using the combined oral contraceptive pill, both of which cause benign hyperplasia of the endocervical glands. This appearance may be recognised on visualising the cervix as a bright red vascular area. It is termed cervical ectopy.

Excessive vaginal discharge is a common gynaecological complaint, which should always be investigated. Careful examination of the vulva for signs of inflammation and discharge should be followed by a vaginal speculum examination to enable swabs to be taken for microbiological identification of any infective organism, and to visualise the cervix to look for a carcinoma.

Pathological causes of vaginal discharge

Common infectious causes
- *Candida albicans*
- *Trichomonas vaginalis*
- *Gardnerella vaginalis*
- *Chlamydia trachomatis*.

Other infectious causes
- Beta-haemolytic streptococcus
- *Neisseria gonorrhoeae*
- Herpes simplex virus
- Human papillomavirus
- Childhood vulvovaginitis.

Other pathological causes
- Chemical vaginitis
- Foreign body
- Chronic cervicitis
- Cervical polyps
- Cervical tumours
- Urinary or faecal fistulae.

Candidiasis

Candidiasis is the most common cause of infective vaginal discharge. *Candida albicans* is a yeast which thrives in moist skin folds. It is frequently found in asymptomatic women and it can often be isolated from the bowel. It is not usually sexually transmitted but may be carried by the uncircumcised male. The usual symptoms are vulval pruritus and vaginal soreness. Predisposing factors are diabetes, poor hygiene, nylon underwear and use of broad spectrum antibiotics. The diagnosis is made on the clinical grounds of finding a thick white cheesy discharge together with the culture of the organism from a swab. Treatment is with clotrimazole vaginal pessaries, together with clotrimazole cream if vulvitis is present, or with oral fluconazole. Recurrent infection is a common problem. This is thought to occur as a result of reinfection from a persistent bowel reservoir of organisms. Treatment is then with long-term courses of antifungal drugs. Advice should be given to wear loose cotton underwear and skirts to prevent excessive perspiration, and any predisposing factors such as diabetes should be identified and remedied.

Trichomonas

This causes a yellowish-green vaginal discharge, and a characteristic 'strawberry cervix' due to the prominent appearance of blood vessels. Trichomonas may also be carried asymptomatically in the vagina. It can be sexually transmitted so both partners should be screened for other sexually transmitted diseases. Diagnosis can be made by dark ground microscopic examination of a sample from the posterior vaginal fornix. The protozoa can be seen swimming around by whipping movements of their flagellae (Fig. 22). Treatment is with metronidazole. This should be given to both partners, with the advice to avoid alcohol during treatment. The dose is 400 mg 8-hourly for 5 days, or 2 g as a single dose.

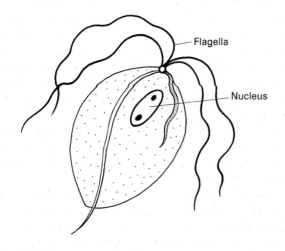

Fig. 22 *Trichomonas vaginalis*.

Bacterial vaginosis

Bacterial vaginosis is a common vaginal infection among women of reproductive age. It is caused by the anaerobic bacterium *Gardnerella vaginalis*. It causes a grey discharge and a fishy odour, although many women are asymptomatic. Microscopic examination of the discharge reveals typical 'clue cells', which are vaginal epithelial cells exhibiting surface dimpling from attached bacteria. Treatment is with metronidazole.

Untreated vaginal infection with gardnerella increases the risk of ascending infection resulting in pelvic inflammatory disease. In pregnancy, gardnerella infection is associated with both premature rupture of the membranes and chorioamnionitis.

Chlamydia

Chlamydia is an important cause of pelvic inflammatory disease. Screening has identified the organism in 8% of women attending for termination of pregnancy, and it is frequently found in association with other sexually transmitted diseases. In common with gonorrhoea, infection in the female may be asymptomatic. Cervical infection with chlamydia presents with vaginal discharge secondary to cervicitis. The organism is difficult to isolate by culture, but the diagnosis can be made by fluorescent monoclonal antibody or polymerase chain reaction testing. Women giving a history of a recent change in sexual partner together with a vaginal discharge should be referred to a genitourinary clinic for full genital microbiological screening, contact tracing and follow-up. Treatment is with a tetracycline such as doxycycline 100 mg 12-hourly for 14 days, or a single 1 g dose of azithromycin. Successful control of infection depends on investigation and treatment of the sexual partner.

Vulvovaginitis

Vulvovaginitis presents with an offensive vaginal discharge, and is seen in all age groups.

Childhood vulvovaginitis usually occurs due to under-oestrogenisation of the vagina. Oestrogen cream and attention to hygiene are indicated.

In women of reproductive age the common causes of vaginal discharge are infections with thrush, gardnerella and trichomonas. Rarer causes include a chemical vaginitis from an allergic reaction to detergents, douches, bath salts or deodorants. A foreign body in the vagina such as a forgotten tampon is an unusual cause, which may result in the toxic shock syndrome. This is a severe systemic infection with circulatory collapse due to release of staphylococcal toxins.

Vaginal discharge in post-menopausal women is usually due to bacterial vaginitis. The long-term effect of low oestrogen levels results in the vaginal skin becoming thin and easily traumatised, and lacking in glycogen. Colonisation with the Lactobacillus thus decreases and the pH rises, allowing pathogenic bacteria to infect the vagina. The possibility of a carcinoma should be remembered in this age group, particularly if the discharge is blood-stained.

12.3 Infections of the cervix

Learning objective

You should:

- know how to investigate suspected cervical infection

Acute infection of the cervix may be chlamydial, gonococcal or herpetic in origin. It may present with vaginal discharge, but is also commonly asymptomatic. The cervix usually looks red and may bleed easily on contact. Cervical swabs, colposcopy and cervical biopsy are all helpful in diagnosis.

Gonorrhoea

Gonorrhoea is a sexually transmitted infection caused by the Gram-negative diplococcus *Neisseria gonorrhoeae*. The incubation period is 2–5 days. It infects the mucous membranes of the cervix, urethra, anus, rectum and oropharynx. It may present with generalised malaise, vaginal discharge and dysuria, but some cases are asymptomatic. Untreated infection can persist as a chronic cervicitis or progress to a more severe and generalised illness. The potential sequelae of gonorrhoea infection include infertility, chronic pain and menstrual dysfunction.

If gonorrhoea infection is suspected, swabs should be taken from the urethra, cervix and rectum, put onto Stuart's transport medium, and screening undertaken for other STDs.

Complications of gonorrhoea
- Pelvic inflammatory disease
- Bartholin's abscess
- Joint pains
- Skin rash
- Endocarditis.

Treatment
A single dose of a long-acting penicillin is given by intramuscular injection. In cases of penicillin allergy, spectinomycin is effective. Tetracycline is often given in addition to eradicate possible chlamydial infection. Follow-up with repeat swabs is essential to confirm eradication, as some strains of the gonococcus have acquired penicillin resistance.

Chronic cervicitis

Chronic cervicitis causes a chronic persistent vaginal discharge. Cervical and vaginal swabs should be taken to exclude infection. In chronic cervicitis there is often no specific infection isolated. The cervix just appears enlarged and has copious mucous secretion from the glands. Obstruction of the gland openings results in mucous retention cysts, called Nabothian follicles. The naked eye appearance is of an enlarged irregular cervix with cystic lesions. Together with a firm irregularity on digital examination this can lead to a clinical suspicion of cancer. If there is doubt about the clinical appearance of the cervix a cervical smear and urgent referral for colposcopy is indicated. Provided specific infections and neoplasia have been excluded, destruction of the inflamed columnar epithelium by cauterisation or cryotherapy may produce a cure.

12.4 Acute pelvic inflammatory disease

Learning objectives

You should:

- understand the implications of pelvic inflammatory disease

- know how to manage suspected pelvic inflammatory disease

- be able to construct a differential diagnosis from the symptoms and signs in a case of suspected pelvic inflammatory disease

Pelvic inflammatory disease refers to infection involving the upper genital tract. It usually results from ascending sexually-acquired infection of the lower genital tract. Once pathogens gain access to the peritoneal cavity via the fallopian tubes a severe pelvic peritonitis may result. Common pathogens include chlamydia, *N. gonorrhoeae* and anaerobic bacteria. Any sexually active woman is at risk of pelvic inflammatory disease, but precipitating factors include the intra-uterine contraceptive device, multiple sexual partners and instrumentation of the cervix in the presence of pathogenic organisms. The risk is reduced by the use of barrier methods of contraception and by limiting the number of sexual partners.

Early diagnosis and treatment is essential to prevent permanent damage to the fallopian tubes. This is sometimes difficult because infections can be asymptomatic and some women unfortunately become infertile in this way (see p. 202). In severe cases the fimbrial ends of the tubes become occluded, allowing them to become distended with inflammatory exudate. This is called a hydrosalpinx (Fig. 23). If the tube becomes distended with pus it is called a pyosalpinx. This indicates severe irreversible damage.

Clinical findings

Presentation is typically with bilateral lower abdominal pain and fever, accompanied by a vaginal discharge and deep dyspareunia. Examination reveals guarding and rebound tenderness over the lower abdomen and a tender uterus. Moving the cervix on vaginal examination causes severe pain called excitation. An adnexal mass with a high fever and leucocytosis suggests a pyosalpinx or tubo-ovarian abscess. Transperitoneal infection occasionally spreads to the upper abdomen, causing upper abdominal pain and perihepatic adhesions.

Symptoms and signs of acute pelvic inflammatory disease

- Acute lower abdominal pain
- Vaginal discharge
- Fever
- Pelvic tenderness
- Adnexal mass.

Investigation of suspected acute pelvic inflammatory disease

A white cell count and erythrocyte sedimentation rate (ESR) should be taken together with swabs from the cervix, urethra, vagina and rectum. An important differential diagnosis here is ectopic pregnancy, so a pregnancy test should always be sent. If positive, ultrasound can help to distinguish between an ectopic and an intra-uterine gestation. Acute appendicitis, adnexal torsion and a bleeding corpus luteum cyst can all produce similar symptoms. Laparoscopy is therefore useful for diagnosis and is indicated in patients who do not respond to antibiotics. Laparoscopy allows assessment of tubal damage and culture of fluid from the fallopian tubes and pouch of Douglas. The typical findings in acute pelvic inflammatory disease are hyperaemia of the fallopian tubes with oedema and a sticky exudate on their peritoneal surface.

Treatment

Hospital admission is required for severe cases, for bed rest, intravenous antibiotics and analgesia. If an intra-uterine contraceptive device (IUCD) is present it should be removed. Combination antibiotic therapy is started immediately and is reviewed when bacteriological culture results are available. However, causative organisms are only isolated in about 30% of cases. Metronidazole covers anaerobic organisms, whilst tetracyclines should be given for chlamydial infections. Treatment is given for 10–14 days. A single intramuscular dose of 4.8 megaunits of procaine penicillin with 1 g oral probenecid will treat gonococcus.

Long-term morbidity from pelvic inflammatory disease

- Recurrent attacks of infection
- Chronic pelvic pain
- Dyspareunia
- Ectopic pregnancy
- Infertility
- Menstrual disturbance.

Chronic pelvic inflammatory disease

Recurrent attacks of pelvic inflammatory disease may result in chronic pelvic pain, menstrual disturbance, dyspareunia and infertility. The uterus and adnexae may become fixed due to tethering by adhesions. The best option for future fertility is by in vitro fertilisation. Tubal reconstructive surgery is rarely of value. Relief from chronic pelvic pain and menstrual irregularity is often eventually sought by hysterectomy and bilateral salpingo-oophorectomy.

12.5 Pelvic abscess

Learning objectives

You should:

- understand the different pathophysiologies leading to a pelvic abscess

- understand the principles of management of a pelvic abscess

A collection of pus may accumulate in the pelvis to form an abscess. This is usually a tubo-ovarian abscess resulting from pelvic inflammatory disease. The features are a swinging fever, pelvic pain and a tender pelvic mass, with tenesmus if there is pressure on the rectum. Occasionally an abscess will spontaneously discharge into the posterior vaginal fornix or rectum, resulting in a prompt relief of pain. If there is no clinical improvement after 48 hours of intravenous antibiotics, drainage is required. This may be achieved by posterior colpotomy if the abscess is filling the pouch of Douglas. Otherwise, laparoscopic drainage and irrigation will be necessary. Major surgery to excise the pelvic organs is rarely neces-

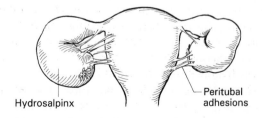

Hydrosalpinx

Peritubal adhesions

Fig. 23 Acute pelvic inflammatory disease: hydrosalpinx.

sary and carries a risk of bowel injury and deep vein thrombosis.

Causes of pelvic abscess
- Pelvic inflammatory disease
- Appendicitis
- Postoperative
- Illegal abortion
- Diverticulitis.

12.6 HIV infection

Learning objectives

You should:

- understand the implications of HIV infection

- understand the principles of HIV prevention

- be aware how disease presentation may vary

The human immunodeficiency virus (HIV) is a retrovirus which causes acquired immune deficiency syndrome (AIDS). It may be transmitted by unprotected penetrative sexual intercourse, infected blood, and from mother to baby during pregnancy, labour or by breast feeding. It selectively infects T lymphocytes with the CD4 antigen, which decreases the host immune defences. Antibodies are produced 4–8 weeks after exposure, and are detectable in blood. Of those infected with HIV, 50% develop AIDS within 10 years. Many individuals will have acquired HIV infection unknowingly and can therefore be expected to develop AIDs in the future. By 1994 over 10 000 AIDS cases had been reported in the UK, most of whom have now died. Of the registered HIV-seropositive patients, 11% are female. As no cure or vaccine is currently available, disease prevention is the main method of controlling spread of HIV. Screening of blood, use of condoms and limiting the number of sexual partners all reduce the risk of infection.

Acute infection with HIV is usually subclinical, but there may be a transient non-specific illness. This is followed by a chronic infection, characterised in one third of patients by a persistent generalised lymphadenopathy. When this is accompanied by non-specific constitutional symptoms such as fever, weight loss and malaise, coupled with minor opportunistic infections such as oral candidiasis, it is called AIDS-related complex.

Full-blown AIDS develops after a median incubation period of 8–10 years. It is defined by the presence of certain reliably diagnosed diseases in the absence of any other cause of immune deficiency (Box 53). The patient will be seropositive. The clinical presentation varies according to the presenting disease. Symptoms include weight loss, dry cough, purple skin lesions of Kaposi's sarcoma, diarrhoea, perianal ulceration, headache and dementia. Death occurs within 2 years of diagnosis. Treatment with zidovudine has been shown to improve survival and decrease the incidence of opportunistic infections.

12.7 Rare causes of pelvic sepsis

Learning objectives

You should know:

- that rare chronic granulomatous pelvic infections exist

- that TB and actinomycosis are rare causes of infertility

Actinomycosis

Actinomycosis is caused by the anaerobic obligate fungal parasite *Actinomyces israeli*. It is a very uncommon cause of chronic pelvic infection, and thus rarely suspected on clinical grounds. It causes a characteristic granulomatous tissue reaction with the formation of hard masses and multiple discharging sinuses, which can result in bowel or ureteric obstruction. Extensive abdominal actinomycosis may occasionally be mistaken for malignancy, with the associated risk of inappropriate surgery. This emphasises the fundamental importance of obtaining a tissue diagnosis prior to undertaking treatment. Diagnosis is made by anaerobic culture of pus, when typical yellowish 'sulphur granule' colonies are seen. Treatment is with penicillin.

Actinomyces is sometimes reported in a cervical smear in a healthy woman in association with the IUCD. In such cases the coil can be changed and a course of penicillin given.

Box 53 Diseases indicative of cellular immune deficiency seen in AIDS

- Opportunistic infections
- Pneumocystis pneumonia
- Cryptococcosis
- Cytomegalovirus
- Herpes simplex virus
- Toxoplasmosis
- *Mycobacterium kansasii* or *avium*
- Candidiasis — oesophageal or pulmonary
- Progressive multifocal leucoencephalopathy
- Malignancies
  - Kaposi's sarcoma
  - primary cerebral lymphoma
  - non-Hodgkin's lymphoma

Tuberculosis

Tuberculosis (TB) infects one third of the world's population. Pelvic tuberculosis is usually secondary to a primary lung infection, but it is a rare cause of infertility in this country. The fallopian tube is the most commonly affected site in the pelvis. It becomes thickened and filled with caseous material, with tubercles on the peritoneal surface. The diagnosis is rarely suspected on clinical grounds and is usually made on TB culture of uterine curettings. Treatment is with rifampicin, isoniazid and ethambutol.

Pyometra

Pyometra is a collection of pus in the uterus. It is usually secondary to a necrotic endometrial carcinoma or a cancer of the sigmoid colon which has eroded into the uterus.

Self-assessment: questions

Multiple choice questions

1. Which of the following are common causes of vaginal discharge?
   a. Herpes virus
   b. Candidiasis
   c. Trichomonas
   d. Lactobacillus
   e. Gardnerella

2. Concerning HIV/AIDS:
   a. AIDS may present with recurrent vaginal candidiasis
   b. Drug abusers sharing infected needles are a high risk group
   c. Antenatal screening should be offered to all pregnant women
   d. There is an increased risk of cervical intraepithelial neoplasia (CIN)
   e. The majority of cases of AIDS in the UK occur in heterosexual men

3. Which of the following are true regarding *Candida albicans*?
   a. It is commonly carried in the gastrointestinal tract
   b. It always produces symptoms when present in the vagina
   c. The male partner may be a carrier
   d. Recurrent attacks of vaginal candidiasis are associated with diabetes insipidus
   e. The combined oral contraceptive pill predisposes to recurrent vaginal candidiasis

4. Genital warts:
   a. Are caused by a virus which is usually sexually transmitted
   b. May grow in pregnancy
   c. Usually need to be treated under general anaesthetic
   d. Have a characteristic clinical appearance
   e. In pregnancy can be treated with podophyllin

5. Acute pelvic inflammatory disease:
   a. Rarely results in infertility due to tubal damage
   b. Is always sexually transmitted
   c. Is commonly caused by chlamydia
   d. may be asymptomatic
   e. Pelvic ultrasound is more useful than laparoscopy in diagnosis

6. Which of the following are risk factors for pelvic inflammatory disease?
   a. Avoidance of barrier contraception
   b. Use of the oral contraceptive pill
   c. Multiple sexual partners
   d. Pregnancy
   e. Clip sterilisation

7. Which of the following organisms are correctly matched with the lesion?
   a. Human papillomavirus — Condylomata lata
   b. Scabies mite — Pearly white skin papules
   c. Herpes virus — Genital ulceration
   d. Actinomycosis — Granulomatous peritonitis
   e. *Molluscum contagiosum* — Pruritic skin burrows

Short notes

What is the normal vaginal pH during reproductive years and how is this maintained? What changes occur in the vaginal pH after the menopause, and what is the significance of this?

Case histories

Case history 1

A 17-year-old sexually active woman has a 10-day history of lower abdominal pain, increased vaginal discharge and pain on micturition. On examination the cervix is hyperaemic and there is tenderness on bimanual palpation. There is a low grade pyrexia.

What is the differential diagnosis and what investigations are indicated?

Case history 2

A 38-year-old woman complains of an offensive odour after sexual intercourse. Examination reveals a greyish vaginal discharge. A sample of fluid is taken from the posterior fornix and mixed with 10% potassium hydroxide, which produces a fishy odour. On microscopy there are numerous squamous cells with stippled borders.

What are these cells called? Name the diagnosis and the correct treatment.

OSCE questions

OSCE 1

A 20-year-old woman has recently been treated in hospital for acute salpingitis. She now has a few questions for you:

1. The hospital told her the swabs were all negative, so did she really have an infection?
2. How could she have caught the infection?
3. Why was she treated with three different antibiotics?
4. Why was it necessary for the hospital to contact all her recent sexual partners?

5. Is she likely to have difficulty getting pregnant in the future?
6. Some of her friends want to know if there is any screening for chlamydia?

OSCE 2

A 16-year-old girl presents with genital warts. She wants to know:

1. What treatments are available?
2. Will treatment eradicate the virus from her?
3. Will using condoms reduce her chances of further genital warts?
4. Should her partner have any treatment?

Self-assessment: answers

Multiple choice answers

1. a. **False.**
   b. **True.**
   c. **True.**
   d. **False.** Lactobacilli are the dominant bacteria in the healthy vagina. They produce lactic acid by metabolising glycogen. This maintains the vaginal pH at around 4, which inhibits the growth of undesirable organisms such as Gardnerella.
   e. **True.**

2. a. **True.**
   b. **True.**
   c. **True.**
   d. **True.** Women with HIV have an increased incidence of CIN and should be offered colposcopy.
   e. **False.** The majority of cases of AIDS in the UK occur in homosexual men.

3. a. **True.**
   b. **False.** Asymptomatic vaginal colonisation with Candida occurs in 10% of women.
   c. **True.**
   d. **False.** Diabetes mellitus should be excluded by checking a random blood sugar in women with recurrent vaginal candidiasis.
   e. **False.**

4. a. **True.**
   b. **True.** Warts tend to grow rapidly in the third trimester of pregnancy.
   c. **False.** Treatment is usually with local application of podophyllin or trichloracetic acid. Surgical excision or laser ablation is only required for extensive areas.
   d. **True.** The diagnosis is usually made on clinical appearance, but large or persistent warty lesions should always be biopsied to exclude a carcinoma.
   e. **False.** Podophyllin is contraindicated in pregnancy because it is teratogenic.

5. a. **False.** Infertility due to tubal damage is a significant risk from even a single chlamydial infection.
   b. **False.** Most cases are sexually transmitted but infection can spread to the fallopian tubes from another septic focus in the peritoneal cavity, such as a perforated appendix.
   c. **True.**
   d. **True.**
   e. **False.** Laparoscopy is much more useful than ultrasound in diagnosis.

6. a. **True.**
   b. **False.** Women who use the oral contraceptive pill have a lower incidence of pelvic inflammatory disease mainly because the cervical mucus is thicker, which forms a more effective barrier to bacteria.
   c. **True.**
   d. **False.** In pregnancy the presence of a gestation sac and the increased blood flow to the pelvic organs reduces the risk of pelvic inflammatory disease.
   e. **False.** Clip sterilisation impedes bacterial access to the peritoneal cavity so prevents spread of infection.

7. a. **False.** HPV causes condylomata acuminata. Condylomata lata are seen in secondary syphilis.
   b. **False.** Scabies mite causes pruritic skin burrows.
   c. **True.**
   d. **True.**
   e. **False.** *Molluscum contagiosum* causes pearly white skin papules.

Case history answers

Case history 1

The symptoms and clinical findings are suggestive of infection with either chlamydia or gonorrhoea. Endocervical and urethral swabs should be taken, and urine should be sent for culture to exclude a urinary tract infection. The patient should be immediately referred to a genito-urinary clinic for full STD screening and contact tracing.

Case history 2

These are the so-called clue cells, which are epithelial cells with numerous bacteria adherent to them. Together with the fishy odour on addition of potassium hydroxide, this is characteristic of Gardnerella infection. Treatment is with metronidazole.

Short notes answers

The normal vaginal pH is around 4.5 during the reproductive years. This is due to the metabolism of glycogen to lactic acid by the numerous lactobacilli. After the menopause, decreasing oestrogen levels lead to glycogen depletion in the vaginal cells. This reduces the numbers of lactobacilli so the pH rises. The significance of this is that the reduced vaginal acidity after the menopause renders it more susceptible to infection.

OSCE answers

OSCE 1

1. The sensitivity of currently available laboratory tests is such that a negative result does not exclude a diagnosis of acute salpingitis. Diagnosis and treatment is thus often based on clinical findings.

2. The infection is usually sexually transmitted.

3. A number of different organisms can cause acute salpingitis, such as *Chlamydia trachomatis, Neisseria gonorrhoea* and anaerobes. A tetracycline such as doxycycline covers chlamydia, penicillin or a cephalosporin covers gonorrhoea, and metronidazole covers the anaerobes, so three drugs are often given simultaneously.

4. Contact tracing and treatment of sexual partners is vital to prevent reinfection and chronic salpingitis occurring.

5. Although even one episode of acute salpingitis can result in tubal damage, with resultant infertility and increased risk of ectopic pregancy, she should be reassured that prompt and appropriate antibiotic treatment reduces the risk.

6. It is likely that screening and treating asymptomatic chlamydia infections in high risk groups, such as single women under the age of 25 years, would decrease the incidence of long-term complications such as infertility, ectopic pregnancy and pelvic pain. However, this is not possible currently, as there is a lack of a simple, cheap and rapid diagnostic test with sufficient sensitivity and specificity.

OSCE 2

1. Painting the warts with podophyllin solution or trichloracetic acid. Cryotherapy using liquid nitrogen. Diathermy or surgical excision under anaesthetic for large warts, or those resistant to the other treatments.

2. The virus is often found on histological examination of clinically normal tissue adjacent to the warts, and as such, it is unlikely that any physical treatment completely eradicates the virus.

3. Although condoms do afford some protection from sexually transmitted diseases, they do not appear to reduce the risk of recurrence after treatment.

4. Yes, her partner should be examined, and offered treatment if any warts are found.

13 Pelvic pain and endometriosis

Overview

There are many and widely differing causes of pelvic pain in women. Pain of gynaecological origin may result from normal physiological events, such as ovulation and menstruation, or may alternatively result from a pathological process, such as torsion of an ovarian cyst. Accurate diagnosis is therefore important in the management, but this can sometimes be difficult. For example, ectopic pregnancy remains as a cause of maternal death in this country. Endometriosis is a disease characterised by pelvic pain, and in the more severe cases, can cause significant morbidity.

Introduction

Pelvic pain is a common complaint, particularly amongst women of reproductive age. It may be caused by diseases in the gynaecological, urinary, gastrointestinal or musculoskeletal systems. However, many cases of chronic pelvic pain have no obvious organic cause. Clues to the diagnosis may be provided by the character of the pain, and its relationship to menstruation, ovulation or sexual intercourse. For example, the pain from ovulation occurs at mid-cycle and is short-lived, whereas the pain in advanced pelvic malignancy is usually chronic and deep-seated.

13.1 Gynaecological causes of acute pelvic pain

Learning objectives

You should:

- understand the pathophysiological principles of pelvic pain
- be able to construct a differential diagnosis based on the clinical features

Causes include:

- ectopic pregnancy
- mittelschmerz
- rupture, torsion or haemorrhage of an ovarian cyst
- acute pelvic inflammatory disease
- miscarriage
- degeneration of uterine fibroids
- trauma.

Ectopic pregnancy

Pain initially arises due to stretching of the visceral peritoneum covering the fallopian tube. This has an autonomic nerve supply and the resulting pain is poorly localised in the lower abdomen. Later, leakage of blood from the fimbrial end of the tube causes irritation of the parietal peritoneum. This has a somatic nerve supply, so the pain becomes both more severe and localised. Shoulder tip pain results from blood tracking up the paracolic gutter to the under-surface of the diaphragm.

Mittelschmerz

Pain in the iliac fossa lasting anything from a few hours to 2 days is regularly experienced by many women at the mid-cycle. It is called mittelschmerz (literally, 'middle pain'). It is thought to be caused by bleeding from the surface of the ovary following ovulation.

Rupture of ovarian cyst

Rupture of a corpus luteum cyst occasionally presents with acute pelvic pain due to intraperitoneal bleeding. The blood loss is rarely significant. Haemorrhage into a cyst without rupture will also cause acute pain.

Torsion of ovarian cyst

An ovarian cyst may twist on its pedicle, initially giving rise to a poorly localised pain. Examination reveals a tender pelvic mass. If strangulation and infarction occur the pain will become severe and localised, and be accompanied by pyrexia.

Acute pelvic inflammatory disease

Acute pelvic inflammatory disease produces severe bilateral lower abdominal pain due to pelvic peritoneal inflammation. Guarding and rebound tenderness are accompanied by fever and vaginal discharge.

Miscarriage

Severe cramping lower abdominal pain accompanied by vaginal bleeding and passage of products of conception is characteristic of miscarriage in early pregnancy. There is usually a preceding history of amenorrhoea.

Degeneration of uterine fibroids

Fibroids may rapidly enlarge during pregnancy and outgrow their blood supply, due to the stimulatory effects of oestrogen. This results in infarction of the fibroid, which is called red degeneration. A localised tender uterine mass is usually palpable.

Trauma

Accidental perforation of the uterus causes a dull pelvic ache. This can occur when an intra-uterine contraceptive device is being fitted or during hysteroscopy. If the perforation is recognised the patient should be closely observed for signs of peritoneal bleeding, but this is rarely severe.

Chronic pelvic pain

There are many gynaecological causes of chronic pelvic pain, and some of these are discussed elsewhere. Chronic pelvic inflammatory disease (Ch. 12) may cause deep dyspareunia, chronic pelvic aching and low back pain together with infertility and menstrual dysfunction. On examination the uterus may be tender and fixed, and in severe cases there are bilateral hydrosalp-

inges and a pelvis frozen by adhesions. Uterovaginal prolapse (Ch. 18) characteristically causes a dragging pelvic discomfort and lower backache, which is relieved by lying flat.

Gynaecological causes of chronic pelvic pain include:

- dysmenorrhoea
- pelvic pain syndrome
- mittelschmerz
- pelvic inflammatory disease
- endometriosis
- adenomyosis
- pelvic venous congestion
- uterovaginal prolapse
- pelvic neoplasm
- psychogenic pelvic pain.

13.2 Dysmenorrhoea

Learning objectives

You should:

- be able to interpret the degree to which dysmenorrhoea is affecting a woman
- understand the mechanisms of action of the drug treatments

Some degree of discomfort during menstruation is experienced by most women, and is considered physiological. This consists of cramping lower abdominal pains which radiate to the upper thighs and lower back. It is typically worst on the first and second day of menstruation and is relieved by simple analgesics.

However, a significant proportion of women are incapacitated by dysmenorrhoea, and are unable to attend work or school for several days each month.

Clinically, it is useful to distinguish between primary and secondary dysmenorrhoea.

Primary dysmenorrhoea

Severe primary dysmenorrhoea occurs in 5% of young women. It often occurs during the teens, starting a year or two after the menarche when ovulatory cycles have become established. The pain is due to powerful uterine contractions caused by high levels of endometrial prostaglandins and leukotrienes. The pain radiates to the back and legs and is often accompanied by nausea and diarrhoea. Symptoms are worst at the onset of menstruation and rarely persist beyond 48 hours. The diagnosis can usually be made from the history and examination alone.

Treatment of primary dysmenorrhoea

Explanation and reassurance are essential. Simple analgesics may suffice, but in more resistant cases hormonal therapy may be indicated, combined with stronger analgesics.

Drug treatment for primary dysmenorrhoea

- Paracetamol
- Prostaglandin synthetase inhibitors
- Combined oral contraceptive pill
- Progestogens.

Prostaglandin synthetase inhibitors. Drugs such as mefenamic acid, ibuprofen and naproxen inhibit the endometrial synthesis of prostaglandins, in addition to having a direct analgesic effect. They are cheap, effective, and only need to be taken immediately before and during menstruation. Side-effects are listed in Box 54.

Combined oral contraceptive pill. The low-dose combined oral contraceptive pill inhibits ovulation and reduces both endometrial growth and prostaglandin concentrations. It provides effective treatment for primary dysmenorrhoea and is especially useful if contraception is also required. It may be prescribed in combination with prostaglandin synthetase inhibitors for the treatment of severe primary dysmenorrhoea. If initial medical therapy is unsuccessful, alternative causes of cyclical pain such as endometriosis should be considered.

Secondary dysmenorrhoea

Secondary dysmenorrhoea usually affects women of an older age group. The pain starts several days before menstruation approaches. It is often sited in the pelvis and lower back, and is constant in nature. Less is known about the aetiology but it is often secondary to organic disease such as fibroids, endometriosis, adenomyosis or chronic pelvic infection. Sometimes all that is found is a bulky uterus with thickened uterosacral ligaments. Treatment is aimed at the cause, and if childbearing is complete hysterectomy is an option. In the absence of

pelvic pathology, treatment with progestogens should be tried first.

13.3 Pelvic pain syndrome

Learning objectives

You should:

- know which investigations to use in the diagnosis of pelvic pain
- understand the different management options for pelvic pain syndrome
- recognise the importance of excluding serious pathology as a cause of pelvic pain

Pelvic pain syndrome is used to describe chronic pelvic pain when no obvious organic cause can be identified. The pain is usually a long-standing dull ache in one or other iliac fossa, and is accompanied by deep dyspareunia, post-coital ache and abdominal bloating. Headache, backache and vaginal discharge may also be present. It occurs during the reproductive years, and is frequently accompanied by both sexual problems and depression.

Diagnosis

A diagnosis of pelvic pain syndrome can only be made following exclusion of pelvic pathology. Both pelvic ultrasound and laparoscopy are useful in this respect. There is some evidence that the pain may be caused by congestion of pelvic veins, as demonstrated by pelvic venography, whereby radio-opaque dye is injected into the myometrium via a long needle passed through the cervix. These veins are characteristically seen in the broad ligaments and pelvic sidewall. They are often larger on the side of any developing ovarian follicle, which suggests that they are under the cyclical influence of ovarian hormones. In clinical practice, however, pelvic venography is rarely performed.

Management

Simple reassurance. Reassuring a woman that her pelvis is free of serious disease can have a beneficial therapeutic effect and may be all that is required. In other cases treatment with progestogens such as medroxyprogesterone acetate in a daily dose of 50 mg can be helpful. This will suppress ovarian oestrogen production and thereby induce narrowing of the dilated pelvic veins.

Box 54 Prostaglandin synthetase inhibitors: side-effects

Common
- Gastrointestinal – nausea, diarrhoea, heartburn
- Central nervous – headache, dizziness, drowsiness

Rare
- Renal failure
- Blood dyscrasias
- Bronchospasm

Psychological treatment. This approach has an important role to play, particularly when there is a large anxiety component. Relaxation therapy, stress avoidance and non-directive counselling have all been shown to produce long-term benefits when compared to control groups.

Surgery. Surgical procedures such as transection of the uterosacral ligaments or resection of the superior hypogastric nerve plexus have been advocated for treating unexplained pelvic pain, but they are rarely used in current practice. Hysterectomy and bilateral salpingo-oophorectomy followed by hormone replacement therapy is reserved for older women who have completed their families. Attempts should be made to identify the pain-dependent personality type before resorting to surgery, as such women do not generally benefit.

13.4 Endometriosis

Learning objectives

You should:

- understand the principles of management of endometriosis

- appreciate why endometriosis may present in several different ways

Endometriosis is a benign but troublesome gynaecological condition. It is characterised by deposits of functioning endometrial tissue outside the usual location in the uterine cavity. These deposits respond to stimulation by ovarian hormones in a similar manner to the endometrium. Cyclical bleeding thus occurs, which causes local inflammation and adhesion formation. This may give rise to clinical symptoms, and in particular pelvic pain. Endometriosis does not occur before puberty, and tends to regress after the menopause because of declining oestrogen levels.

Aetiology of endometriosis

There are several proposed aetiological theories. The most popular is that of backward flow of menstrual fluid through the fallopian tubes and into the peritoneal cavity, with subsequent implantation onto dependent peritoneal surfaces. This would explain the predilection of endometriosis for the pouch of Douglas. Certainly retrograde menstruation is a commonly observed phenomenon at laparoscopy. Other aetiological theories include embolism via pelvic veins or lymphatics, and coelomic metaplasia.

Clinical features of endometriosis

Endometriosis is most common in nulliparous Western women. Parity appears to confer protection. Interestingly, the symptoms of endometriosis depend more on the site of disease than the extent (see Box 55). It may occasionally be an incidental finding at laparoscopy, and sometimes even the most extensive endometriosis is asymptomatic.

The classic symptoms are cyclical pelvic pain, dysmenorrhoea and dyspareunia. Pain is caused by extravasation of blood. This causes intense inflammation, followed by scarring and adhesion formation. Bleeding may occur into the peritoneal cavity, into the substance of the ovaries to form chocolate cysts, or into the lumen of the bowel or bladder. Rare symptoms thus include cyclical haematuria and cyclical rectal bleeding. Endometriosis involving the rectovaginal septum, uterosacral ligaments or vaginal fornices causes dyspareunia. Sometimes endometriosis is discovered during the course of investigations into infertility, when the fallopian tubes and ovaries may be distorted and scarred with endometriotic deposits. Endometriosis found deep within the myometrium is called adenomyosis. This presents with severe dysmenorrhoea. Rarely endometriotic deposits obstruct the bowel or ureter, when it can be mistaken for a carcinoma due to the extensive tissue induration.

Clinical signs of endometriosis

- Nodular thickening and tenderness in the uterosacral ligaments or pouch of Douglas
- Fixed tender retroverted uterus
- Adnexal swelling or tenderness.

A diagnosis of endometriosis may be suspected on clinical grounds, but confirmation requires laparoscopy, as many of the symptoms, such as dysmenorrhoea, may be of physiological rather than pathological origin. Similarly a normal pelvic examination does not exclude a diagnosis of endometriosis. Laparoscopy permits a thorough assessment of the extent of disease, with respect to the

---

Box 55 Sites of occurrence of endometriosis

Common	**Rare**
• Ovaries	• Bowel
• Uterosacral ligaments	• Implantation in scars
• Peritoneum lining pouch of Douglas	• Rectovaginal septum
• Myometrium	• Bladder
	• Vaginal vault
	• Lung

sites, size of deposits and presence of adhesions. The typical clinical appearance of endometriosis is of small scattered pigmented spots.

Treatment of endometriosis

This may be medical, surgical or a combination of the two. Treatment is only necessary if symptoms are present. The choice of treatment depends on the age and parity of the patient, her desire for fertility and the extent of disease present. Surgery is preferred in women with large endometriotic cysts or gross adhesions, whereas superficial peritoneal implants respond better to hormonal therapy. The success of treatment is assessed by relief of symptoms, appearance on repeat laparoscopy or by measurement of the subsequent pregnancy rate. Serial CA 125 measurements are sometimes used (see p. 240).

Medical treatment

In addition to analgesics, hormonal therapy is the treatment of choice for younger women with relatively small lesions. This avoids the risks of surgery and the development of further post-operative adhesions. The aim is to induce a hypo-oestrogenic state or a pseudo-pregnancy state, both of which suppress endometriotic lesions. Treatment needs to be for 6–9 months, and should be given in a dose sufficient to suppress menstruation. Hormonal treatments are potentially but not reliably contraceptive, so barrier methods should also be used.

Drugs used to treat endometriosis are:

- Continuous combined oral contraceptive pill
- progestogens
- danazol
- gestrinone
- gonadotrophin-releasing hormone analogues.

Continuous combined oral contraceptive pill. This is given continuously for 3 months in order to suppress all bleeding. Side-effects include weight gain, headaches and breast tenderness.

Progestogens. Continuous progestogen therapy for 6–9 months is first line medical treatment. Medroxyprogesterone acetate 30–100 mg daily is effective. Side-effects include breakthrough bleeding and weight gain.

Danazol. This synthetic derivative of testosterone can be given in a daily dose of 200–800 mg. It is widely used in the treatment of endometriosis, and improves symptoms in up to 85% of patients. Side-effects are androgenic and dose-related. They include weight gain, acne, oily skin, hirsutism and muscle cramps.

Gestrinone. This drug is similar to danazol but has a longer half-life, so is taken only twice a week.

Gonadotrophin-releasing hormone (GnRH) analogues. GnRH analogues differ from the endogenous decapeptide LHRH in one or two amino acids. This confers an increased resistance to enzymatic degradation, with the result that they act as superactive agonists with a long half-life. Continuous administration causes an initial stimulation of pituitary gonadotrophin release for a few days, followed by down-regulation due to desensitisation. This results in low levels of luteinising hormone (LH) and follicle-stimulating hormone (FSH), leading to reversible ovarian suppression with low oestrogen levels. Administration is either by monthly subcutaneous depot injection or by nasal spray. GnRH analogues are as effective as danazol in relieving symptoms and inducing resolution of endometriotic deposits, but are considerably more expensive. Side-effects are hypo-oestrogenic and include hot flushes, vaginal dryness and dyspareunia. There is also a loss of bone calcium which limits their long-term use because of the risk of osteoporosis.

Surgery

There is no definitive hormonal treatment capable of completely eradicating endometriosis, so many patients eventually come to surgery.

Conservative surgery. Conservative surgery (see Box 56) is indicated in those patients with symptomatic disease who wish to preserve their fertility. It can be carried out by laparotomy or laparoscopy. Superficial endometriotic deposits can be destroyed by electrocoagulation or laser. Deposits situated on the uterosacral ligaments causing dyspareunia are suitable for treatment in this way. Laser ablation has the advantage of being able to vaporise tissue precisely, which is then evacuated as smoke. There is minimal thermal damage to surrounding tissues, and the wounds heal with virtually no scarring. Division of adhesions is undertaken to restore normal pelvic anatomy. Removal of ovarian endometriomata is a more extensive procedure as severe anatomical distortion from extensive fibrosis is frequently present. The aim is to conserve as much ovarian tissue as possible and minimise subsequent adhesion formation.

Radical surgery. In cases where chronic pelvic pain persists and childbearing is complete a permanent surgical cure can be considered. This is by total abdominal

---

Box 56 Conservative surgery for endometriosis

- Adhesiolysis
- Excision of endometriotic cysts
- Electrocautery
- Laser

hysterectomy and bilateral salpingo-oophorectomy, together with excision or destruction of all visible endometriotic deposits. In severe cases the ovaries are involved with deep-seated disease. Ovarian conservation therefore carries a risk of compromising treatment outcome in terms of pain relief. Without ovarian function, any small remaining deposits of endometriosis will tend to regress, and this is not usually affected by the small amounts of oestrogen present in hormone replacement therapy.

More extensive surgery is required rarely, for instance when endometriosis has resulted in bowel or ureteric obstruction, or when there is a painful deposit in the rectovaginal septum. These can be extremely difficult operative procedures due to obliteration of tissue planes by scarring.

13.5 Non-gynaecological causes of pelvic pain

Learning objectives

You should:

- be able to interpret the features of the history in order to construct a likely differential diagnosis

Non-gynaecological causes include:

- irritable bowel syndrome
- constipation
- urinary tract infection or calculus
- acute appendicitis
- diverticulitis
- colonic cancer
- lumbosacral disc prolapse.

Irritable bowel syndrome

This is a common cause of pelvic pain in young women. It appears to have a large psychosomatic element, and is often exacerbated by stress and emotional upset. It is a diagnosis of exclusion, as similar symptoms may also be caused by serious gynaecological pathology (see Box 57). Treatment is directed towards symptoms. This usually involves bowel antispasmodics, increasing dietary fibre, and lifestyle changes directed at stress reduction.

13.6 Investigation of pelvic pain

Learning objectives

You should:

- understand how to use investigations appropriately to the clinical pattern

History

A carefully directed history may provide clues as to the origin of the pain (Table 15). Recurrent cyclical pain is usually of gynaecological origin. It is helpful to make a distinction between acute and chronic pain. The severity can be ascertained by asking about interference with work or sleep, and by enquiry into analgesic use.

Examination

Observation of affect and body language may be helpful. Women with pelvic pain syndrome often appear

---

Box 57 Common symptoms of irritable bowel syndrome

- Lower abdominal cramping pain
- Constipation
- Diarrhoea
- Abdominal bloating
- Flatulence
- Dyspareunia

Table 15 Pelvic pain: history and interpretation

Feature of history	Likely cause of pain
Occurs with menses	primary dysmenorrhoea
Precedes and persists after menses	secondary dysmenorrhoea
Occurs at midcycle	mittelschmerz
Associated with bowel symptoms	irritable bowel syndrome
Associated with dyspareunia	endometriosis
History of sexually transmitted disease	pelvic inflammatory disease
Sudden onset of severe pain	acute accident to pelvic organ
Associated amenorrhoea	ectopic pregnancy or miscarriage
Chronic unremitting pain	pelvic malignancy

mildly depressed. Anaemia, weight loss, ascites or a pelvic mass are suggestive of malignancy. A palpable noisy caecum in a nervous young woman is typical of irritable bowel syndrome. An enlarged or immobile uterus will focus attention on to that organ as a likely source of symptoms. Thickened nodular uterosacral ligaments are suggestive of endometriosis.

Investigations

The history and examination findings may be all that are required to make a diagnosis. If further investigations are needed, the following are the most useful:

- full blood count
- pregnancy test
- midstream specimen of urine
- plain abdominal X-ray
- pelvic ultrasound
- laparoscopy.

13.7 Dyspareunia

Learning objective

You should:

- have an understanding of the many different causes of dyspareunia

Dyspareunia means painful sexual intercourse. The pain may be felt at the beginning of penetration when it is called superficial dyspareunia, or deeply in the pelvis when it is called deep dyspareunia. It may persist after intercourse as a post-coital ache. Dyspareunia may be organic or psychological in origin (see Box 58).

All organic causes must be excluded before psychogenic dyspareunia can be diagnosed.

13.8 Psychogenic pelvic pain

Learning objective

You should:

- be aware that investigation may not always uncover a physical cause for pelvic pain

Psychogenic pelvic pain should only be diagnosed when all other causes of pain have been excluded. The typical patient has had frequent hospital admissions, and multiple operations to remove normal organs such as the appendix, ovaries or uterus. The patient is often reluctant to accept advice that nothing physically wrong can be found, and it may be difficult to establish rapport during a consultation. A history of poor relationships and an unhappy childhood are typical, resulting in a lack of self-esteem and a negative attitude towards sex. Antidepressants are often prescribed but psychosexual counselling is more useful.

13.9 Psychosexual problems

Learning objectives

You should:

- appreciate why psychosexual problems are often not mentioned by patients
- understand how they may arise within a relationship
- understand the principles of psychosexual counselling

Both the frequency and importance of psychosexual problems are easily underestimated in gynaecological practice. Both patient and doctor often take the easier option of concentrating on the purely physical problems, with the result that emotional problems are either unrecognised or ignored. Sympathy and understanding on the part of the doctor are essential. If the woman senses that the doctor is unaware or uninterested she will feel unable or reluctant to express her real concerns.

Commonly encountered psychosexual problems:

- Loss of libido – loss of the desire for sex
- Vaginismus – spasm of the perivaginal muscles making penetration difficult

---

Box 58 Dyspareunia: organic causes

Superficial dyspareunia	Deep dyspareunia
• Vaginal infection	• Endometriosis
• Vaginal atrophy	• Pelvic inflammatory disease
• Painful episiotomy scar	• Scarred retroverted uterus
• Intact hymen	• Ovary adherent to vaginal vault
• Vaginal septum	• Vagina shortened by surgery
	• Chronic constipation
	• Irritable bowel syndrome

- Orgasmic failure
- Premature ejaculation.

Physical causes such as vaginal infection or atrophy must be excluded. Within a relationship one partner may hold the other entirely responsible for the problem or even deny that any difficulty exists. The underlying cause of most psychosexual problems is disharmony and poor communication within the relationship, and this may arise due to differences in social, religious or cultural beliefs, or a difference in attitudes, preferences or expectations towards sex. The resulting hostility towards the partner may be subconsciously expressed by an unwillingness to become aroused, so that sex is withheld as a form of punishment.

Common causes of psychosexual problems include:

- anxiety
- emotional immaturity
- feelings of guilt or resentment
- ignorance
- failure of communication.

Specialised psychosexual counselling is usually only successful if both partners are willing to attend and share ownership of the problem. This is not always the case as one partner may be deriving secondary gain from the situation and be reluctant to accept help. Counselling involves identification and exploration of sexual problems followed by re-education and retraining. Behaviour therapy is sometimes used, with the aims of improving physical arousal and reducing sexual anxiety. The woman must be encouraged to accept pleasure without guilt, and to take an active part in love-making. The woman is encouraged to teach her partner which areas of her body are most responsive and to what type of stimulation. Long-term success depends on motivation and commitment of both partners, and an interested and sensitive doctor with the necessary training in these techniques.

13.10 Premenstrual syndrome

Learning objectives

You should:

- be able to recognise the symptoms of the premenstrual syndrome
- be able to construct a simple patient information leaflet regarding premenstrual syndrome

Some degree of premenstrual symptoms such as pelvic discomfort, breast tenderness and irritability are experienced by most women in the week to 10 days before their period. The onset of menstruation brings about relief from these symptoms. The term premenstrual syndrome (PMS) is used when symptoms are severe enough to produce significant life disruption, and this occurs in a small percentage of women.

Premenstrual symptoms (see Box 59) result from the combined cyclical effects of both oestrogen and progesterone. Central nervous system symptoms are less easy to explain and may be mediated by a central deficiency of serotonin. The symptoms are abolished by pregnancy, and by surgical removal or medical suppression of the ovaries. Symptoms may be reproduced by the cyclical administration of hormone replacement therapy after the menopause.

Treatment of PMS

Reassurance and explanation are needed. Self-help groups, relaxation techniques and stress management can all enable a woman to cope more easily with her symptoms. Simple analgesics may be sufficient when the predominant symptom is pain or headache. Many drug therapies have been claimed to be useful but few have been proven by randomised controlled study. What has been demonstrated is the large placebo effect of many different treatments, so any new therapy should ideally be tested against a placebo.

When symptoms are severe, suppression of the ovarian cycle with exogenous oestrogen in the form of implants is effective, but this needs to be given in combination with progestogens in order to prevent endometrial hyperplasia. The combined low-dose oral contraceptive pill would also seem a logical choice, particularly when contraception is required, because ovulation is suppressed. Treatment of PMS with progestogens has been advocated on the basis that there might be a progesterone deficiency in the luteal phase of the cycle, although evidence for this is lacking. Selective serotonin uptake inhibitors such as fluoxetine may be useful where psychological symptoms predominate. Gonadotrophin-releasing hormone analogues are only useful for short-term therapy because of the long-term risks of osteoporosis and cardiovascular disease which result from oestrogen lack. They may be

---

Box 59 Symptoms of premenstrual syndrome

Physical	Psychological/behavioural
- Abdominal bloating	- Tension
- Breast tenderness	- Irritability
- Headache	- Depression
- Fluid retention	- Tiredness
	- Poor concentration
	- Aggression
	- Clumsiness

used for 6 months as a therapeutic trial when uncertainty exists as to the true extent of the premenstrual component of symptoms. Diuretics are often prescribed but there is no controlled evidence in their support. Oil of evening primrose, danazol and bromocriptine may all be effective in relieving cyclical mastalgia.

Drugs commonly used to treat premenstrual syndrome include:

- oral contraceptive pill
- oestrogen implants
- progestogens
- oil of evening primrose
- vitamin B_6
- selective serotonin reuptake inhibitors
- GnRH analogues
- bromocriptine.

Self-assessment: questions

Multiple choice questions

1. Which of the following may cause pelvic pain?
   a. Haematocolpos
   b. Ovarian hyperstimulation
   c. Primary syphilis
   d. Fractured coccyx
   e. Retroverted mobile uterus

2. Which of the following may be aggravated premenstrually?
   a. Epilepsy
   b. Primary dysmenorrhoea
   c. Genital herpes
   d. Suicidal tendencies
   e. Hirsutism

3. Which of the following can be caused by endometriosis?
   a. Haemoptysis
   b. Haemochromatosis
   c. Infertility
   d. Renal failure
   e. Cancer

4. Regarding endometriosis:
   a. Asymptomatic deposits of endometriosis are found in 20% of women of reproductive age
   b. Once found it should always be treated
   c. May present with a painful nodule in a surgical scar
   d. It always persists until the menopause
   e. The ovaries are the most commonly involved sites

5. Side-effects of treatment for endometriosis include:
   a. Acne
   b. Hot flushes
   c. Decrease in breast size
   d. Endometrial hyperplasia
   e. Vaginal dryness

6. Which of the following statements are true?
   a. Removal of both ovaries cures premenstrual syndrome
   b. Visceral pain from the uterus, fallopian tubes and ovaries is transmitted via the autonomic nervous system (T10–L1)
   c. A raised white cell count is useful in the differential diagnosis of pelvic infection from that of red degeneration of a fibroid
   d. Cone biopsy of the cervix can cause secondary dysmenorrhoea
   e. Pelvic pain syndrome is a psychological disorder

7. Which of the following are true?
   a. Urinary stone disease is an important non-obstetric cause of abdominal pain in pregnancy
   b. Abdominal X-irradiation in pregnancy is most harmful between 4 and 8 weeks' gestation
   c. Ultrasound is useful in the investigation of an adnexal mass
   d. Laparoscopy is useful in the investigation of pelvic pain accompanied by hypovolaemic shock
   e. Laparoscopy is normal in up to 30% of women with pelvic pain

8. An area of calcification may be seen in the pelvis on a plain abdominal X-ray with which of the following?
   a. Gallstones
   b. Uterine fibroids
   c. Dermoid cyst
   d. Ureteric calculus
   e. Osteoid osteoma

9. Which of the following may cause bowel obstruction?
   a. Endometriosis
   b. Acute porphyria
   c. Congenital band adhesion
   d. Post-surgical adhesions
   e. Rectus sheath haematoma

Short notes

1. How is a diagnosis of adenomyosis made?
2. What are the clinical features of a ruptured endometriotic cyst? What is the differential diagnosis and treatment?

Case histories

Case history 1

A 24-year-old woman complaining of cyclical pelvic pain and deep dyspareunia is found to have several small scattered deposits of endometriosis on the peritoneum of the pouch of Douglas. She does not wish to conceive at present.

1. What would be the most appropriate treatment?

> Three years later her symptoms have improved, but she has been trying to conceive for 6 months without success. Repeat laparoscopy again shows multiple small endometriotic deposits, with normal, patent fallopian tubes and healthy ovaries. There are no other infertility factors present in either partner.

2. What is the appropriate management now?

Case history 2

> A 42-year-old lady has recently undergone total abdominal hysterectomy and bilateral salpingo-oophorectomy for treatment of endometriosis. She is experiencing troublesome hot flushes and asks you about hormone replacement therapy.

What advice would you give?

Case history 3

> A healthy 32-year-old woman complains of severe pain on sexual intercourse with her husband. This has now become so severe that they are unable to achieve penetration. Her general practitioner has been unable to find anything wrong.

1. Describe the initial management.
2. Investigations reveal no physical cause for the pain. What is the management now?

Case history 4

> A 26-year-old woman had been admitted 3 days ago to a medical ward following her third overdose. She is making a satisfactory recovery, but you are asked to come and give a gynaecological opinion because of her long-standing complaint of chronic pelvic pain. She has previously undergone cholecystectomy, and also suffers from asthma, low back pain and depression. She had a normal laparoscopy 6 months ago.

What is the most likely diagnosis?

Self-assessment: answers

Multiple choice answers

1. a. **True.** Haematocolpos is a condition in which menstrual fluid cannot escape from the vagina due to an imperforate hymen or vaginal atresia. Soon after the menarche, cyclical cramping pain occurs in the absence of menstruation. Blood may accumulate in the vagina, resulting in a tense mass.
   b. **True.** Hyperstimulation of the ovaries can result from exogenously administered gonadotrophins in the treatment of infertility, causing massive cystic enlargement of the ovaries, ascites, abdominal distension and pain.
   c. **False.** The chancre of primary syphilis is painless.
   d. **True.** A fracture of the coccyx may result in long-term pain. This is called coccydynia.
   e. **False.** Uncomplicated uterine retroversion in the absence of pelvic pathology does not cause pain. Fixed retroversion caused by disease such as endometriosis may.

2. a. **True.** Epilepsy and migraine may both become significantly worse premenstrually, possibly due to an increased responsiveness of the central nervous system (CNS).
   b. **False.** Pelvic pain may be a feature of the premenstrual syndrome but primary dysmenorrhoea describes cramping pelvic pain which coincides with the onset of menstruation.
   c. **True.**
   d. **True.** Suicide attempts, criminal activity and psychiatric admissions are all more common during the premenstrual period. This is possibly mediated via the high luteal phase levels of progesterone.
   e. **False.**

3. a. **True.** Endometriosis may rarely occur in the lungs, possibly as a result of transport via the lymphatic or vascular system. Cyclical haemoptysis may then occur.
   b. **False.**
   c. **True.** Up to 30% of women with endometriosis may suffer from infertility.
   d. **True.** Renal failure may rarely result from bilateral ureteric obstruction secondary to pelvic endometriosis.
   e. **False.** Endometriosis is a benign disease.

4. a. **True.** Accurate assessment of the incidence of endometriosis is difficult to establish but it is an asymptomatic finding in up to 20% of women undergoing laparoscopy for other reasons such as sterilisation.
   b. **False.** Endometriosis only requires treatment if it is causing troublesome symptoms.
   c. **True.** Endometriosis can be found in any surgical scar, probably as a result of direct implantation, when a painful nodule is noticed. Typical examples are laparoscopy and episiotomy scars.
   d. **False.** It may regress in pregnancy or before the menopause.
   e. **True.** Ovarian involvement occurs in 65% of cases of endometriosis, making it the most common site of disease.

5. a. **True.** Acne may be caused by the androgenic component of both danazol and progestogens.
   b. **True.** Hot flushes are a consequence of oestrogen deficiency, which is caused by GnRH analogues.
   c. **True.** as for answer b.
   d. **False.** Endometrial hyperplasia usually results from unopposed oestrogen stimulation of the endometrium.
   e. **True.** as for answer b.

6. a. **True.** Although surgery is rarely undertaken for severe premenstrual syndrome, removal of both ovaries is curative.
   b. **True.** The pelvic organs have a visceral innervation from the autonomic nervous system (T10–L1). The sensation of visceral pain in these organs is produced by distension, chemical irritation, ischaemia and inflammation, but they are insensitive to tactile and thermal stimulation.
   c. **False.** The white cell count is raised in both pelvic infection and red degeneration.
   d. **True.** Cone biopsy occasionally causes cervical stenosis and retention of menstrual fluid, resulting in secondary dysmenorrhoea.
   e. **False.** Psychological disorders and pelvic pain syndrome often coexist, but a cause and effect is difficult to establish. Indeed any psychological effect may be a consequence rather than a cause of chronic pain.

7. a. **True.** Urinary calculi typically cause pain in the flank. Early diagnosis is important in pregnancy because of the risk of septic obstruction of the kidney, which may lead to premature labour.
   b. **True.** Abdominal X-irradiation during pregnancy is most harmful to the fetus when organogenesis is most rapid, and this is between the 4th and 8th week of gestation.
   c. **True.** Ultrasound is a useful non-invasive tool in the investigation of a pelvic mass, when a differentiation can be made between cystic and solid lesions. However, laparoscopy or laparotomy is usually needed for precise diagnosis.
   d. **False.** Laparoscopy is contraindicated in patients with hypovolaemic shock. Laparotomy is required.
   e. **True.** Laparoscopy often shows normal pelvic organs. This usually means the pain is of physiological rather than pathological origin.

8. a. **False.** Gallstones would be seen in the right hypochondrium.
   b. **True.** Fibroids may become calcified.
   c. **True.** A dermoid cyst may contain teeth, bone or cartilage.
   d. **True.** A calculus lying in the pelvic ureter may show up as calcification.
   e. **True.** An osteoid osteoma of the pubic ramus would show up as an area of calcification on X-ray.

9. a. **True.**
   b. **False.**
   c. **True.**
   d. **True.**
   e. **False.**

Short notes answers

1. A diagnosis of adenomyosis can only be made on histological examination of the uterus after hysterectomy, when endometrial glands are found deeply penetrating the myometrium. It may be suspected on the clinical grounds of dysmenorrhoea, dyspareunia and menorrhagia in a woman with an enlarged tender uterus.
2. Rupture or leakage of an endometriotic cyst results in the escape of old blood into the peritoneal cavity. This causes acute lower abdominal pain. The differential diagnosis is acute pelvic inflammatory disease, ruptured ectopic pregnancy or a torted ovarian cyst. Examination in all of the above may reveal a tender mass, and ultrasound is unlikely to be diagnostic. A negative sensitive pregnancy test

would make a diagnosis of ectopic pregnancy unlikely. Laparoscopy or laparotomy will be necessary for diagnosis. Treatment is by peritoneal irrigation and ovarian cystectomy.

Case history answers

Case history 1

1. The most appropriate treatment would be a 9-month course of the continuous combined oral contraceptive pill. Continuous administration without the usual 7-day break would provide amenorrhoea for 9 months and thus encourage regression of the endometriotic deposits. Contraception would also be provided.
2. Expectant management is indicated over the next 6 months, as between 60 and 70% of such women will become pregnant within a year. Treatment of small deposits of endometriosis which are not causing anatomical distortion does not improve fertility and merely delays the couple from trying.

Case history 2

The surgically-induced menopause is responsible for the symptoms, which are due to oestrogen deficiency, and in the long term this puts her at increased risk of both heart disease and osteoporosis. Oestrogen replacement therapy should therefore be given, at least until the age of 50 years. There is a theoretical risk that this could stimulate residual endometriotic deposits, but in practice this is extremely rare.

Case history 3

1. A case history is vital here. Organic causes must be excluded but it is not uncommon for dyspareunia in this situation to be psychosomatic. Sometimes, for example, a family history is obtained which reveals anxiety relating to recent severe gynaecological illness in a close relative.

   Examination should be directed towards detection of physical causes such as vaginal infection, abrasions or atrophy. If candida is suspected a vaginal swab should be sent for culture. A painful or poorly-healed episiotomy scar may be tender. A relative oestrogen deficiency can occur with breast feeding, resulting in vaginal dryness. Pelvic examination should assess the presence and degree of any deep pelvic pain or masses. Tender uterosacral ligaments would suggest endometriosis. If no local cause is found, pelvic ultrasound and laparoscopy are indicated. If pelvic disease is found which is felt to be causing or contributing to the

problem this should be treated as appropriate. Occasionally an episiotomy scar needs revision to excise a tender skin bridge, or unsuspected pelvic endometriosis may be found.

2. If no physical cause is found this should be carefully explained to the woman. At this stage it is appropriate to interview both partners in more depth with particular emphasis on the sexual history. The assistance of a psychosexual counsellor may be useful. Introducing the idea that the symptoms may not be due to a physical problem is frequently met with resistance from either or both partners. Feelings of resentment, disloyalty and lack of communication should be explored, and enquiry made of any previous traumatic experiences or recent childbirth. There may, for example, be resentment towards a partner's excessive work commitments or drinking habits. If the problem is of recent origin with a previously satisfactory sex life, resolution may be relatively simple, but if there have always been difficulties within the relationship there may be a more fundamental problem rooted in childhood which may be more difficult to resolve.

If vaginismus is diagnosed, relaxation therapy and graduated vaginal dilators can be used. The woman is instructed on how to use progressively larger dilators, and from there to a resumption of regular sexual intercourse. The aim is to reduce sexual anxiety and turn love-making into an actively enjoyable event again for both partners.

Case history 4

This type of patient represents a difficult problem. The most likely diagnosis here is psychogenic pelvic pain, but it can only be made after exclusion of organic disease such as chronic pelvic infection and endometriosis. Acute exacerbations of pain and frequent hospital admission is the usual pattern, and there is a real danger of overlooking genuine pathology if it does arise. There are usually deep-rooted psychological problems, and a reluctance to accept the absence of a demonstrable physical cause.

14 Family planning

Overview

Despite the availability of a wide variety of different contraceptive methods, 30% of babies born in the UK are the result of unplanned pregnancies. In addition, many unplanned pregnancies are terminated. In the UK, the combined oral contraceptive pill is the most popular contraceptive method, but breast feeding remains an important method in the developing world. It is important to take a detailed history before prescribing the combined oral contraceptive pill because there are some absolute contraindications.

Some contraceptive methods have additional non-contraceptive therapeutic effects which may be beneficial to some users, for example, the significantly decreased menstrual blood loss with the levonorgestrel – containing intrauterine device.

Introduction

Most couples have a need for contraception at some time in their reproductive lives. A wide range of methods are available, each having individual merits and disadvantages. Couples may choose different methods at different times in their lives depending on their age, medical needs and desire for children. The effective provision of information, education and advice regarding all aspects of contraception and sexual health is an important role of family planning clinics, general practitioners and schools.

Different methods of contraception include:

- hormonal
- intra-uterine devices
- barrier methods
- natural methods
- sterilisation.

The ideal contraceptive would be 100% reliable, fully reversible, free from all side-effects, easy to use and cost-effective. No single method fulfils all these criteria, but many come close. The effectiveness of a contraceptive is usually expressed by the Pearl index, which is the number of unwanted pregnancies that would theoretically occur if 100 women used that particular method for 1 year (Table 16).

14.1 Hormonal methods of contraception

Learning objectives

You should

- understand the mode of action of hormonal methods of contraception

- understand why the combined oral contraceptive pill has some absolute contraindications

- understand why different hormonal methods may suit different women

There are three types: combined oestrogen/progesterone pills, progestogen only pills, and injectable progestogens.

Table 16 Contraceptive methods: Pearl index ratings

Method of contraception	Pearl index
Hormonal	0.1–3
Intra-uterine devices	1
Barrier	3–20
Natural	20–30

The combined oestrogen/progesterone oral contraceptive pill

The combined oral contraceptive pill (COC) contains both an oestrogen and a progestogen. It is the most popular contraceptive for women under the age of 30 years, and it is extremely effective if taken regularly. The oestrogen component is usually ethinyl oestradiol, in a dose of between 20 and 35 micrograms, whilst a variety of different progestogens are used (Table 17).

Most preparations contain a mixture of oestrogen and progestogen in a fixed ratio, but the so-called phasic preparations employ a varying ratio of doses in an attempt to correspond more closely to the normal hormonal cycle.

Pills are usually supplied in a pack of 21. The first pill is normally taken on day 1 of the cycle. This provides immediate contraception. If started on day 5, additional precautions such as the sheath need to be used for the next 7 days. If a pill is forgotten by more than 12 hours past the usual time of taking, additional precautions should be used for the next 7 days. A pill is taken every day for 21 days, followed by a 7-day break before starting on the next packet. During this break most women will have a withdrawal bleed, which is lighter than a period.

Mode of action

The COC inhibits ovulation. This is achieved by a negative feedback of oestrogen on the hypothalamus and pituitary. Production of gonadotrophin-releasing hormone (GnRH) is thus inhibited and follicle-stimulating hormone (FSH) and luteinising hormone (LH) secretion is reduced. The progestogen component renders cervical mucus hostile to sperm and the endometrium unfavourable for implantation, which further adds to the contraceptive effect.

Advantages of COCs

The main advantages of the COC is that compared with barrier methods the woman has complete control of her own contraception, and the mode of action is unrelated to the act of sexual intercourse. The reduction in both menstrual blood loss and dysmenorrhoea are useful therapeutic effects, whilst changes in the cervical mucus confer increased protection against pelvic inflammatory disease. Withdrawal bleeds can be avoided altogether if desired by omitting the 7-day break from pills and starting immediately on the next packet. This results in a greater total monthly dosage of hormones but this is unlikely to be significant.

Side-effects are listed in Box 60.

Suppression of ovulation by the COC confers protection against:

- benign ovarian cysts
- ectopic pregnancy
- benign breast disease
- ovarian and endometrial cancer.

Breakthrough bleeding occurs when the blood levels of hormones are too low. This may be helped by switching to a pill with a higher progestogen dose. Side-effects such as acne and hirsutism can be overcome by changing to a pill containing a less androgenic progestogen such as desogestrel or gestodene.

Adverse effects and risks of COC

Circulatory disease

The COC causes a small increase in the risk of stroke, myocardial infarction and thromboembolic disease, and a slight increase in blood pressure. For pills containing levonorgestrel or norethisterone the risk of thromboembolic disease is 5 to 10 cases per 100 000 women per year. The risk of thromboembolic disease is doubled with pills containing the progestogens gestodene and desogestrel, and in 1995 the Committee on Safety of Medicines advised that pills containing these progestogens should only be used by women who were intolerant of other combined oral contraceptives and prepared to accept an increased risk of thromboembolism. Smoking, hypertension and immobility substantially increase the risk of both thromboembolic and arterial disease in COC users.

All women using the COC therefore need regular blood pressure reviews, and should be advised to stop taking it 6 weeks prior to major elective surgery.

Breast cancer

For women under 25 years who take the COC for more than 4 years there may be a small increase in the risk of breast cancer. There is no increased risk for women between the ages of 25 and 45 years.

Table 17 Progestogens used in COC pills, and dosage	
Progestogen	**Dose**
• Norethisterone	0.5–1.5 mg
• Levonorgestrel	150–250 µg
• Desogestrel	150 µg
• Gestodene	75 µg

Box 60 Side-effects of COCs

Common	Rare
• Nausea	• Hirsutism/acne
• Headache	• Weight gain
• Breakthrough bleeding	• Vaginal dryness
• Breast tenderness	• Facial skin pigmentation

Cervix cancer

There is an association with COC use but this is more likely to be due to the link between cervix cancer and sexual activity.

Drug interactions

Additional contraceptive precautions need to be used during and for 7 days following any course of antibiotics. Broad spectrum antibiotics such as penicillin impair the absorption of oestrogen, resulting in sub-therapeutic blood levels, breakthrough bleeding and a reduced contraceptive effect. Drugs such as anticonvulsants induce liver enzymes, which increase the metabolism of both oestrogen and progesterone, so a higher dose pill is required.

Contraindications to COC

Enquiry about diabetes, hypertension or previous thromboembolism is essential before prescribing COCs (see Box 61). Women over the age of 35 years who smoke should be advised about other methods of contraception. Pregnancy must be excluded by a menstrual history and if necessary a vaginal examination and pregnancy test.

Progestogen-only pills

The progestogen-only pill (POP) accounts for 10% of oral contraceptive use. It is taken continuously without the 7-day break, and this must be to within 3 hours of the same time each day. If a pill is taken more than 3 hours late, the next one should be taken on time, and additional contraceptive precautions such as the sheath should be used for the next 48 hours. The POP is particularly suitable for women in whom oestrogen is contraindicated.

Progestogens used in POPs are:

- norgestrel
- levonorgestrel

- norethisterone
- ethynodiol diacetate.

Mode of action

- Makes cervical mucus hostile to sperm
- Makes endometrium unsuitable for implantation
- Interferes with ovulation in 60% of users
- Reduces tubal motility.

The POP should be started on day 1 of the cycle, when it provides immediate contraceptive protection.

Advantages of POP include:

- no age limit
- minimal metabolic effects
- no interference with breast feeding
- no interference from broad spectrum antibiotics.

Disadvantages of POP include:

- irregular bleeding and amenorrhoea
- higher failure rate than combined pill
- requires user motivation to ensure correct timing
- increased risk of ectopic pregnancy.

Side-effects of POP

Irregular bleeding and amenorrhoea occur in up to 50% of users. Weight gain, breast tenderness, headache and acne are less common.

Progestogen injections and implants

Long-acting slow-release depot progestogen preparations (Table 18) are ideal for women who are forgetful with pill taking. In contrast to the POP, injections inhibit ovulation due to higher serum levels of progestogen. As with implants, they also thicken cervical mucus which inhibits sperm motility, and render the endometrium thinner which inhibits implantation.

Box 61 Contraindications to COC

Circulatory disorders
- Thromboembolic predisposition
- Ischaemic heart disease
- Focal migraine
- Transient ischaemic attacks or stroke
- Hyperlipidaemia
- Hypertension
- Arteritis
- Diabetes with arterial or renal complications
- Heavy smoking

Others
- Gross obesity
- Liver disease or impaired liver function
- Breast cancer
- Undiagnosed abnormal genital tract bleeding
- Pregnancy
- Hyperprolactinaemia

Table 18 Injectable progestogens: administration, duration

Type of progestogen	Route of administration	Duration
Depot medroxyprogesterone acetate	Intramuscular injection	12 weeks
Norethisterone enanthate	Intramuscular injection	8 weeks
Etonogestrel implant	Subcutaneous implant	3–5 years

Advantages of injectable progestogens

- Highly effective
- Reduced menstrual blood loss
- Good compliance.

Disadvantages

Injectable preparations are irreversible until their effects have worn off. Resumption of regular menstruation and fertility takes an average 6 months after stopping progestogen injections. Side-effects include unpredictable bleeding or amenorrhoea. The degree of protection against sexually transmitted disease, via the effect on cervical mucus, is less than that provided by condoms.

An implant is a small flexible tube which is inserted subcutaneously under local anaesthetic. The inner upper arm is the usual site. A small amount of hormone is released continuously, and this confers contraception via the effect on cervical mucus and endometrium. Ovulation may also stop. Normal fertility and menstruation return as soon as the implant is removed.

14.2 Intra-uterine devices

Learning objectives

You should:

- be able to explain how the intra-uterine device works

- advise a woman about the relative merits and assess her suitability to it.

The contraceptive effect of intra-uterine objects was long ago recognised in the form of stones placed in the camel uterus. The intra-uterine device (IUD) produces a high level of contraceptive reliability, and is particularly suitable for the older woman who has contraindications to the combined pill. The main advantage is that following insertion no further motivation is required by the user, and the contraceptive action is unrelated to sexual intercourse. Removal is usually straightforward and is effected by pulling on the threads of the device, which project into the vagina. This brings about an immediate reversal of the contraceptive action. The design (see Fig. 24) consists of a small pliable plastic frame of variable shape either coated with spirals of copper or containing levonorgestrel. The Orth Gyne T380 Slimline has a total surface area of copper of 380 mm². It has a Pearl index of less than 1 and provides effective contraception for 4 years. Older devices consisting purely of plastic, such as the Lippes loop, are now rarely used.

Fitting of IUDs

Fitting of IUDs requires a specifically trained nurse or doctor. Pelvic examination is required to assess the size and position of the uterus. Genital tract infection should be screened by taking swabs.

Fitting should be either during menstruation or within 7 days from the beginning of the period. When the cervix has been visualised and cleaned, a thin flexible tube containing the IUD is passed into the uterus after sounding. The tube is then withdrawn leaving the IUD in place. The threads are then trimmed.

Mode of action

IUDs produce a mild inflammatory reaction in the endometrium. The viability of gametes is reduced, and both fertilisation and implantation are impeded. The local release of copper adds to the contraceptive efficiency and allows a smaller size of device to be used.

The levonorgestrel-containing IUD releases a small continuous amount of progestogen from a reservoir, which causes endometrial atrophy. This frequently causes amenorrhoea, which is a useful therapeutic

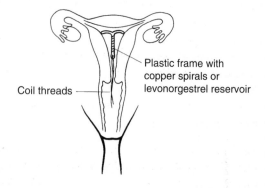

Plastic frame with copper spirals or levonorgestrel reservoir

Coil threads

Fig. 24 Intra-uterine contraceptive device (IUCD).

effect in women with menorrhagia. It is effective for 5 years.

Side-effects of intra-uterine devices

Lost threads

If the threads are not visible the device may have been expelled. Alternatively they may have been drawn up into the uterine cavity. If gentle sounding of the cervical canal with a specially-designed thread retriever is unsuccessful, an ultrasound scan is indicated to ascertain if the device is still present. It can also be seen on X-ray. The possibility of a pregnancy should always be remembered.

Pain

There is usually transient pain on insertion. Persistent pain may signify a device which is too large. Pain with pyrexia signifies pelvic infection.

Pelvic infection

The IUD is not suitable for women with multiple sexual partners, who are at increased risk of pelvic inflammatory disease.

Bleeding

Menstrual loss may be heavier or irregular in the first few months after insertion. This is less of a problem with the smaller copper-containing devices. The levonorgestrel containing IUD usually reduces menstrual blood loss. Approximately one in 10 women have the device removed because of problems with bleeding.

Expulsion

Expulsion occurs in under 5% of cases. It is due to uterine contractions and usually occurs within 3 months of insertion. All women wearing the IUD should be advised to feel occasionally for the threads which project through the cervix to check the device is still in place. The Multiload Cu 250 has the lowest expulsion rate of any device, due to small protuberances on the side arms which impart a fundal-seeking effect. In practice asymptomatic expulsion is rare.

Uterine perforation

Perforation is rare, and usually occurs at the time of insertion. It should be suspected if the threads are not seen at the routine 6-week check. An ultrasound scan will detect if the device is in an extra-uterine location, when it will require removal from the peritoneal cavity. This is usually achieved by laparoscopy.

Pregnancy

The IUD provides more protection against intra-uterine than ectopic pregnancy. If pregnancy occurs in the presence of an IUD there is a 1:30 chance of this being extra-uterine. Ectopic pregnancy should therefore be suspected if lower abdominal pain or irregular bleeding occur. The viability and location of a pregnancy should be confirmed by an ultrasound scan. If it is intra-uterine, gentle attempts at IUD removal should be made if the threads are visible, as this reduces the risk of both second trimester abortion and premature labour. Alternatively the woman may request a termination of pregnancy.

Contraindications to the intra-uterine device

Pregnancy, undiagnosed irregular genital tract bleeding, pelvic inflammatory disease and previous ectopic pregnancy are absolute contraindications to the IUD. Relative contraindications include nulliparity, menorrhagia and multiple sexual partners.

14.3 Barrier methods of contraception

Learning objective

You should:

● understand the advantages and disadvantages of barrier methods of contraception

Barrier methods of contraception (see Box 62) prevent contact between sperm and ovum, thereby preventing fertilisation. They are the most widely used contraceptive method worldwide. They comprise:

● diaphragm
● spermicides
● male condom
● female condom.

Diaphragm

Various types of occlusive caps are available, but the diaphragm is the most popular. This consists of a hemispherical dome of latex rubber with a stiffened rim

> **Box 62** Advantages and disadvantages of barrier methods
>
> | **Advantages** | **Disadvantages** |
> |---|---|
> | • Safety | • High user motivation required |
> | • Low failure rate if used correctly | • Messy |
> | • Protection against sexually transmitted infection | • Interference with sexual intercourse |
> | • Reduced risk of cervical epithelial neoplasia | |

that can be compressed for insertion and removal (see Fig. 25). It fits between the posterior vaginal fornix and the anterior vaginal wall just above the symphysis pubis. Measurement for size of diaphragm and education regarding insertion and removal are carried out in the family planning clinic. The diaphragm should always be used in conjunction with a spermicidal cream or jelly. The smaller thimble-like cervical cap and the vault cap are rarely used.

Spermicides

Spermicides should be used as adjuncts to other barrier methods of contraception rather than relied upon on their own. They come as creams, jellies, pessaries and foams. The usual chemical constituent is nonoxynol-9, which causes the rapid death of sperm. The contraceptive sponge is a small sponge impregnated with nonoxynol-9 which is inserted into the vagina to cover the cervix. Although convenient and available for purchase over the counter it has a relatively high failure rate.

Male condom

Most male condoms are made from thin latex rubber and are prelubricated with a spermicide. They are rolled onto the erect penis prior to coitus. Effective contraception depends greatly on correct technique and the motivation of the user, and failure rates are higher with young inexperienced couples. The condom and the COC are sometimes used in combination to provide maximum protection against both pregnancy and sexually transmitted disease.

Female condom

The female condom consists of a lubricated polyurethane sheath that fits inside and lines the vagina. Few couples use this method on a regular basis.

14.4 Natural methods of family planning

> ### Learning objectives
>
> You should:
>
> • understand how natural methods of family planning work
> • understand why there are limitations with these methods

Natural methods of family planning rely on avoidance of sexual intercourse at the fertile time of the cycle. Sperm can survive in the female genital tract for up to 5 days and the egg can be fertilised up to 48 hours after ovulation, so the fertile time is thus from day 10 to 16 in a 28-day cycle, assuming ovulation occurs on day 14. Fertility is relatively low from day 1 to day 10 of the cycle when the ovarian follicles are growing, and from 48 hours after ovulation until the end of the cycle. Relying on natural methods is generally unreliable, with pregnancy rates in excess of 10 per 100 woman years.

Fig. 25 Insertion and removal of the diaphragm.

A   B   C   D

Much better results may be obtained if the couple are highly motivated.

Calendar calculation

Simple calendar calculation of the safe times in the cycle is called the rhythm method. Used in isolation it is too unreliable to be recommended for most couples.

Mucus assessment

This is called the Billings method, and entails regular inspection of cervical mucus. When ovulation is imminent, the cervical mucus is thin and watery, and intercourse should be avoided. After ovulation the mucus becomes thick and viscid due to the effect of progesterone, signifying the fertile time is over.

Temperature measurement

Daily temperature taking on waking can be used to detect the small rise which accompanies ovulation. Fertility is low from 3 days after the rise, by which time the ovum will have perished. This method has severe limitations as it cannot predict the end of the safe time in the follicular phase of the cycle.

14.5 Sterilisation

Learning objectives

You should:

- be able to counsel a couple regarding sterilisation
- understand why pre-operative counselling is important

Sterilisation offers a permanent and reliable contraceptive option to couples who have completed their family. This is achieved either by male vasectomy, which is usually done under local anaesthetic, or by female tubal occlusion, when small clips are placed on the fallopian tubes via laparoscopy. Careful counselling of both partners is essential to minimise the chances of later regret. The procedure must be considered permanent and irreversible, and couples should also be aware of the small but definite incidence of failure.

Vasectomy

In general vasectomy is marginally safer and easier to perform than tubal occlusion, but sterility is not achieved until about 3 months after the operation when negative sperm counts have been obtained. Complications include scrotal bruising and painful sperm granuloma.

Tubal occlusion

This has the advantage of being immediately effective. The failure rate is increased when the operation is performed at the time of caesarean section or termination of pregnancy, as the tubes are thicker.

Reversal of sterilisation

Careful counselling prior to sterilisation will minimise the chance of later regret. Young women who undergo sterilisation at the time of termination of pregnancy are at particular risk. A new relationship is a common reason for request for a reversal. The success rate for reversal of female sterilisation is dependent on the length of fallopian tube destroyed by the initial operation and the microsurgical skills of the surgeon. Success rates of 75% are reported, but the risk of subsequent tubal pregnancy is also increased.

14.6 Post-coital contraception

Learning objectives

You should know:

- the options available for post-coital contraception
- how their mode of action dictates when they can be used

There are two methods of emergency contraception which can be used following unprotected sexual intercourse. Neither should be used on a regular basis and they are no substitute for proper long-term contraception.

The post-coital pill

The regimen consists of 100 µg of ethinyl oestradiol and 500 µg of levonorgestrel, repeated after 12 hours. If given within 72 hours of unprotected intercourse ovulation is delayed and implantation is inhibited.

The IUD

If an IUD is inserted within 5 days of unprotected intercourse, implantation will be prevented.

Follow-up is essential after emergency contraception, both to exclude an ongoing pregnancy and to give advice regarding future contraception.

14.7 Contraception and the menopause

Learning objectives

You should:

- understand why contraception is an important issue in the perimenopause

- understand why it can sometimes be a problem

Although fertility gradually declines during the peri-menopausal years, many women wish to know when they may safely stop contraception altogether without risking pregnancy. Pregnancy is rarely welcome at this age, and has a higher risk of both miscarriage and chromosomal abnormalities. A diagnosis of the menopause can only be made retrospectively, and is often difficult in women using the COC or hormone replacement therapy, when periods may be artificially prolonged. The usual advice is that contraception should be continued for 12 months after the last menstrual period if it occurs over the age of 50 years, and for 2 years if it occurs earlier. Many couples opt for sterilisation as a permanent method of contraception around this time. This has the advantage over hormonal methods that there is no interference with menstruation and thus with identification of the menopause. The intra-uterine device has the advantage that if it is fitted after the age of 40 years it does not require changing or removal until after the menopause.

14.8 Termination of pregnancy

Learning objectives

You should:

- understand the implications of termination of pregnancy

- understand why earlier termination is safer

- appreciate the importance of sex education

Despite the widespread availability of contraceptives in this country a large number of pregnancies remain unplanned, and 150 000 abortions are performed each year because of unwanted pregnancy. There is a continuing need for young people to be provided with good advice regarding contraception, including both local availability and post-coital contraception. Sex education should begin at an early age in schools, and should include the complex emotional issues around relationships as well as more basic information.

The Abortion Act

The 1967 Abortion Act (amended in 1990) permits termination of pregnancy by a registered medical practitioner subject to certain conditions. Two doctors are required to certify that the abortion is justified under one or more of the grounds listed in the Act, and the Chief Medical Officer must be informed within 7 days of the procedure.

Clauses of the Abortion Act

A The continuance of the pregnancy would involve risk to the life of the pregnant woman greater than if the pregnancy were terminated

B The termination is necessary to prevent grave permanent injury to the physical or mental health of the pregnant woman

C The pregnancy has not exceeded its 24th week and the continuance of the pregnancy would involve risk, greater than if the pregnancy were terminated, of injury to the physical or mental health of the pregnant woman

D The pregnancy has not exceeded its 24th week and the continuance of the pregnancy would involve risk, greater than if the pregnancy were terminated, of injury to the physical or mental health of any existing child(ren) of the family of the pregnant woman

E There is a substantial risk that if the child were born it would suffer from such physical or mental abnormalities as to be seriously handicapped.

Methods of abortion

- Up to 9 weeks' gestation: medical termination
- Up to 14 weeks' gestation: suction evacuation of uterus
- Over 14 weeks' gestation: prostaglandin induction, or less commonly dilatation and evacuation, or rarely hysterotomy.

Medical termination consists of oral administration of 600 mg of the anti-progesterone mifepristone (RU 486), followed 48 hours later by 1 mg gemeprost inserted into the vagina. Within 8 hours, 96% of women will have aborted. This is a safe and effective method of inducing miscarriage without the need for surgical intervention

Suction evacuation is normally carried out under general or local anaesthetic. The cervix is dilated, and the products of conception are aspirated via a plastic cannula inserted into the uterine cavity.

Above 14 weeks, termination becomes more difficult to procure and the complications are greater (see Box 63).

Counselling and contraceptive advice should be given prior to abortion. Women who are Rhesus negative should be given anti-D to prevent Rhesus immunisation. The risks from pelvic infection can be minimised by screening for chlamydia beforehand, or by prophylactic antibiotic cover during the procedure.

Box 63 Complications of abortion

Immediate
- Haemorrhage
- Infection
- Trauma, e.g. cervical tear, uterine perforation, bowel injury
- Incomplete abortion with retained products

Late
- Cervical incompetence
- Infertility
- Regret

Self-assessment: questions

Multiple choice questions

1. Which of the following statements regarding the POP are true?
   a. It works mainly by inhibiting ovulation
   b. Contraceptive efficacy is highly dependent on the motivation of the user
   c. The dose of progestogen is higher than that in the combined pill
   d. It is suitable for both diabetic and hypertensive women
   e. It is best avoided in women following ectopic pregnancy
   f. It does not appear in breast milk
   g. Additional precautions should be taken if antibiotics are prescribed

2. Which of the following statements are true?
   a. Hypoallergenic condoms are available for people with allergy to rubber
   b. The HIV virus can penetrate latex condoms
   c. Coitus interruptus (withdrawal of the penis prior to ejaculation) is almost as effective as using a condom
   d. Condoms are free of charge from family planning clinics
   e. Condoms have a 'use by' date

3. Which of the following are ture regarding the diaphragm?
   a. It should be replaced every 5 years
   b. It should be left in for 6 hours after intercourse
   c. Some users notice an increased frequency of urinary tract infections
   d. A larger size may be needed after a vaginal delivery
   e. Diaphragms are suitable for women with utero-vaginal prolapse

4. Which of the following are true regarding the IUD?
   a. Serum copper levels are unchanged
   b. The levonorgestrel-containing IUD is associated with a small increase in the haemoglobin level
   c. The copper-containing IUD is associated with a small decrease in the haemoglobin level
   d. The plastic frame of the levonorgestrel-containing IUD contains barium so that it can be seen on X-ray.
   e. The risk of ectopic pregnancy is increased

5. Regarding the combined oral contraceptive pill:
   a. The incidence of iron deficiency anaemia is reduced by 50%
   b. The incidence of benign breast disease is increased by 30%
   c. The COC is protective against both ovarian and endometrial cancer
   d. It carries a small increased risk of venous thromboembolism
   e. It has no effect on the risk of breast cancer

6. Which of the following are true?
   a. The levonorgestrel-releasing IUD increases menstrual blood loss
   b. Injectable progestogens do not inhibit lactation
   c. The injectable progestogen depo-provera inhibits ovulation
   d. Post-coital IUD insertion is effective if fitted within 7 days of unprotected intercourse
   e. Return of fertility may be delayed following removal of a contraceptive implant

7. Regarding contraception and the menopause:
   a. Measurement of FSH is an accurate indicator of fertility
   b. The low dose COC can be used up to the menopause in healthy non-smoking women
   c. Contraception should be continued for 6 months after the last period in a woman over the age of 50 years
   d. Women taking HRT do not need additional contraception
   e. Sterilisation has no effect on the timing of the menopause

Short notes

1. What contraceptive advice should be given to a 28-year-old non-smoking epileptic woman wishing to use the COC?

2. How does the COC work? How long can a woman stay on the COC? What effect does the COC have on the menstrual cycle? What is meant by breakthrough bleeding, and what are the common causes?

3. A woman telephones your surgery for advice. She forgot to take her pill last night and is worried about the risks of pregnancy. She is on a COC.

4. What is meant by the Pearl index? Which contraceptive methods have the lowest index? What are the criteria for an ideal contraceptive?

5. Outline the different methods of contraception available, giving the relative merits and disadvantages of each.

6. A woman wearing an IUCD has missed her last period. She did a pregnancy test which she bought from a chemist and this was positive. What is the correct management?

7. What are the risks associated with termination of pregnancy?

OSCE question

A 32-year-old woman who is being delivered by caesarian section next week asks if she could be sterilised at the same time. In the past, she has been advised not to take the COC because she smokes. She actually fell pregnant this time whilst taking the POP, because she often forgot to take her pills on time.

1. Would you agree to her request, and if not, why not?
2. On further questioning, the woman explains that she wants to be sterilised because she finds it difficult to remember to take a daily pill. What other contraceptive options should you discuss with her?
3. The couple decide to use the sheath for now, but return 6 months later, certain that they wish to have permanent contraception, and do not, under any circumstances, want any more children. What are the two options here?
4. They decide on female laparoscopic sterilisation. What are the main implications of this procedure, and what are the specific risks involved?
5. You explain to her that the chance of requiring a laparotomy to do the procedure is slightly higher in view of her previous caesarian section. Why is this?

Self-assessment: answers

Multiple choice answers

1. a. **False.** About 40% of women continue to ovulate on the POP. The contraceptive action is mainly via effects on cervical mucus and the endometrium.
    b. **True.** Effective contraception is dependent on the user taking the POP within 3 hours of the same time every day.
    c. **False.** The dose of progestogen is lower than that used in combined pills.
    d. **True.** Although progestogens cause impairment of glucose tolerance, this is minimal with the small amounts contained in the POP, and it is a good choice for diabetic women. Blood pressure may be slightly raised by the POP but much less so than with the combined pill.
    e. **True.** Ectopic pregnancy occurs in about 1 in 1000 POP users, probably because tubal function is impaired by progestogens. If future fertility is desired following an ectopic pregnancy, the POP should be avoided.
    f. **False.** Most drugs taken by the mother appear in small amounts in breast milk, and the POP is no exception. Although this understandably causes concern to some mothers, there is no evidence that it causes any harm. Unlike the combined pill it does not interfere with the quantity of breast milk.
    g. **False.** Antibiotics only interfere with the absorption of oestrogen, so no additional precautions are needed with the POP.

2. a. **True.**
    b. **False.**
    c. **False.** Relying on the male partner to withdraw prior to ejaculation is a highly ineffective method of contraception. Even if he possesses the necessary degree of self-control, sperm are often released prior to ejaculation.
    d. **True.**
    e. **True.**

3. a. **False.** The diaphragm should be replaced every year.
    b. **True.**
    c. **True.**
    d. **True.** Variation in size may occur with age, pregnancy and weight change.
    e. **False.** It is unsuitable in women with utero-vaginal prolapse, poor perineal muscle tone or congenital abnormalities such as a septate vagina. The symptoms of prolapse may be treated with a

vaginal ring pessary which sits in the vagina in a similar position to the diaphragm, but this has no contraceptive effect.

4. a. **True.** Copper acts locally. Systemic absorption is minimal and serum levels are unchanged.
    b. **True.** The levonorgestrel-containing IUD reduces menstrual blood loss which results in a rise in haemoglobin levels.
    c. **True.** By contrast, menstrual blood loss is increased in users of the copper-containing IUD, which results in a slight reduction in haemoglobin levels.
    d. **True.**
    e. **False.** There is no evidence that the IUD actually increases the risk of ectopic pregnancy. It merely provides more protection against intra-uterine than extra-uterine pregnancy, so that a higher proportion of the pregnancies that occur in women wearing IUDs are ectopic.

5. a. **True.** Iron deficiency anaemia is less common because of the reduction in menstrual blood loss.
    b. **False.** The incidence of benign breast disease is reduced by up to 75% in COC users.
    c. **True.**
    d. **True.** The risk of deep vein thrombosis in women not taking hormones is 5 per 100 000 per year. In women taking the COC pill, the risk is dependent on the type of progestogen. In women taking levonorgestrel or norethisterone-containing pills it is 15 per 100 000 per year. In women taking gestodene or desogestrel-containing pills it is 30 per 100 000 per year.
    e. **False.** The risk of breast cancer is slightly raised with COC use below the age of 25 years, or before the first full-term pregnancy. After the age of 25 years, the risk does not seem to be increased.

6. a. **False.** In contrast to copper-containing IUDs, the levonorgestrel-releasing IUD reduces menstrual blood loss.
    b. **True.**
    c. **True.** The injectable progestogen depo-provera is almost 100% effective because it inhibits ovulation. This contrasts with the progestogen-only pill, which does not rely on inhibition of ovulation for its contraceptive effect.
    d. **False.** Post-coital IUD insertion is effective up to 5 days following unprotected intercourse.
    e. **False.** Fertility is restored immediately.

7. a. **False.** FSH levels can fluctuate greatly at the time of the menopause, and ovulation may occur many months after a raised level.
   b. **True.** It is safe to continue low-dose COC pills up to the age of 50 years in fit, normotensive, non-smoking women with no family history of cardiovascular disease.
   c. **False.** Contraception should be used for 12 months after the last period in this situation
   d. **False.** Women who start hormone replacement therapy (HRT) before the last period remain fertile so need contraception. Non-hormonal methods are preferred in this situation.
   e. **True.** A disadvantage of the COC is that the occurrence of the menopause may be masked because withdrawal bleeds may continue for as long as the pills are taken. Sterilisation avoids this confusion as it has no effect on menstruation.

Short notes answers

1. The COC can be used by epileptic women but higher dose pills containing 50 µg oestrogen are usually required in order to provide both effective contraception and cycle control. This is because most anticonvulsants, with the exception of sodium valproate and clonazepam, interfere with the metabolism of the pill by their effect on induction of liver enzymes. She should be advised to start on day 1 of the cycle, when contraception is provided immediately, or on day 5, when additional precautions are needed for the next 7 days. If breakthrough bleeding occurs with a 50 µg pill, the dose should be increased still further by giving two 35 µg pills a day. The woman should also be advised that control of epilepsy is sometimes reduced by the COC, although some individuals actually get fewer attacks. If she was multiparous, she could be advised to try an IUD as a more suitable alternative contraceptive. If her family was complete she should be informed about both male and female sterilisation as a permanent and effective alternative.

2. The COC provides contraception primarily by reducing pituitary gonadotrophin secretion, thereby suppressing ovulation. The progestogenic component also contributes to the contraceptive effect by making cervical mucus thick and hostile to sperm, and by causing the endometrium to be inactive.

   A healthy woman may continue to take a low-dose COC until 50 years of age, provided there are no contraindications such as smoking, obesity, or family history of cardiovascular disease. Regular supervision including 6-monthly checks of blood pressure is required. A woman who smokes, even in the absence of other risk factors, should stop the COC by the age of 35 years because of the increased risk of both cardiovascular and thromboembolic disease.

   The menstrual cycle is regulated by the COC, so that withdrawal bleeds occur during the pill-free week. These may be much lighter and less painful than normal periods. If pills are taken continuously without a break, no bleeding should occur.

   Breakthrough bleeding describes irregular vaginal bleeding on days when pills are taken. It usually occurs when the serum levels of oestrogen become too low to sustain the endometrium. The most common cause is forgotten pills. Other causes include diarrhoea or vomiting, which result in malabsorption of pills, and interaction with other drugs such as antibiotics. It is important to exclude unrelated causes of irregular vaginal bleeding such as carcinoma of the cervix and threatened miscarriage.

3. If she is less than 12 hours late, she needs to take the forgotten pill immediately, and the next one on time. If she is more than 12 hours late, she will also need to use additional contraceptive precautions such as the sheath for the next 7 days.

4. The Pearl index is a measurement of contraceptive efficacy. It is the number of pregnancies that would occur in 100 women using that particular contraceptive method for 1 year. The COC has a Pearl index of only 0.1–3, making this a very effective contraceptive. Moreover, it is likely that a proportion of the COC failures are user-related, resulting from forgotten pills, rather than a failure of the method itself. For the intra-uterine device the Pearl index is around 1, and it is even lower for the progestogen-containing IUD.

   An ideal contraceptive would fulfil the following criteria: completely safe, with no side-effects; 100% effective; fully reversible; easy to use; cheap; controllable by the woman.

5. This answer should outline the different contraceptive methods available as detailed in the preceding chapter. The main methods can be grouped under the headings Hormonal, Barrier, Intra-uterine devices, Natural methods and Sterilisation. A mention should also be made of post-coital contraception. The relative merits of the different contraceptives that will appeal to different couples depending on factors such as age, desire for further children, medical conditions and sexual

habits should be discussed. For example, sterilisation may be an attractive option for a couple in a stable relationship who have completed their family, whilst the COC is a reliable reversible method for a healthy non-smoking woman, with the additional therapeutic benefit of a reduction in menstrual blood flow. A woman who finds it difficult to remember to take a pill on a regular basis may be better suited to an implant or injection, or an IUD. Barrier methods require user motivation and education for the best results, but offer a degree of protection against sexually transmitted diseases.

6. The pregnancy and its location must be urgently confirmed because of the risk that it may be ectopic. In addition the presence and location of the intra-uterine device must be established. The possibilities for the device are that it has been expelled or wrongly inserted, or that it is in the uterine cavity but has failed to prevent implantation of a pregnancy. A history should be taken to ascertain the date of the last menstrual period, when any symptoms of pregnancy first appeared, and whether any abdominal pain has been experienced. Pain which precedes vaginal bleeding is suggestive of an ectopic pregnancy. On examination an enlarged uterus compatible in size with the duration of amenorrhoea would suggest an intra-uterine location for the pregnancy. The threads of the coil should be palpable if it is in the uterine cavity. Adnexal swelling or tenderness are suggestive of ectopic pregnancy. Investigations should include a repeat pregnancy test if there is any doubt, and a pelvic ultrasound scan to locate the pregnancy and establish viability.

    If the pregnancy is intra-uterine, the coil should be gently removed by pulling on the threads to reduce the risks of miscarriage and infection. If the woman does not wish to continue with the pregnancy, termination should be discussed. If the coil is in an extra-uterine location it will need to be retrieved, which can usually be accomplished by laparoscopy. If the pregnancy is in an ectopic location this is most commonly in the fallopian tube. Urgent hospital admission is required because of the risk of tubal rupture and haemorrhage. Treatment is usually by removal of the ectopic pregnancy by laparoscopy or laparotomy. Following treatment the woman should be advised against the use of an intra-uterine device in the future.

7. Complications of termination of pregnancy can be divided into early and late. Early ones include bleeding, uterine and cervical trauma, infection, retained products of conception. Serious complications are rare but include bowel trauma from uterine perforation, and septicaemia from severe intra-uterine infection. Late complications include infertility resulting from tubal infection, cervical incompetence, and psychological problems stemming from regret.

OSCE answer

1. Although it may seem an attractive option, sterilisation performed at the time of caesarian section carries a slightly higher failure rate from tubal reanastomosis. It also carries a risk of later regret if her unborn child is found to have a problem such as a severe congenital abnormality or metabolic disease shortly after delivery. For these reasons, sterilisation is usually deferred for at least 3 months.

2. It is important with any sterilisation request to establish whether a permanent method of contraception is genuinely sought, or if the couple have just been unable to find a reversible method that suits them. Both the IUD or an implant may be acceptable reversible options, and should be discussed.

3. Female sterilisation, by laparoscopic clip occlusion of the fallopian tubes, and male sterilisation by vasectomy. Both should be discussed.

4. The main implication is that it should be considered permanent, although future tubal reanastomosis can be undertaken to reverse it. This is not, however, always successful. There is a small failure rate with sterilisation, and a small risk of laparotomy if either bowel trauma or major haemorrhage are caused by the laparoscopic instruments.

5. Because of the increased chance of adhesions obscuring an adequate view of the pelvic organs.

15 Infertility

Learning objectives

You should understand:

- how ovulation is controlled
- how mature sperm are produced

Overview

Ovulation normally occurs on day 14 in a 28 day cycle. It is controlled by hormones secreted from the anterior pituitary. Spermatogenesis is a temperature dependent process occurring in the seminiferous tubules, which leads to the production of mature sperm.

Infertility may arise due to problems in either partner, and has a variety of causes. Anovulation, tubal disease and endometriosis are the common female causes. Infection, undescended testes and anti-sperm antibodies can all cause male infertility.

The chances of pregnancy occurring for a given couple having unprotected intercourse are 80% after 1 year. Investigations are therefore usually only started after this time. The simplest and least invasive tests should be performed first, such as confirmation of ovulation by measurement of day 21 serum progesterone and seminal fluid analysis.

Most forms of ovulatory failure can be corrected with clomifene (clomiphene) treatment. Assisted reproduction techniques, such as in vitro fertilisation, are useful in the treatment of endometriosis, tubal disease and clomifene-resistant ovulatory failure. Intracytoplasmic sperm injection (ICSI) is a useful treatment for severe male factor infertility.

15.1 General principles

Infertility is defined as the inability to conceive after 1 year of unprotected intercourse. It affects 15% of all couples, but the incidence is increasing, largely because of a developing trend towards delayed childbearing. The average time fertile couples take to conceive is 6 months, with 90% conceiving within 1 year. Investigations into infertility are therefore not normally commenced until after 1 year of trying.

Female fertility is highest in the age range 20–24 years, and declines gradually after the age of 35 years. In men, ageing has only a minor effect on fertility.

Infertility can be divided into:

- Primary infertility – no previous pregnancies of any kind
- Secondary infertility – previous pregnancy, but current difficulty in conceiving.

Normal sperm production and function

Spermatozoa are produced in the seminiferous tubules and undergo further maturation in the seminal vesicles. Production of mature spermatozoa takes around 70 days. Normal spermatogenesis requires an environment of 1°C below normal body temperature, which is why the testicles hang outside the body in the scrotum. In cryptorchidism where the testis is undescended, the higher temperature impairs spermatogenesis, resulting in male infertility. Cervical mucus undergoes changes at the time of ovulation from being thick and tenacious, to becoming thin and watery. This enables spermatozoa to penetrate readily through it. When the mucus is favourable it will exhibit 'spinnbarkeit', which means it can be stretched out into a long thread, and will dry on a microscope slide into a characteristic ferning pattern. After swimming through the favourable cervical mucus, spermatozoa are transported to the ampullary portion of the fallopian tube by a combination of uterine contractions and the wafting action of the cilia which line the tube. Penetration and fertilisation of the oocyte takes place in the tubal ampulla.

Normal ovulation

Ovulation occurs on a regular monthly basis, on around day 14 in a 28-day cycle. The ovaries are controlled by gonadotrophin hormones secreted from the anterior pituitary gland, called luteinising hormone (LH) and follicle-stimulating hormone (FSH). These in turn are controlled by the pulsatile secretion of gonadotrophin-releasing hormone (GnRH) from the hypothalamus. GnRH travels to the anterior pituitary via the hypothalamo-hypophyseal portal circulation, where it stimulates the secretion of FSH and LH. These gonadotrophins are released into the blood stream, and target the ovary. FSH acts on the granulosa cells, whilst LH acts on the theca, stroma, granulosa and luteal cells. The combined action of FSH and LH stimulates the development of ovarian follicles and the production of oestrogen from the granulosa cells. Oestrogen initially exerts a negative feedback effect on gonadotrophin secretion, but as levels rise a positive feedback develops, which culminates in a large surge of LH. This LH surge triggers maturation and ovulation of the dominant follicle. After ovulation the follicle becomes luteinised to form the corpus luteum, which secretes progesterone. The released oocyte undergoes spontaneous demise within 48 hours in the absence of fertilisation.

15.2 Causes of infertility

Learning objective

You should understand:

- the mechanisms by which infertility may be caused

Common causes of infertility are:

- male infertility   20%
- defective ovulation   20%
- tubal disease   25%
- endometriosis   10%
- unexplained infertility   20%
- hostile cervical mucus   5%

It should be remembered that several causes may co-exist.

Male infertility

Male infertility accounts for 20% of cases and can arise from a wide variety of causes (see Box 64). Most infertile men are otherwise entirely healthy, and it is unusual to find a serious underlying cause such as a chromosomal disorder or an anatomical problem such as an undescended testes. Gonadotrophin insufficiency and testicular trauma are rare causes of male infertility.

Box 64 Male infertility

Common causes
- Oligospermia
- Antisperm antibodies
- Undescended testes
- Varicocele
- Scrotal hyperthermia
- Erectile failure

Rare causes
- Testicular trauma
- Chromosomal abnormality, e.g. Klinefelter's
- Azoospermia
- Epididymal or vasal obstruction
- Retrograde ejaculation
- Endocrine disorder, e.g. pituitary tumour
- Infections, e.g. mumps, chlamydia, gonorrhoea

Box 65 Factors associated with male infertility

- Smoking
- Marijuana
- Excessive alcohol consumption
- Environmental toxins
- Drugs, e.g. anabolic steroids, cytotoxins

Erectile failure may result from neurological problems or performance anxiety. Ejaculatory failure may be due to sympathetic denervation.

Defective ovulation

Absent or irregular ovulation is another common cause of infertility. Associated clinical manifestations of anovulation include oligomenorrhoea, amenorrhoea and the polycystic ovary syndrome (see Ch. 11. p. 145).

Anovulation usually results from a reversible dysfunction of some part of the hypothalamic/pituitary/ovarian (HPO) axis. This may be associated with an abnormal body mass index. A woman needs to have between 26 and 28% of her body weight as fat in order to have regular fertile ovulatory cycles. Body for percentage above or below this range may result in a reversible hypothalamic dysfunction. Oestrogen and gonadotrophin levels often remain in the normal range, but because of a lack of coordination between ovary and pituitary, ovulation becomes sporadic. In severe weight loss there tends to be a greater degree of hypothalamic dysfunction with both gonadotrophin and oestrogen levels being low. This is called hypogonadotrophic hypogonadism. Other typical examples of HPO axis dysfunction include the polycystic ovary syndrome, where high LH levels interfere with normal follicular development, and hyperprolactinaemia, where raised prolactin levels interfere with the pulsatile secretion of gonadotrophins.

Anovulation rarely results from irreversible failure of the hypothalamus, pituitary or ovaries. Premature ovarian failure may occur secondary to anti-ovarian antibodies, or may occur when the ovaries become pre-maturely exhausted of ovarian follicles.

Tubal disease

Damage to the delicate cilial lining of the fallopian tubes interferes with transport of both oocyte and spermatozoa. Sexually transmitted pelvic infection is the usual cause of the damage, with chlamydia and gonorrhoea being the common pathogens. In severe cases the fimbrial ends of the tube adhere together and become sealed. Other causes of tubal damage include previous pelvic surgery and endometriosis, both of which may cause tubal adhesions and scarring.

Endometriosis

In severe cases, endometriosis causes mechanical distortion of the fallopian tubes and destruction of the ovaries. However, even minor degrees of endometriosis are associated with infertility although the exact mechanism is unknown.

Hostile cervical mucus

In this condition the cervical mucus is unreceptive to spermatozoa, causing agglutination or immobilisation. It may be associated with the presence of antisperm antibodies.

Unexplained infertility

In 20% of couples no satisfactory explanation for infertility can be found. In this situation, all tests of fertility are normal, but the couple are still having difficulty in achieving a pregnancy.

Rare causes of infertility include fibroids distorting or impinging on the uterine cavity and thereby preventing implantation, and psychosexual problems resulting in decreased coital frequency.

15.3 Investigation of infertility

Learning objective

You should:

- be able to use infertility investigations selectively, according to the history and clinical findings

General

Wherever possible a couple should be seen and investigated together, since either or both partners may have an underlying cause for the infertility. The history must be taken with sensitivity. Although infertility is not a life-threatening or physically painful disease the emotional distress and bereavement experienced by childless couples can be great. Specific details should be sought regarding the duration of infertility, any previous pregnancies and relevant past illnesses (see Box 66).

The male is examined, looking for any hernia or varicocele. The presence and size of the testes is noted. The prostate gland should be palpated by rectal examination for any tenderness, which would be suggestive of prostatitis. Female pelvic examination is done to confirm normal anatomy, exclude pregnancy, and detect the rare occurrence of a congenital anatomical malformation such as vaginal atresia.

The nature of any investigations to be performed should be explained to the couple. Unless the history and examination findings point strongly to a particular cause, it is usual to commence tests with a seminal fluid analysis and confirmation of ovulation with a day 21 serum progesterone level. Rubella antibodies should be checked, and immunisation recommended if indicated.

If the duration of infertility is short, the sperm count is normal and ovulation is confirmed, there may be no need to investigate further at this stage as the majority of couples will achieve a pregnancy within 2 years. Conversely, many couples will be concerned about their age and be keen to have further investigations as soon as possible. Specialist referral is then necessary for tests of tubal patency (see below).

Seminal fluid analysis

Seminal fluid analysis provides information about the numbers of sperm and their motility. Two semen speci-

---

Box 66 Relevant points about the history

Female history
- Coital frequency
- Menstrual details
- History of pelvic infection or pelvic surgery
- Contraceptive history such as previous use of IUCD

Male history
- Recent illness
- Drugs, smoking, excessive alcohol
- Mumps orchitis
- Previous testicular surgery
- Problems with erection or ejaculation
- Exposure to toxins or radiation

mens should be collected, 6 weeks apart and after 3 days' abstinence, by masturbation into a sterile container. Specimens should be kept at room temperature and handed in to the laboratory within 2 hours of production. A normal analysis shows a volume of between 2 and 6 ml, a sperm density of 20–250 million per ml, an abnormality rate of less than 30% and a motility of 60% at 1 hour. Oligospermia is defined as less than 20 million spermatozoa per ml, and azoospermia as complete absence of spermatozoa. Large numbers of white cells in the semen are suggestive of genital tract infection. The presence of antisperm antibodies in serum or semen is suggestive of immunological infertility.

More sophisticated tests of sperm function such as the swim-up test and computer-assisted seminal analysis are generally only performed in tertiary referral centres. There is no satisfactory test of the actual fertilising ability of sperm, but the ability of human sperm to penetrate oocytes from the golden hamster gives some correlation with fertility, but it is rarely used in practice.

Other male investigations

If azoospermia or severe oligospermia are found, measurement of FSH levels and karyotyping will be required. If these are normal, vasal or epididymal obstruction is likely. In this situation, a testicular biopsy can be useful to confirm normal spermatogenesis, prior to consideration of exploratory surgery. Occasionally clinical signs of a chromosomal disorder such as Klinefelter's syndrome may be seen. This can present with male infertility, small testes and gynaecomastia.

Tests for ovulation

There are several indicators of ovulation (see Box 65). A history of regular monthly periods is suggestive, as anovulation usually results in oligomenorrhoea. A simple method which the woman can undertake herself at home is daily temperature recording, as mentioned in Chapter 14. The oral temperature is taken every morning before rising, and recorded on a special chart. A rise of 0.5°C over the last 14 days of the cycle is suggestive of ovulation. However, these indicators are unreliable, and the gold standard is measurement of a day 21 serum progesterone level. If ovulation has occurred this should be greater than 30 nmol/L. Timing of the test is crucial as the corpus luteum produces progesterone during the luteal phase of the cycle with a peak 7 days before the next period. This would be on day 21 in a 28-day cycle, or 7 days before the next period in a cycle of any other length.

If ovulation is not confirmed, the hypothalamic/pituitary/ovarian endocrine axis will require further investigation. FSH and LH are measured in the early follicular phase of the cycle, together with testosterone, prolactin and thyroid function. Low gonadotrophin levels are suggestive of a hypothalamic disorder, whilst grossly elevated levels suggest primary ovarian failure. Elevated prolactin levels would suggest a pituitary tumour. An LH:FSH ratio greater than 3:1 accompanied by a slightly raised testosterone level suggests polycystic ovary syndrome.

Tests for tubal patency

Tests of tubal patency are usually delayed until last as they are both more invasive and carry a small risk of pelvic infection. They should be performed during the first 10 days of the cycle to prevent disruption of an early pregnancy.

Hysterosalpingogram

A hysterosalpingogram (Fig. 26) entails injecting radio-opaque dye through the cervix under radiographic control. The dye demonstrates the internal contours of the uterus and fallopian tubes, and should be seen to spill freely into the peritoneal cavity from the fimbrial ends.

Box 67 Indicators of ovulation

- Luteal phase progesterone > 30 nmol/L
- Temperature charts
- Spinnbarkeit
- Secretory change on endometrial histology

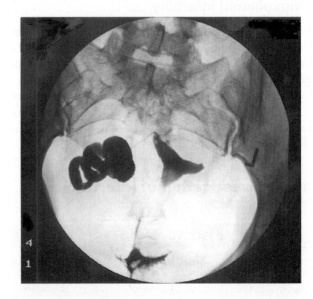

Fig. 26 Hysterosalpingogram. Radio-opaque dye is injected through the cervix under radiographic control.

Fimbrial occlusion of the tubes results in distension with dye but no spillage. Müllerian duct abnormalities such as bicornuate uterus, and intra-uterine pathology such as polyps, may also be detected.

Laparoscopy

This allows a full visual inspection of the abdomen and pelvis via a telescope inserted through a small sub-umbilical incision under general anaesthetic. The peritoneal surfaces of the uterus, tubes and ovaries can be inspected for the presence of adhesions or endometriosis, and follicular development in the ovaries can be assessed. Previous acute salpingitis may result in fine peritubal adhesions and clubbing of the delicate fimbrial ends. A solution of methylene blue dye is then injected through the cervix. This normally fills and then spills from the fimbrial ends of the tubes without resistance. Hysteroscopy may be undertaken at the same time to visualise the uterine cavity, and an endometrial sample can be sent for histology and culture if required.

Hysterosalpingo-contrast sonography

This new technique involves transcervical injection of an echo-contrast medium, which allows tubal patency to be visualised with ultrasound imaging via a trans-vaginal probe.

Tests for sperm/mucus compatibility

The ability of sperm to penetrate cervical mucus can be assessed using the post-coital test. This has to be done at the mid-cycle when the mucus is favourable. It involves taking a sample of cervical mucus from the endocervical canal 6–12 hours after sexual intercourse. This is placed on a slide and examined under the microscope, when large numbers of progressively motile sperm should be seen.

15.4 Treatment of infertility

Learning objective

You should understand:

- how and why different treatment options are used in infertility

General

Simple advice regarding the optimum timing for intercourse is usually helpful. The couple should be reassured and advised that pregnancy may still occur naturally even if the duration of infertility has been many years. This is especially so if investigations have all been normal. When a problem has been identified, accurate information should be given about the possible treatment options. Some couples will need time to adjust and express their feelings, and if emotional difficulties arise the assistance of an understanding professional counsellor may be helpful.

The option of adoption should also be discussed at an early stage. However, few babies are now available for adoption due to the changing social attitude towards single parenthood.

Disorders of ovulation

Correction of an abnormal body mass index will often restore ovulation. Under- or overweight women should therefore be advised that their fertility will be substantially improved by weight normalisation.

If infertility persists despite efforts at weight correction, ovulation can be induced with drugs. This is usually successful, but there are some possible drawbacks, including an increased risk of multiple pregnancy. Drugs used for induction of ovulation include:

- clomiphene
- gonadotrophins
- gonadotrophin-releasing hormone
- dopamine agonists.

Clomiphene

Most forms of ovulatory failure can be successfully treated with anti-oestrogens, of which clomiphene is the most frequently used. It is a straightforward and inexpensive treatment with few side-effects. Clomiphene stimulates follicular maturation by an anti-oestrogenic action. This blocks the normal negative feedback of oestrogen on pituitary gonadotrophin secretion, which occurs in the early follicular phase of the cycle. Clomiphene is given in a dose of 50 mg daily from day 2 to day 6 of the cycle. Intercourse should be planned to coincide with ovulation at mid-cycle. 70% of women will ovulate in response to clomiphene, and this can be monitored by measurement of a day 21 progesterone level. A pregnancy rate of 50% can be achieved if treatment is continued for up to six cycles. If pregnancy does not occur despite confirmation of ovulation, other problems such as tubal disease should be suspected. If ovulation does not occur, clomiphene can be given in a higher dose, and in combination with human chorionic gonadotrophin (HCG). This should only be done with careful ultrasound monitoring of follicular growth because of the increased risk of ovarian hyperstimulation. When a follicle reaches 16–18 mm in diameter an injection of 3000 IU of HCG is given. This simulates the LH surge and triggers ovulation. If this fails, therapy with gonadotrophins should be considered.

Side-effects of clomiphene include hot flushes and breast tenderness. Ovarian hyperstimulation with cyst formation is rare. The incidence of multiple pregnancy is 6%.

Gonadotrophins

Gonadotrophins are much more powerful drugs for inducing ovulation. They are highly effective for hypothalamic/pituitary/ovarian dysfunction which has not responded to clomiphene. They are also used in normally ovulating women during in vitro fertilisation (IVF) and gamete intra-fallopian transfer (GIFT) cycles where the aim is to induce multiple ovarian follicles for egg collection. They are also expensive.

Gonadotrophin preparations were originally obtained from cadaver pituitary extracts, but they are now prepared from the urine of post-menopausal women. Commercial preparations of human menopausal gonadotrophin contain both FSH and LH. Pure preparations of FSH are also available. They are usually given by daily intramuscular injections early in the follicular phase of the cycle. Multiple follicles develop with exogenously administered FSH and LH, whereas only one follicle becomes dominant in natural cycles. Careful monitoring is important to allow adjustment of dosage and to avoid ovarian hyperstimulation. HCG may be given to trigger ovulation when the dominant follicle is 16–18 mm in diameter. In IVF and GIFT cycles, the oocytes are harvested just prior to ovulation.

Gonadotrophin-releasing hormone

Gonadotrophin-releasing hormone (GnRH) is effective in inducing ovulation in selected patients with hypogonadotrophic amenorrhoea characterised by low levels of LH, FSH and oestrogen. It is given subcutaneously or intravenously via a pulsatile infusion pump, usually in the arm. There is a lower rate of multiple pregnancy than with gonadotrophin therapy.

Dopamine agonists

Some 15% of women with ovulation disorders have increased serum prolactin concentrations. The underlying cause should be investigated prior to treatment. Common causes include drugs such as phenothiazines, primary hypothyroidism, and pituitary tumours. One third of cases are idiopathic. Treatment with dopamine agonists such as cabergoline or bromocriptine aims to restore ovulation. In cases where a pituitary macroadenoma is present, pregnancy carries the small risk of causing tumour enlargement with compression of the optic chiasma. Regular monitoring of visual fields during pregnancy is therefore required.

Hyperstimulation

Ovarian hyperstimulation is a serious complication of ovulation induction. Women with polycystic ovarian disease appear to be at particular risk. It is characterised by ovarian cyst formation, accompanied by the escape of fluid and protein from the vascular space into the peritoneal and pleural cavities. This results in painful abdominal distension. If pregnancy has occurred, secretion of endogenous HCG causes further stimulation. Hyperstimulation is minimised by careful ovarian monitoring during ovulation induction regimens. Treatment consists of fluid replacement and correction of electrolyte imbalance.

Treatment of tubal disease

The choice lies between tubal microsurgery and in vitro fertilisation (IVF). In general the results of tubal microsurgery are poor, with subsequent pregnancy rates of only 20%. Gross tubal disease destroys the cilia so tubal function will not return even if patency is restored. When the tubes are not severely damaged, microsurgery is a useful treatment. The principles of tubal microsurgery are magnification, minimal tissue handling, and meticulous haemostasis. Subsequent adhesion formation is minimised by covering all raw peritoneal surfaces, using fine monofilament sutures, and irrigating with intraperitoneal steroids. Poor prognostic factors include dense and extensive tubal adhesions, bilateral hydrosalpinges, previous tubal surgery and age over 35 years. The decision to offer tubal surgery will be influenced by the presence or absence of these factors, and the availability of IVF treatment.

Types of tubal microsurgery

Salpingolysis
Salpingolysis involves division and removal of tubal adhesions in order to restore normal anatomy.

Cuff salpingostomy
Cuff salpingostomy involves opening up the blocked fimbrial end of the tube and securing the edges back to prevent them closing again. This may be achieved using laser laparoscopy.

Cornual re-anastomosis
Occlusion of the interstitial portion of the tube which runs in the uterine wall can be treated by cornual reanastomosis. This involves dividing the tube close to the uterus, cutting out the blocked segment, and anastomosing the fresh ends. It is a rarely performed procedure.

Reversal of sterilisation
Some of the best results from tubal surgery are in sterilisation reversal, because the tube, with the exception of

the occluded portion, is healthy. The occluded part is excised and the cut ends are anastomosed with the aid of an operating microscope and fine monofilament sutures. Success rates of 90% have been achieved.

Other operations

Procedures such as myomectomy or removal of tubal polyps are only indicated if the uterine cavity or tubal anatomy is grossly distorted. Fibroids are often present in fertile women, and surgical removal may cause unwanted adhesions, and scars which may weaken the uterus.

Endometriosis

Surgery is indicated for endometriosis when it is causing mechanical distortion of the fallopian tubes, when the aim is to restore normal anatomy. If unsuccessful, IVF can be offered, providing the ovaries are accessible and capable of yielding eggs. Small asymptomatic deposits of endometriosis should not be treated, as this will not improve fertility, but merely delays attempts at conception still further.

Treatment of male infertility

General measures

Treatments to improve a poor sperm count are generally disappointing. A healthy lifestyle, reducing consumption of alcohol and stopping smoking is advised. Excessive scrotal temperature has a detrimental effect on spermatogenesis, so advice to wear loose fitting pants and avoid very hot bathing is usually given. Men with azoospermia, atrophic testes and increased FSH concentrations will have irreversible seminiferous tubular failure and usually be sterile. These couples should be counselled regarding the option of donor insemination.

Surgery

Surgical ligation of a varicocele is advised if it occurs in association with male infertility. However, both the mechanism of fertility impairment by a varicocele and the beneficial effect that ligation has are unclear. Pregnancy rates of 70% have been reported following ligation but other studies have been unable to show any increase in pregnancy rates compared with similar patients who were not treated. Only a prospective controlled trial of varicocele ligation will clarify this.

Azoospermia and severe oligospermia resulting from blockage of the vas deferens may be treatable by microsurgical anastomosis of the vas to the epididymis, but the success rate is low. Testicular biopsy is usually performed beforehand to confirm normal spermatogenesis. Vasectomy reversal by re-anastomosis of the vas deferens has a 50% success rate.

Drug treatment

Numerous drug treatments have been advocated for the treatment of idiopathic oligospermia, including gonadotrophins, androgens, clomiphene, vitamin C and zinc. None have withstood evaluation by randomised controlled trial.

Specific disorders may benefit from drug treatment. Active genital tract infection such as chlamydia, or a documented semen infection, should be treated with an appropriate antibiotic for a minimum of 2 weeks. Hypogonadotrophic hypogonadism can be treated with HCG injections over a 6-month period.

Sperm antibodies

These can be treated by immunosuppression with prednisolone, but there is little evidence of treatment efficacy. Intra-uterine insemination is usually preferred.

Intra-uterine insemination

Intra-uterine insemination (IUI) involves injecting semen through the cervix via a small cannula at the time of ovulation. This is especially useful in cases of retrograde ejaculation, whereby semen is ejaculated backwards into the bladder. Under these circumstances, spermatozoa can be collected by centrifugation of urine. Frozen semen which has been stored prior to chemotherapy can be used for IUI, as spermatogenesis does not always recover. IUI is also used to treat sperm/mucus incompatibility due to antisperm antibodies, but it appears to be little better than normal sexual intercourse. Intra-uterine insemination using donor semen is very successful in the treatment of oligospermia, azoospermia and sperm/mucus incompatibility. This technique can be used in conjunction with gonadotrophins to induce follicular growth if the woman has an irregular cycle. Donor semen is occasionally used when a couple have had an abnormal baby and counselling suggests a high risk of recurrence due to an inherited male genetic disorder. Fertile healthy anonymous donors have to be carefully selected. Medical, family and social histories are obtained, and details such as height, weight, eye colour, hair colour and race are recorded to enable the recipient couple to have some choice regarding these characteristics. Semen is frozen to allow time for screening for sexually transmitted disease, hepatitis, and human immunodeficiency virus (HIV).

In vitro fertilisation (IVF)

Many forms of male infertility respond well to in vitro fertilisation (IVF). Spermatozoa that are unable to reach the oocyte due to poor motility may be perfectly able to achieve fertilisation once they are brought into close contact with an egg in vitro. Gamete intra-fallopian transfer (GIFT) is a simpler but less reliable alternative.

Semen is collected by masturbation. The first part of the ejaculate is collected separately as this contains a higher concentration of spermatozoa. A culture medium is then added, into which the most active spermatozoa will swim. This effectively removes the abnormal, poorly motile and dead sperm, leaving a sample containing a high concentration of motile, viable ones. The aim is to prepare a suspension containing 50 000 active spermatozoa per ml, for fertilisation of several embryos. The remainder of the IVF technique is described below. The results of IVF in the treatment of male infertility vary between different centres but pregnancies can be obtained in up to 40% of treatment cycles.

The advent of intracytoplasmic injection of sperm (ICSI) has greatly improved the outlook for men with both oligospermia and obstructive azoospermia. This technique consists of the micro-injection of a single spermatozoon directly into the oocyte cytoplasm.

15.5 Assisted conception

Learning objective

You should:

- understand how and why IVF is a useful infertility treatment option

There are two main forms of assisted conception: in vitro fertilisation (IVF) and gamete intra-fallopian transfer (GIFT).

IVF

In vitro fertilisation involves removal of an egg from the ovary, exposing it to sperm under laboratory conditions to allow fertilisation, and then placing the resulting embryo directly into the uterus. It is a sophisticated and expensive technique which is used only when more simple treatments have failed.

Situations in which IVF may be useful include:

- tubal disease
- male factor infertility
- endometriosis
- sperm/mucus incompatibility
- unexplained infertility
- egg donation.

Stages in IVF treatment

Ovarian stimulation

Several eggs are needed to ensure the best chance of a successful pregnancy. Controlled ovulation induction is performed using gonadotrophin injections. These must be started early in the cycle before the development of a dominant follicle. Sometimes a short period of pituitary suppression with GnRH analogues is used to prevent follicular development before gonadotrophin treatment is begun. Follicular growth is closely monitored with regular ultrasound examination and serum oestradiol measurements. The aim is to produce several follicles of about 20 mm in diameter. An injection of HCG is then given to promote further oocyte maturation. Larger follicles are associated with high spontaneous abortion rates, and smaller ones generally contain immature ova. Occasionally the cycle has to be abandoned if follicular developments is too rapid, because of the risk of hyperstimulation.

Egg collection

Egg collection is carried out just prior to ovulation. This is done by transvaginal ultrasound-guided needle aspiration, or more rarely by laparoscopy.

Fertilisation

The eggs are mixed with a prepared sample of semen, which the male partner has been asked to produce. Fertilisation should take place within a few hours. If the sperm count is very low or when the sperm have difficulty penetrating the egg, a technique called intracytoplasmic sperm injection (ICSI) may be used, whereby a single sperm is injected directly into the egg.

Embryo transfer

When an embryo has reached the four cell stage, it is placed inside the uterus by gentle injection through the cervix using a fine plastic tube. This needs no anaesthetic, but the woman is advised to rest for a few hours afterwards. Progesterone injections may be given following embryo transfer in order to help implantation. Serial serum HCG measurements over the next 2 weeks are used to monitor progress. Rising levels are an early indicator of a successfully implanted pregnancy, at a stage before ultrasound can detect fetal heart activity. Up to three embryos are placed in the uterus. This increases the pregnancy rate because a high percentage will fail to implant. It also, however, increases the risk of multiple pregnancy.

Success rates of IVF

The success rate varies between different centres, but around 20% of women treated by IVF will have a child to take home.

GIFT

GIFT is a much simpler technique than IVF, requiring fewer laboratory facilities. Eggs are collected by laparoscopy following ovarian stimulation, and immediately placed in the fallopian tube together with a sample of semen. Fertilisation then takes place in vivo. GIFT is not suitable when there has been tubal damage because of the increased risk of ectopic pregnancy. It is used in the treatment of unexplained and male factor infertility.

15.6 Ethical problems in infertility

Learning objective

You should:

* understand how and why there are profound ethical issues in infertility

Funding

The provision of expensive infertility treatments such as IVF within the National Health Service places considerable demands on limited health care resources. The prioritisation of resource allocation by different health authorities has led to unequal funding of infertility services throughout the country. As a result IVF is only available either on a private basis or under strict eligibility criteria in some areas.

High multiple pregnancy

Triplets and higher order multiple pregnancies can result from the placement of three or more embryos into the uterus during IVF treatment. This is done to improve the chances of a single successful implantation. The high incidence of premature delivery in high order multiple pregnancies results in increased perinatal mortality and morbidity, and places enormous demands on special care baby units. Early selective fetal reduction is a controversial technique whereby a number of fetuses are deliberately aborted at an early stage in order to improve the survival chances of the remaining ones.

Donor insemination

Couples need to be aware of the possible impact of donor insemination on their relationship, and consider their future plans with regard to telling the child. Under current law the anonymity of the donor is maintained, although this is currently under discussion. Donor insemination has been used in single women who wish to have a family but choose to be without a male partner.

Surrogate mothers

A surrogate mother carries a pregnancy on behalf of a commissioning couple, usually as a result of artificial insemination with semen from the male partner or by placement of a fertilised embryo into the uterus. Following birth the baby is given to the commissioning couple. The ethical dilemma is whether or not exploitation takes place, but it can be argued that the surrogate mother is fully aware of what she is doing and in many cases gains financially from the process. The law in this country currently forbids the setting up of an agency to provide surrogate mothers for commissioning couples on a commercial basis.

Research involving embryos

The practice of IVF has been developed by research and the results are continually being improved by incorporation of research findings into clinical practice. Such research inevitably involves the use of human embryos. IVF generates more embryos than can be implanted, so the 'spares' can either be destroyed, frozen or used to further develop our understanding of the reproductive process. Research using human embryos is permitted in this country subject to strict guidelines and controls.

Age and IVF

The success rate of IVF is greatly reduced in women over 38 years of age. Successful pregnancies have been achieved in women much older than this, but they have a significantly increased risk of chromosomal abnormalities, and the mother is less able to tolerate the profound physiological changes of pregnancy.

Preimplantation diagnosis

This is achieved by removing one cell from the embryo at the four cell stage, prior to implantation during IVF treatment. The cell can then be used for antenatal diagnostic testing. As the embryonic cells at this stage are pluripotential, normal fetal development is unaffected.

Self-assessment: questions

Multiple choice questions

1. Which of the following statements are true?
   a. Infrequent ejaculation improves the sperm count in oligospermic men
   b. Certain coital positions improve the chance of conception
   c. Conception is more likely with an increasing frequency of intercourse
   d. Artificial insemination using the husband's semen (AIH) is a useful treatment for unexplained infertility
   e. Male factors account for 10% of infertility

2. Regarding the post-coital test:
   a. It must be done on day 21 of the cycle
   b. It can detect anovulation
   c. It can detect tubal problems
   d. It can detect azoospermia
   e. Ovulatory mucus is essential for interpretation

3. Which of the following provide evidence of ovulation?
   a. Day 14 progesterone level
   b. Endometrial biopsy
   c. A rise in the basal body temperature
   d. Menstruation
   e. Gonadotrophin levels

4. Which of the following investigations are correctly matched with the condition?
   a. Hysterosalpingogram — Detection of blocked tubes
   b. Serum prolactin — Investigation of anovulation
   c. Karyotype — Azoospermia
   d. Endometrial culture — Pelvic tuberculosis
   e. Laparoscopy — Endometriosis

5. Which of the following measures can be used to correct anovulation?
   a. Bromocriptine
   b. Weight loss
   c. Low-dose oestrogen
   d. HCG injection
   e. Clonidine

6. A couple have a 2-year history of infertility. The male partner is healthy with no past serious illnesses, and has one child from his previous marriage. The female partner has a regular 29-day menstrual cycle and has a normal body mass index. Her only previous pregnancy was an ectopione. Which of the following investigations is most likely to reveal the cause of the infertility?
   a. Semen analysis
   b. Pelvic ultrasound examination
   c. Hormonal profile
   d. Laparoscopy
   e. Hysteroscopy

7. Which of the following may cause male infertility?
   a. Gonorrhoea infection
   b. Cystic fibrosis
   c. Hydrocele
   d. Prolactinoma
   e. Cytotoxic chemotherapy

Short notes

1. Why do women become less fertile after the age of 35 years?

2. When should infertility be investigated? What are the most commonly used investigations?

3. Why are two semen samples collected, 3 months apart, in the investigation of infertility?

4. What are the possible reasons for unexplained infertility?

5. What points in a woman's history would suggest a tubal problem causing infertility?

6. What are the risks of treatment with gonadotrophin therapy? How can these be minimised?

7. (i) Which patients are unsuitable for IVF treatment?
   (ii) Why might an IVF cycle be unsuccessful?

OSCE question

Patricia and her husband have been trying for a baby for 18 months. Patricia has just seen her GP, and following this inital consultation, she has some questions to ask you:

1. Why has she been advised to have her rubella status checked?
2. Why has she been advised to start taking 0.4 mg folic acid daily?

3. Why have they been advised to have regular intercourse throughout the cycle, and not bother with temperature charts?

4. The doctor said that because she has a regular 28 day cycle, it is only necessary to measure one hormone on the 21st day. What about the other hormones, such as thyroid hormones, and prolactin?

5. If she falls pregnant, how much alcohol can she safely drink?

Self-assessment: answers

Multiple choice answers

1. a. **False.** There is no evidence that infrequent ejaculation improves the sperm count in oligospermic men.
   b. **False.**
   c. **True.** The more frequent the intercourse, the more likely conception is to occur.
   d. **False.** AIH is only of value where intercourse is impossible because of some major sexual dysfunction, or where retrograde ejaculation is occurring due to a bladder neck disorder. Both of these are rare causes of infertility.
   e. **False.** Male factors account for up to 25% of infertility.

2. a. **False.** The post-coital test must be performed on day 14 of the cycle when cervical mucus is most receptive to sperm motility. Poor sperm motility will be seen if it is performed at other times in the cycle.
   b. **False.** The test cannot detect ovulatory problems.
   c. **False.** The test cannot detect tubal problems.
   d. **True.**
   e. **True.**

3. a. **False.** Progesterone secretion reaches a maximum 7 days before menstruation, so should be measured on day 21 in a 28-day cycle.
   b. **True.** Following ovulation the endometrium undergoes secretory change, and if this is seen on histological examination it provides indirect evidence of ovulation.
   c. **True.**
   d. **False.** Menstruation may occur in the absence of ovulation.
   e. **False.** Gonadotrophin levels are not clinically useful in confirming ovulation. The LH surge occurs prior to ovulation.

4. a. **True.** Hysterosalpingography is used to assess tubal patency.
   b. **True.** Hyperprolactinaemia from any cause may result in anovulation.
   c. **True.** An abnormal karyotype, such as Klinefelter's syndrome, is a rare cause of azoospermia.
   d. **True.** Pelvic tuberculosis is a rare cause of infertility in the UK, but if suspected, endometrial curettings should be sent for TB culture.
   e. **True.** Diagnostic laparoscopy is used in suspected cases of endometriosis. It also allows assessment of the site and size of any deposits.

5. a. **True.** Bromocriptine is used to restore ovulation in the treatment of hyperprolactinaemia.
   b. **True.** Weight loss to within a normal body mass index in obesity will usually allow a return of ovulation.
   c. **False.** Low dose oestrogen is occasionally used to improve the quality of cervical mucus but it does not cause ovulation.
   d. **True.** HCG injections are used to stimulate ovulation when clomiphene alone fails.
   e. **False.** Clomiphene, not clonidine, is the most commonly used agent for induction of ovulation.

6. a. **False.**
   b. **False.**
   c. **False.**
   d. **True.** The history of a previous ectopic pregnancy makes a tubal problem the most likely cause of infertility in this case, and laparoscopy is the best way of assessing this.
   e. **False.**

7. a. **True.** Gonorrhoea may result in post-infection obstruction in the vas deferens.
   b. **True.** Most males with cystic fibrosis have azoospermia due to abnormal development and obstruction of the vas deferens and epididymis.
   c. **False.**
   d. **True.** A pituitary tumour such as a prolactinoma is a treatable cause of male infertility.
   e. **True.**

Short notes answers

1. The prime reason that female fertility declines with age is that ovulation occurs less frequently due to depletion in the number of oocytes. Other reasons include decreasing coital frequency with age, thus reducing the chances of conception, and the increased incidence of miscarriage from chromosomal abnormalities. With increasing age the uterus is more likely to harbour fibroids which may interfere with implantation. Male fertility also declines very slightly with age.

2. It is usual to begin investigations after 1 year of infertility, but it may be appropriate after 6 months if there is particular concern about the woman's age. It is preferable to perform the investigations in a logical order, beginning with the simplest and least invasive, and with correct timing in the cycle. The

common investigations include: semen analysis, post-coital test, day 21 progesterone, laparoscopy and hysteroscopy. More intensive cycle monitoring with ultrasound scan, LH, FSH and prolactin measurement is only indicated where anovulation is suspected.

3. The production of two semen analyses 3 months apart is required because of the large natural variation in the sperm count in any individual. This is due to the long maturation process of spermatozoa, during which time any minor illness such as a viral infection can produce a temporary depression of the sperm count which may persist for several months.

4. There are many possible reasons for unexplained infertility. In many cases there is likely to be a subtle abnormality present which has eluded detection. For example, there is no easy method of assessing the fertilising ability of sperm. Only in IVF cycles where gametes are observed in vitro can fertilisation be definitely confirmed.

   Tests of tubal patency are also relatively crude assessments. They are unable to confirm oocyte pick-up by the fimbria, or demonstrate normal ciliary action which is necessary for oocyte transport.

   Confirmation of ovulation by measurement of the luteal phase progesterone may not be 100% reliable. Minor abnormalities of both the follicular and luteal phases of the ovarian cycle can result in a condition called the luteinised unruptured follicle syndrome, whereby the oocyte is not released but luteal progesterone levels are normal.

   Unexplained infertility could also be due to unrecognised or unvolunteered sexual dysfunction. It is not possible to accurately judge the frequency of sexual intercourse, which in some cases may be a most infrequent event despite claims to the contrary. Alternatively the problem may be one of recurrent subclinical pregnancy loss rather than a failure to conceive. Despite all these factors many patients with unexplained infertility will become pregnant within 3 years.

5. Any history of pelvic surgery makes a tubal cause for the infertility more likely. Examples include ectopic pregnancy, ovarian cystectomy or even appendectomy, which may all result in tubal adhesions. Recurrent bouts of pelvic inflammatory disease, post-abortal sepsis or past problems with an intra-uterine device are similarly suggestive of a tubal problem. Chronic pelvic pain and dyspareunia may indicate endometriosis or past pelvic infection.

6. Gonadotrophins are powerful drugs used in ovulation induction, which can be unpredictable in their effects. Careful monitoring of ovarian function by ultrasound examination and serial plasma oestradiol estimations are essential because of the risk of ovarian hyperstimulation. Treatment cycles have to be abandoned if the developing follicles become too large. The other main risk is of high-order multiple pregnancy, accompanied by an increased likelihood of pre-term delivery, higher perinatal morbidity and mortality.

   There is also concern regarding a possible small increased risk of ovarian cancer associated with ovulation induction. For this reason treatment duration should not normally exceed 6 months.

7. (i) There are some women for whom IVF is of no help. Very scarred ovaries or severe bowel adhesions can make egg collection dangerous or impossible, because of poor access. Donor eggs could then be used. Women who have had a hysterectomy, or those with severe uterine abnormalities or uterine tuberculosis are unsuitable for IVF. Women over the age of 42 years have a very low success rate with IVF.

   (ii) Common reasons for failure of IVF cycles are failure of fertilisation, failure of the embryos to develop normally, and failure of the replaced embryos to implant. More rarely the ovaries resist all attempts to induce suitable follicular development, or conversely become overstimulated with large cysts. Very occasionally it proves impossible to harvest the oocytes. Finally, a pregnancy may occur but be in an ectopic location.

OSCE answer

1. Maternal rubella infection in the first 8–10 weeks of pregnancy results in severe fetal abnormalities in up to 90% of cases. The rubella status of the female partner should therefore be checked, and if seronegative, rubella vaccination should be offered.

2. Folic acid supplementation is advised both whilst trying to conceive and during the first 12 weeks of pregnancy, in order to prevent fetal neural tube defects.

3. There is no evidence that the use of temperature charts improves outcome so their use is discouraged. Advice to time intercourse has been evaluated by patients as being the most emotionally stressful element of infertility management.

4. In the presence of regular menstruation, ovulation can be confirmed with a day 21 serum progesterone level. There is no value in measuring thyroid function, prolactin or any other hormones in the absence of symptoms, if the progesterone confirms ovulation.

5. Excessive alcohol consumption reduces female fertility. The safe limit for consumption in pregnancy is not known. The usual advice is not to drink more than one or two units of alcohol once or twice a week when trying to become pregnant.

16 Early pregnancy loss

Overview

Spontaneous miscarriage in early pregnancy is a relatively common event. In 50% of cases, it is due to a foetal chromosomal abnormality. Great care and compassion are needed in order to manage this condition, as it is usually a highly traumatic and emotional event for the woman concerned. The prognosis for a subsequent pregnancy following early miscarriage is usually good. There are a variety of causes of recurrent early pregnancy loss, including both endocrine and congenital uterine abnormalities, but in many cases, no obvious cause can be found.

Ectopic pregnancy occurs when the fertilised ovum implants outside the uterine cavity. The commonest site is the fallopian tube. The usual cause is tubal damage, from previous pelvic inflammatory disease which has impaired tubal transport.

16.1 General principles

Learning objective

You should understand:

- the events which occur during the establishment of pregnancy

The establishment of a viable pregnancy requires success at several stages in the reproductive process:

- Fertilisation of the oocyte to form a zygote
- Hatching of the blastocyst from the zona pellucida
- Transport of the blastocyst to the uterine cavity
- Differentiation of the blastocyst into an outer trophoblast and the inner cell mass
- Adherence and penetration of the endometrial lining by the trophoblast – implantation
- Establishment of direct contact with maternal circulation – haemochorial placentation.

Fertilisation takes place in the fallopian tube. This must occur within 48 hours of ovulation because after this time the egg becomes unviable. The fertilised ovum is surrounded and held together by a protective layer, called the zona pellucida. By day 7 it has hatched out from the zona pellucida, and consists of about 60 cells. It is now called a blastocyst. The blastocyst is transported to the uterine cavity, where the endometrium has been carefully prepared for implantation under the control of oestrogen and progesterone. These hormones are thought to mediate their actions on the endometrium via locally-produced paracrine regulators such as epidermal growth factor and insulin-like growth factor. Implantation occurs by the ninth day. This process requires close cell-to-cell interaction between the trophoblast and the endometrium, and must occur during a relatively short receptive window in the endometrial cycle. Even though the embryo contains paternally-derived foreign antigens it is not rejected by the maternal immune system, and appears to be protected by locally-acting immunosuppressive mechanisms. The process of placentation in humans is called haemochorial, meaning that direct contact is established with the maternal blood circulation. Such contact secures a ready supply of nutrients for the developing embryo.

16.2 Early pregnancy loss

Learning objective

You should understand:

- why and how there is a 25% rate of early pregnancy loss

A high proportion of early pregnancies fail. A rate of 25% is usually quoted, but the true incidence is probably much higher as very early pregnancy loss may pass unrecognised. Most pregnancy loss occurs within 6 weeks of ovulation. The causes can be divided into three broad categories: embryo defects, uterine defects, and maternal disorders. In addition to these, many potentially harmful environmental agents have been implicated in early pregnancy loss. These include glue solvents, insecticides, lead, alcohol and smoking. There is no good evidence that microwave ovens or computer screens cause pregnancy loss. Finally, miscarriage may occasionally be iatrogenic, following chorionic villus sampling or amniocentesis.

Embryo defects

Chromosomal abnormalities in the embryo account for the majority of early pregnancy loss. The incidence correlates with maternal age, particularly for trisomy 21. Only a minority of chromosomally abnormal embryos survive beyond the first trimester.

Hydatidiform mole is a rare embryonic cause of pregnancy loss. It arises when a sperm fertilises an ovum from which the maternal genetic material has been lost. The chromosomes are thus totally paternally-derived, and there is no embryonic tissue present. The most common symptom is vaginal bleeding in the first trimester. This may be accompanied by hyperemesis gravidarum. The uterine size is often larger than dates, but no fetal heart sounds are present. Ultrasound examination shows a characteristic snowstorm appearance. Treatment is by suction evacuation of the uterus. Molar pregnancy is further discussed in Chapter 17.

Uterine defects

- Congenital malformations of the uterus, cervical incompetence and uterine fibroids are all rare causes of miscarriage.
- An endometrium that is unfavourable for implantation due to inadequate hormonal stimulation is a potential but unproven cause of early pregnancy failure. Low levels of luteinising hormone (LH), progesterone and human chorionic gonadotrophin (HCG) have been documented in association with miscarriage, but this is more likely to be the result, rather than the cause, of a failing pregnancy.

Maternal disorders

Maternal infection

Any acute febrile maternal illness is a rare cause of both miscarriage and premature labour. However, there are some specific infections which are more commonly associated with pregnancy loss. These include listeriosis, toxoplasmosis, parvovirus and brucellosis.

Maternal disease

The presence of circulating maternal antiphospholipid antibodies is associated with both recurrent early pregnancy loss and unexpected late fetal loss. The mechanism is by immune-mediated placental microvascular damage. These antibodies may occur in isolation or as a feature of systemic lupus erythematosus.

Immunological factors

Rejection of the paternally-derived fetal antigens by the maternal immune system has been suggested as a cause for miscarriage. There is no definitive proof or effective treatment for this.

16.3 Clinical manifestations

Learning objective

You should understand:

- the different ways in which early pregnancy loss can present

Early pregnancy loss may present in a variety of different clinical ways.

Threatened miscarriage

Threatened miscarriage is defined as vaginal bleeding before 20 weeks gestation in the presence of a viable fetus. The cervix remains closed and no products of conception have been passed.

Inevitable miscarriage

If the cervix has begun to dilate and products of conception have been passed the terms inevitable or incomplete miscarriage are used. The pregnancy cannot now be saved.

Complete miscarriage

Complete miscarriage is when all the products of conception have been passed, and the uterus has returned to normal size. By this time, the cervix has closed and the pain and bleeding settled.

Silent miscarriage

The demise of an early pregnancy in the absence of vaginal bleeding is called silent or delayed miscarriage. The usual symptoms of pregnancy disappear, and the uterus stops enlarging. Ultrasound examination shows an absence of fetal heart movement. Care is needed to differentiate this condition from a very early viable pregnancy. When there is any doubt the scan should be repeated in 2 weeks, by which time fetal cardiac activity should be apparent.

Anembryonic pregnancy

This diagnosis is usually made by ultrasound examination. An empty gestational sac is seen, with no fetus present.

16.4 Investigation of early pregnancy loss

Learning objective

You should understand:

- why ultrasound has an important role to play in the management of early pregnancy loss

It should be remembered that bleeding in the first trimester may rarely be due to a cause incidental to the pregnancy such as a cervical neoplasm. Inspection of the cervix using a speculum is therefore indicated in all cases of undiagnosed genital tract bleeding.

Ultrasound scanning has revolutionised the management of bleeding in early pregnancy, because fetal viability can quickly be established by demonstrating cardiac activity. Using a transvaginal scan cardiac activity can be detected by 5 weeks' gestation, and by 7 weeks by transabdominal scan. Women with proven viable pregnancies can then be reassured, and the remainder can be spared unnecessary anxiety and diagnostic delays. Many hospitals now provide clinics for rapid assessment and ultrasound in early pregnancy, without the need for hospital admission.

16.5 Treatment of early pregnancy loss

Learning objectives

You should understand:

- why Rhesus status is important

Learning objectives (continued)

- how to use the investigation of ultrasound
- when surgical evacuation of the uterus is indicated
- that care and compassion are important in the management

All non-sensitised Rhesus negative women should be considered for anti-D immunoglobulin, in a dose of 250 IU, to prevent Rhesus isoimmunisation. (See Box 68.)

Threatened miscarriage

If fetal viability has been established by early ultrasound scan the prognosis is good. Only 15% of these pregnancies will subsequently miscarry, and there is no evidence that bed rest is effective in preventing this. If there is continued fresh blood loss, strenuous activity should be avoided. Continued fetal viability can be confirmed by a repeat ultrasound scan. By 12 weeks gestation viability can be checked by auscultating fetal heart sounds using a sonicaid device.

Inevitable miscarriage

Heavy bleeding accompanied by severe lower abdominal cramping pain is suggestive of an inevitable miscarriage. The diagnosis is confirmed by finding a dilated cervix with products of conception coming through the os. These should be removed using sponge-holding forceps, and ergometrine given to stimulate uterine contraction. Bleeding is occasionally severe, necessitating resuscitation with intravenous fluids. Further treatment is by evacuation of the remaining products of conception from the uterus under general anaesthetic.

In cases of anembryonic pregnancy or silent miscarriage, the uterus can be emptied using medical therapy rather than surgical evacuation provided that bleeding is not severe. This has the advantage of avoiding the risks of general anaesthesia and surgical trauma. The usual regimen consists of an oral dose of antiprogesterone, followed 48 hours later by vaginally administered prostaglandin pessary. This induces a complete miscarriage in 90% of cases without the need for surgical evacuation.

Box 68 Indications for anti-D Rhesus negative women

- All miscarriages over 12 weeks
- All miscarriages where the uterus is evacuated
- Threatened miscarriage under 12 weeks in association with pain or heavy bleeding
- Ectopic pregnancy

The other option is expectant management, which aims to avoid both medical and surgical therapy. Resolution may take several weeks, so appropriate counselling is important. There is some evidence that expectant management has a lower rate of pelvic infection, and no adverse effect on future fertility.

If pain and bleeding have stopped by the time the woman is seen, the miscarriage may have progressed to completion. The cervix will be closed and the uterus contracted back to a normal size. No treatment is then necessary.

Coping with early pregnancy loss

Many women experience a profound sense of shock and loss following a miscarriage. Feelings of guilt, anger and remorse are commonly experienced. Because miscarriage is so common, medical and nursing staff working on early pregnancy units need to maintain an awareness of such strong emotions and avoid any attempts to play down the situation. Women should be reassured that they are not to blame, and encouraged to express their feelings. This will help with the grieving process and coming to terms with their loss.

Septic miscarriage

Non-viable products of conception in the uterus may become infected. The common organisms are beta-haemolytic streptococci, chlamydia and coliforms. The early clinical features are a tender uterus with an offensive vaginal discharge. Treatment is by careful evacuation of the uterus under antibiotic cover. A combination of penicillin, doxycycline and metronidazole will cover these organisms. Untreated infection may progress to a severe maternal illness characterised by salpingitis, peritonitis, septicaemia and ultimately death from adult respiratory distress syndrome. This is rarely seen nowadays due to the decline in illegal abortion, which was the major cause.

16.6 Recurrent spontaneous miscarriage

Learning objectives

You should understand:

- how investigations are used to identify the causes of recurrent spontaneous abortion
- how the treatable causes are managed

Recurrent spontaneous miscarriage is defined as two or more consecutive early pregnancy losses. Only in a minority of cases is a recurrent cause identified (see

---

> **Box 69** Causes of recurrent spontaneous miscarriage
>
> - Chromosomal abnormalities
> - Infection
> - Uterine abnormalities
> - Cervical incompetence
> - Antiphospholipid antibody syndrome
> - Activated protein C resistance
> - Polycystic ovary syndrome
> - Chronic maternal illness

Box 69). In most cases, therefore, the prognosis for a successful outcome in the next pregnancy is good.

Although bacterial vaginosis has been implicated, infection is a rare cause, and is more commonly associated with second trimester fetal loss and premature labour.

Congenital anatomical abnormalities of the uterus, or fibroids distorting the uterine cavity, may rarely interfere with implantation on a recurrent basis.

Cervical incompetence resulting from previous cone biopsy or cervical trauma is a rare but treatable cause of recurrent fetal loss. It more usually causes second trimester miscarriage.

Thrombophilic defects such as the antiphospholipid antibody syndrome and activated protein C resistance are an important cause of recurrent pregnancy loss. The underlying pathology is thought to be thrombosis of the uteroplacental vasculature.

Women with polycystic ovary syndrome have a higher than expected incidence of early miscarriage. This is thought to be caused by the high circulating levels of LH.

Finally, there is an increased incidence of balanced chromosal translocations in these couples.

Clinical features of recurrent spontaneous miscarriage

The details relating to any previous admission for suspected miscarriage should be reviewed together with the results of histological examination of tissues removed from the uterus. This enables the diagnosis to be substantiated, and differentiated from a simple missed period in the absence of a pregnancy.

Occasionally the history suggests a likely cause. Cervical incompetence, for example, is characterised by painless second trimester fetal loss or premature labour. The cervix may feel open, and examination show bulging fetal membranes coming through the os.

Investigation of recurrent spontaneous miscarriage

In most cases of recurrent spontaneous miscarriage, clinical examination and investigations are normal.

Table 19 Recurrent spontaneous miscarriage

Investigation	Condition detected
Parental karyotyping	Chromosome abnormality
Vaginal pH	Bacterial vaginosis
Hysterosalpingogram	Uterine anatomical abnormality
Lupus anticoagulant	Thrombophilic defect
Anticardiolipin antibody	
Activated protein C resistance	
Pelvic ultrasound scan	Polycystic ovary syndrome
Day 5 serum LH/FSH	Hypersecretion of LH

However, the investigations set out in Table 19 should be considered.

Treatment of recurrent spontaneous miscarriage

When no cause can be identified the doctor should adopt a sensitive and supporting manner, and an early ultrasound scan in any future pregnancy should be offered. Advice should be given regarding periconceptual folic acid supplementation, and on general measures to improve health such as reducing smoking. The need for continuation of any medications should be reviewed. Hormonal support in early pregnancy with progesterone or human chorionic gonadotrophic injections is sometimes used but there is no evidence of any benefit other than a placebo effect.

Specific measures for specific abnormalities may be indicated (Table 20). Paternal translocations may be associated with a high-risk of affecting future pregnancies. In this situation, artificial insemination using donor sperm is an option. Cervical cerclage is the treatment for cervical incompetence. In this procedure a pursestring suture is placed high in the cervix to help maintain the integrity of the os. Patients with circulating antiphospholipid antibodies may be treated using a combination of low dose aspirin and corticosteroids. The significance of an anatomical abnormality of the uterus should be interpreted with caution in relation to recurrent miscarriage. Successful pregnancy outcome without treatment is common, and corrective surgery is not always helpful. If all other causes have been excluded, hysteroscopic resection of a uterine septum or submucous fibroid may

Table 20 Recurrent spontaneous miscarriage: some causes and treatments

Abnormality	Treatment
Cervical incompetence	Cervical cerclage
Antiphospholipid AB syndrome	Aspirin, ± heparin
Bacterial vaginosis	Metronidazole
Fibroids, uterine septum	Hysteroscopic surgery

sometimes be undertaken. The operation of metroplasty to correct a septate uterus has now been largely replaced by hysteroscopic techniques.

16.7 Ectopic pregnancy

Learning objectives

You should understand:

- why and how ectopic pregnancy remains a cause of maternal death
- why tubal damage is a risk factor for ectopic pregnancy
- how to interpret serial measurements of serum hCG
- why ectopic pregnancy can be managed in a variety of ways
- the implications of an ectopic pregnancy to future fertility

An ectopic pregnancy is one that develops outside the uterus. The vast majority (98%) occur in the fallopian tube, but the ovary, cervix and peritoneal cavity are rare sites. The incidence is 1:150 pregnancies, and this has risen four-fold over the last 20 years.

The significance of ectopic pregnancy is that it is a potentially lethal condition. The most recent confidential enquiry into maternal deaths in the UK reported 19 deaths over a 3-year period which were directly attributable to ectopic pregnancy. Death usually occurred from a combination of diagnostic delay followed by intraperitoneal bleeding and tubal rupture. A diagnosis of ectopic pregnancy should therefore be considered in any woman of reproductive age who presents with abdominal pain.

Aetiology

Previous tubal infection may result in interference with tubal transport mechanisms, because of destruction of the cilial lining and the formation of intratubal adhesions. This increases the chances of the fertilised ovum implanting in the tube rather than the uterus. Any condition causing tubal narrowing will similarly predispose towards ectopic pregnancy. Reversal of sterilisation, tubal endometriosis and tubal polyps are typical examples. The intra-uterine device does not confer protection against ectopic pregnancy, so a high percentage of pregnancies conceived with the device in situ will be ectopic.

Risk factors for ectopic pregnancy include:

- previous ectopic pregnancy
- pelvic inflammatory disease
- tubal surgery
- intra-uterine device
- infertility

- assisted conception techniques such as in vitro fertilisation (IVF) and gamete intra-fallopian transfer (GIFT).

Clinical features

The classical presentation is with abdominal pain, amenorrhoea and vaginal bleeding. Pain usually precedes the bleeding, and results from distension of the fallopian tube by the enlarging pregnancy. If blood leaks into the peritoneal cavity to cause a haemoperitoneum, the pain increases. Shoulder tip pain results from diaphragmatic irritation by blood tracking up the paracolic gutters. Vaginal bleeding is characteristically dark red in colour, and slight.

The typical examination findings are abdominal guarding, cervical excitation and a tender adnexal mass. If the ectopic has ruptured there may be signs of circulatory collapse.

A significant proportion of cases do not present with this classical picture, and the symptoms may easily be mistaken for those of an inevitable miscarriage. A history of amenorrhoea is not always present and the woman may have no suspicion of being pregnant.

Diagnosis

A high index of suspicion is therefore required in any woman with abdominal pain. A sensitive pregnancy test will nearly always be positive but this does not give the location of the pregnancy. Ultrasound examination is only rarely diagnostic, but can nevertheless be useful, particularly in association with serial serum HCG levels. If the pregnancy is intra-uterine, HCG levels double every 48 hours, and it should be visible on USS when the level reaches 6000 IU/L. If a viable intra-uterine pregnancy is seen it makes the possibility of an ectopic pregnancy most unlikely, as the two conditions only rarely coexist. Occasionally, fetal cardiac activity can be demonstrated in the adnexal region, and this is highly suggestive of an ectopic pregnancy. Laparoscopy remains the cornerstone for diagnosis, and is also being increasingly used in the treatment of ectopic pregnancy.

Treatment

Surgery

Patients with ruptured ectopic pregnancy exhibiting signs of shock require immediate resuscitation and urgent laparotomy. All clots and blood are removed from the pelvis, the site of bleeding identified, and the vessels controlled by clamping. The fallopian tube is then excised. Conserving a damaged tube is not recommended because of the high risk of a further ectopic.

In cases where the ectopic has not ruptured it may be possible to perform more conservative surgery, thus preserving the fallopian tube. This is increasingly being performed using laparoscopic techniques because of the considerable advantages in avoiding a laparotomy. However, this requires particular surgical skills and training, and safety must remain the prime consideration. If the surgeon does not have appropriate training in laparoscopic techniques then laparotomy is preferred. In linear salpingotomy a longitudinal incision is made on the antimesenteric border of the tube. The pregnancy is then carefully removed and haemostasis secured using diathermy. The tube is then allowed to heal by secondary intention as surgical closure can result in subsequent narrowing of the lumen. If the tube is damaged, salpingectomy is preferred. Milking the pregnancy out of the fimbrial end of the tube is not recommended because of the risk of persistent trophoblastic tissue causing further bleeding.

The advantages of laparoscopic surgery over laparotomy in treatment of ectopic pregnancy are:

- quicker recovery
- reduced hospital stay
- reduced blood loss
- reduced cost
- fewer adhesions.

Indications for laparotomy in treatment of ectopic pregnancy are:

- ruptured ectopic
- ectopic > 5 cm in diameter
- extensive adhesions
- operator inexperience with laparoscopic surgery.

Non-surgical treatment of ectopic pregnancy

These methods aim to avoid any surgical intervention, and are suitable for small unruptured ectopic pregnancies. Intra-muscular injection of methotrexate causes demise of the pregnancy and thus reduces the need for surgery. Weekly monitoring of serum HCG levels is necessary to confirm that the pregnancy is no longer viable. Rising levels may indicate the pregnancy is still enlarging and are an indication for consideration of surgery.

The disadvantage of conservative treatment is the ongoing small risk of tubal rupture, and the requirement for prolonged surveillance and hospital stay.

Future fertility after ectopic pregnancy

Fertility is reduced following an ectopic pregnancy, largely as a result of tubal damage. Subsequent fertility rates appear to be the same whether salpingotomy or salpingectomy has been performed. The outlook is most favourable in women who have had a previous term pregnancy. In nulliparous women the subsequent intra-uterine pregnancy rate is only 40%. There is a 15% chance that any future pregnancy will be ectopic.

Self-assessment: questions

Multiple choice questions

1. Which of the following are associated with early pregnancy loss?
   a. Sexual intercourse
   b. Wart virus infection
   c. Malaria
   d. Intra-uterine pregnancy with an intra-uterine device in situ
   e. Drinking unpasteurised goat's milk

2. Regarding ectopic pregnancy:
   a. It can always be detected by laparoscopy
   b. It may co-exist with an intra-uterine pregnancy
   c. It cannot survive beyond 16 weeks
   d. It is declining in frequency
   e. The intra-uterine device confers protection against ectopic pregnancy

3. Which of the following are true regarding ectopic pregnancy?
   a. There is an increased chance that a pregnancy occurring in a woman taking the progestogen-only pill will be ectopic
   b. The incidence is reduced in depo-progestogen contraceptive users
   c. There is an increased risk following reversal of sterilisation
   d. There is an increased risk with bilateral tubal occlusion
   e. There is an increased risk in low-dose oral contraceptive users

4. A 28-year-old woman is readmitted with pain and bleeding 10 days following evacuation of the uterus after an incomplete miscarriage. Which of the following are true?
   a. She should be given anti-D if she is Rhesus negative
   b. Clinical examination is more useful in directing management than ultrasound scan
   c. If the cervix is open, retained products are likely
   d. Antibiotics are indicated
   e. Retained products of conception are more likely than infection

Short notes

1. Describe the likely histological nature of material removed from the uterus at evacuation in:
   a. Incomplete miscarriage
   b. Ectopic pregnancy.

2. The on-call gynaecology house officer is asked to see a young woman because she is 5 days late for her period and has lower abdominal pain. She is wearing an intra-uterine contraceptive device. On examination she has a slight pyrexia, and the uterus is tender with a right-sided adnexal mass. Which investigations are indicated, and why?

3. A 34-year-old woman presents with acute onset of severe, constant, right-sided pelvic pain. Her last period was 6 weeks ago. On examination there is guarding in the right iliac fossa. There is no vaginal bleeding. The uterus feels soft but is not significantly enlarged. A pregnancy test is strongly positive. Select the most likely diagnosis from the list below, and explain why the others are less likely:

   Acute appendicitis
   Ureteric colic;
   Threatened miscarriage
   Bleeding corpus luteum cyst;
   Ectopic pregnancy
   Hydatidiform mole.

   What is the single most useful investigation here?

Case history

A 25-year-old woman presents with 7-weeks amenorrhoea, slight cramping lower abdominal pain and vaginal bleeding. Her menstrual cycle is irregular and she has been trying to conceive. She had a positive home pregnancy test 1 week ago. On examination she is not shocked. The uterus is not enlarged, and the cervical os is closed. There is no pelvic tenderness and there are no adnexal masses on vaginal examination. In hospital a sensitive pregnancy test is repeated, and this is again positive. An ultrasound scan shows no evidence of an intra-uterine pregnancy, and no evidence of any adnexal mass.

1. What is the differential diagnosis?
2. What is the correct management?

OSCE question

Catherine is 24 years old, and Alan, her partner, is 26. They want a family, but all three of Catherine's pregnancies have miscarried at between 6 and 8 weeks gestation. She has been to see a specialist, and asks you the following questions:

1. The specialist told her that if she successfully reaches 12 weeks in her next pregnancy, she has a 95% chance of success. Is this true?

2. Why did the specialist ask her if she had ever had a thrombosis?

3. The specialist said if all the tests are normal, this will be reassuring. Surely there must be a problem that will be identified, to enable treatment?

4. Could she not have a stitch put in her cervix to stop the miscarriages?

5. The specialist wants her husband to have a blood test. What is this for?

Self-assessment: answers

Multiple choice answers

1. a. **False.** There is no evidence that sexual intercourse is associated with early pregnancy loss.
   b. **False.**
   c. **True.** Malaria, along with any other febrile illness, may cause miscarriage.
   d. **True.** If pregnancy occurs with an intra-uterine device there is an increased incidence of both miscarriage and infection.
   e. **True.** Drinking unpasteurised goat's milk carries a risk of brucellosis which is associated with miscarriage.

2. a. **False.** Laparoscopy occasionally fails to detect a very early ectopic pregnancy.
   b. **True.** An ectopic pregnancy may occur simultaneously with an intra-uterine pregnancy. This is called heterotopic pregnancy. It is extremely rare, but becoming more common with the use of assisted conception techniques.
   c. **False.** An abdominal ectopic pregnancy may survive to term, although this is rare.
   d. **False.** The incidence of ectopic pregnancy is increasing, mainly due to the increase in pelvic inflammatory disease, assisted conception techniques and earlier diagnosis.
   e. **False.** The intra-uterine device does not confer protection against ectopic pregnancy, so a relatively high percentage of pregnancies conceived with this method are ectopic in location.

3. a. **True.** There is an increased likelihood that a pregnancy conceived whilst using the progestogen-only pill will be ectopic. The contraceptive mode of action is mainly via an effect on cervical mucus, but tubal motility is also reduced. Ovulation is not reliably inhibited, so if fertilisation does take place implantation may occur in the tube.
   b. **True.** Depo-progestogen contraception inhibits ovulation and so reduces the risk of ectopic pregnancy.
   c. **True.** Reversal of sterilisation may result in a patent tube which is narrowed, thus increasing the risk of ectopic pregnancy.
   d. **False.** If the fallopian tubes are occluded, as a result of sterilisation, the chances of any type of pregnancy are greatly reduced. However, in the rare situation when pregnancy does occur after bilateral tubal occlusion, it may be ectopic in location.
   e. **False.** The combined oral contraceptive pill greatly reduces the incidence of ectopic pregnancy as ovulation is inhibited.

4. a. **False.** Anti-D should be given to Rhesus negative women within 72 hours of miscarriage.
   b. **True.** The clinical findings are a better guide to management than ultrasound examination.
   c. **True.** A bulky uterus with an open cervix suggest retained products requiring repeat evacuation under antibiotic cover.
   d. **True.** The presence of a fever, offensive vaginal discharge or pelvic tenderness are all suggestive of infection, which requires treatment with antibiotics.
   e. **False.** Infection is more likely than retained products of conception, although the two may coexist.

Short notes answers

1. The differential diagnosis between an aborting intra-uterine pregnancy and an ectopic pregnancy can sometimes be difficult on clinical grounds. Under these circumstances the nature of material obtained from the uterus at evacuation can help to distinguish between these two conditions.
   a. In an incomplete miscarriage remnants of an intra-uterine pregnancy can usually be seen on histological examination. These consist of chorionic villi and trophoblastic tissue.
   b. In ectopic pregnancy, the uterus will not contain any chorionic villi or trophoblastic tissue because the pregnancy is extra-uterine. Instead the endometrium undergoes a marked decidual change under the influence of rising progesterone levels. On clinical grounds only scanty curettings are obtained from the uterus, and a mistaken diagnosis of complete miscarriage is easily made especially if the possibility of an ectopic pregnancy is not entertained. However, the histological appearance is characteristic and is called the Arias Stella phenomenon. This is suggestive of an ectopic pregnancy, and is sometimes the only clue to the diagnosis.

2. A pyrexia in association with uterine tenderness and an intra-uterine device are suggestive of pelvic infection, so a white cell count is indicated. The

delayed period in association with pain and an intra-uterine device means an ectopic pregnancy is also a possibility, so a pregnancy test should be performed. A pelvic ultrasound scan is indicated to help ascertain the nature of the adnexal mass, which an ectopic pregnancy, or an ovarian cyst could be a tubo-ovarian abscess. If diagnostic difficulty persists, laparoscopy is indicated.

3. The most likely diagnosis here is a bleeding corpus luteum cyst. Acute onset of pain is due to peritoneal irritation by blood. The pregnancy test is strongly positive by 6 weeks, but the uterus will not be significantly enlarged. Ectopic pregnancy should also be considered here, even though it is usually accompanied by some vaginal bleeding, and the pain experienced is initially poorly localised due to tubal distension.

   Acute appendicitis begins with vague colicky central abdominal pain which then localises to the right iliac fossa. The pain of ureteric colic comes in waves radiating from the loin to the groin. Threatened miscarriage characterised by vaginal bleeding. Hydatidiform mole usually presents with vaginal bleeding, hyperemesis or early onset pre-eclampsia. The single most useful investigation is pelvic ultrasound.

Case history answer

1. The differential diagnosis rests between threatened miscarriage, complete miscarriage and ectopic pregnancy. In all three, a sensitive pregnancy test may be positive and remain so for several days. By 7 weeks' gestation an intra-uterine pregnancy should be visible on ultrasound scan as evidenced by a gestation sac or fetal cardiac activity. However, in the presence of menstrual irregularity, ovulation does not reliably occur 2 weeks after the last period, so the pregnancy may not be as old as 7 weeks and therefore may be too small to be detected by USS.

2. In this case the patient can be initially managed conservatively without recourse to surgery. Laparoscopy is only indicated if there is severe pain or signs of shock, suggesting intraperitoneal bleeding from an ectopic pregnancy. Diagnosis in

this case can be made using serial serum measurements of human chorionic gonadotrophin (HCG) in combination with a further ultrasound scan in a week. HCG is produced by the trophoblast tissue, and rising levels would indicate a viable pregnancy. If the location is intra-uterine it will become visible on ultrasound scan by the time the HCG level has reached 6000 IU/L. If the scan is still unable to demonstrate an intra-uterine pregnancy with the HCG at this level, an ectopic pregnancy is extremely likely and laparoscopy is then indicated even in the absence of pain. A fall in HCG level would indicate demise of the pregnancy, but not the location – the same pattern may be seen with an aborting intra-uterine pregnancy.

OSCE answer

1. Although 10–15% of all clinically recognised pregnancies miscarry, these mostly occur before 6 weeks gestation, so yes, this is true.

2. Because the antiphospholipid syndrome may be characterised by recurrent miscarriage, thrombosis or even neurological conditions. Pregnancy loss in this condition may relate to uteroplacental thrombosis, and treatment with aspirin and heparin significantly improves the live birth rate.

3. In a proportion of couples, the recurrent episodes of pregnancy loss will remain unexplained, and all the tests will be normal. The prognosis in this situation is good with regard to future pregnancy, and no specific treatment apart from psychological support is necessary.

4. A cervical stitch should only be used for cervical incompetence, which is a rare cause of second trimester miscarriage.

5. This is looking for a chromosomal problem, most commonly a balanced reciprocal or Robertsonian translocation, which will be found in 3–5% of partners presenting with recurrent miscarriage.

17 Gynaecological neoplasia

Overview

Cancers of the ovary, endometrium and cervix are the commonest gynaecological malignancies. They present with a wide variety of symptoms, and early diagnosis remains a challenge, especially in ovarian cancer. Investigation of suspicious symptoms, such as post-menopausal bleeding, will reveal a cause other than gynaecological cancer in the majority of cases.

Pre-cancerous changes in the cells of the cervix are usually present for many years before cancer develops. These pre-cancerous cells can be detected by cervical smear testing, and treatment of them will significantly reduce the chances of a cancer developing. The introduction of cervical screening has been associated with a fall in the incidence of cervical cancer.

Endometrial cancer usually presents with post-menopausal bleeding. Ovarian cancer has a sinister reputation, largely due to an insidious onset and a tendency to produce symptoms only in advanced disease.

17.1 Incidence of gynaecological cancer

Learning objective

You should understand:

- why deaths from ovarian cancer exceed those from both endometrial and cervical cancer combined

Gynaecological cancer develops in 5% of women. Only breast, lung and bowel cancer are more common. The vast majority of gynaecological cancers arise from the ovary, cervix or endometrium (Table 21).

Lifetime incidence of cancer

- Breast   7.1%
- Ovary   1.4%
- Cervix   1.3%
- Endometrium   1.1%

Both the incidence and mortality rates from ovarian cancer have increased over the last 70 years. Deaths from other female genital tract cancers have generally fallen, apart from cervical cancer in young women.

Five-year survival rates in gynaecological cancer

- Ovary   25%
- Cervix   55%
- Endometrium 66%

Table 21 Gynaecological cancer: new cases and deaths per year in the UK

Site of malignancy	New cases per year	Deaths per year
Ovary	5000	4500
Cervix	4400	2200
Endometrium	4400	1100

17.2 Organisation of gynaecological cancer services

Learning objective

You should:

- understand the reasons for the planned changes in the organisation of gynaecological cancer services

The Calman-Hine report, published in 1995, highlighted the need for changes in the organisation of cancer care in England and Wales because of the relatively poor UK survival rates compared with Europe. The National Cancer Guidance on Gynaecological Cancer was published in 1999, and this guidance signalled significant service changes, with recommendations to centralise large components of the management of gynaecological cancers in fewer, larger centres. Below is a summary of the key points:

- Dedicated diagnostic and assessment services should be established in cancer units, to which all women with possible gynaecological cancers should be urgently referred.
- Specialist multi-professional gynaecological cancer teams should be based in cancer centres. These teams should be responsible for the treatment of all women with ovarian cancer and the majority of women with other gynaecological cancers.
- There should be clear local policies for the management of women with advanced or progressive disease, agreed and co-ordinated between centres, units, palliative care and primary care.
- There should be rapid and efficient communication systems for liaison and cross-referral between all levels of service.
- Audit should take place across the entire service delivery network. It is anticipated that such a national initiative, involving significant service re-configuration, will result in an improved quality of care and better survival rates for women with gynaecological cancer.

17.3 Vulval neoplasia

Learning objectives

You should understand:

- why any suspicious vulval lesion requires biopsy
- the role of surgery and radiotherapy in vulval cancer

Benign vulval tumours

Clinical findings

The finding of a lump in the vulva is a cause for anxiety and requires urgent diagnosis. In most cases, however, these lumps are benign tumours or cysts, and these are not serious. The most common is the sebaceous cyst, which arises as a result of blockage of the gland duct. The characteristic appearance is of a painless firm lump attached to the skin. Sebaceous material can sometimes be extruded from the punctum on the skin surface. Sebaceous cysts are prone to infection causing a painful red swelling, which can result in an abscess. A Bartholin's cyst is diagnosed by its characteristic location on the posterior inner aspect of the labium majus.

Management

Any vulval lump of uncertain nature requires diagnostic biopsy. The treatment of benign swellings is dictated by the degree of symptoms and patient preference. An abscess requires drainage. Bartholin's cysts are treated by marsupialisation, which aims to improve the gland drainage. Most small lumps can be treated by simple excision.

Benign vulval swellings
- Sebaceous cyst
- Lipoma
- Bartholin's cyst
- Warts
- Pigmented mole
- Sweat gland tumour.

Non-neoplastic epithelial disorders of vulval skin

These are a characteristic group of skin conditions affecting the vulva. They were previously called vulval dystrophies. They are chronic non-infective conditions of unknown aetiology, which require long-term surveillance because of their relationship with vulval carcinoma. They must be distinguished from generalised dermatoses which may affect the vulval skin, such as psoriasis and eczema.

There are two varieties: lichen sclerosus and squamous cell hyperplasia. Although the cause is unknown, there is an association with autoimmune disorders.

The histological appearance of lichen sclerosus consists of thinning and atrophy of the epidermis with a lymphocytic infiltration of the dermis. Squamous cell hyperplasia shows thickening and hyperkeratosis, with a mixed picture of both atrophy and hyperplasia.

Clinical features

It is usually seen in post-menopausal women, with vulval itching and irritation. Younger women are occasionally affected, when it presents with superficial dyspareunia. The clinical appearance is characteristic. The vulval skin looks thin, white, shiny, and hairless. In severe cases the entire vulva appears atrophic, with shrinkage of the labia minora and narrowing of the vaginal introitus. The affected area may include the perianal and buttock skin.

Management

The diagnosis must first be confirmed by vulval biopsy. If malignancy is suspected, 'mapping' biopsies from representative areas will be necessary. The condition is a chronic one with no satisfactory cure, and treatment is therefore symptomatic. A short course of topical potent corticosteroid ointment such as clobetasol proprionate will usually control symptoms. Following this, a less potent steroid ointment should be used for long-term control. If treatment is unsuccessful, coexisting fungal infection of the skin should be suspected. Surgical excision of the affected areas of skin is rarely effective in improving symptoms and does not prevent recurrence. Long-term follow-up is required because 3% of patients subsequently develop vulval carcinoma.

Vulval intraepithelial neoplasia (VIN)

Vulval intraepithelial neoplasia (VIN) is a condition in which neoplastic cells are present within the boundaries of the surface epithelium. There is no invasive disease, hence the old terminology 'carcinoma in situ'. The vast majority of cases are of the squamous variety.

Classification of VIN

- Squamous VIN
- Non-squamous VIN (e.g. Paget's disease).

Grades of VIN

- VIN I   cellular abnormality involving the lower third of the epithelium
- VIN II   extension of abnormality into the middle third of the epithelium
- VIN III abnormality extending throughout the entire epithelium.

Aetiology

VIN is strongly associated with previous sexually-transmitted infection with the human papillomavirus (HPV). The deoxyribonucleic acid (DNA) genome of the virus has been extracted from the cells in VIN lesions using in situ hybridisation and the polymerase chain reaction technique.

Clinical features

These are diverse and variable. The usual symptoms are pruritus or soreness, but in many cases VIN is incidentally detected following routine gynaecological examination. Affected skin may look thickened or granular, or there may be a distinct warty, pigmented area.

Examination

The entire vulva should be carefully inspected to allow accurate mapping of affected areas. This is best achieved using magnification with a colposcope. Application of a dilute solution of acetic acid to the vulva accentuates the appearance of lesions. This is very variable however, and the diagnosis must always be confirmed by a biopsy. The cervix and vagina also require colposcopic inspection because of the association with intraepithelial neoplasia of the cervix (CIN) and vagina (VAIN).

Treatment

The natural history of VIN lesions is unpredictable, with both regression or progression to invasive carcinoma being possible. Prolonged colposcopic follow-up is therefore required in all cases. Treatment is individualised because of the wide variation in symptoms, extent of disease and risk of progression to invasive cancer. Small areas can be treated by laser ablation provided a biopsy has been taken, whilst larger areas are better treated by excision. The risk of progression is smallest in younger women, many of whom are asymptomatic. Since surgical excision is no guarantee against either recurrence or development of invasion, treatment in young women tends to be more conservative. Women with multifocal lesions, those who are immunosuppressed, and those over the age of 45 years appear to be at highest risk of developing invasive carcinoma. Complete excision with a margin of normal tissue, combined with long-term surveillance is the treatment for this group.

Treatments for VIN

- Observation
- Laser ablation
- Local excision
- Simple vulvectomy
- Topical 5 Fluorouracil
- Topical alpha-interferon gel.

Paget's disease of the vulva

This is a rare form of non-squamous VIN which arises in the vulval skin. The important feature is the association with an underlying adenocarcinoma of apocrine origin in 20% of cases. Treatment is by wide local excision.

Vulval cancer

Vulval cancer accounts for 5% of all gynaecological malignancies. It is largely a disease of elderly women, characterised by late presentation because symptoms are either ignored by the patient or not fully investigated by the doctor. Vulval cancer is rare in young women but the incidence is increasing. Surgery is the mainstay of treatment.

Aetiology

Changes of lichen sclerosus or squamous cell hyperplasia are often found in the surrounding skin, but it is unknown whether the carcinoma arises directly from these. A small percentage of vulval cancer arises as a result of disease progression of VIN in association with human papilloma virus (HPV) infection. This mechanism may account for the small subset of the disease seen in young women. There is an association between vulval carcinoma and both CIN and cervical cancer. The different pathological types are shown in Box 70.

Natural history

These tumours are usually slow-growing. Infiltration of local tissues produces a firm mass, which may involve the vagina, clitoris, urethra or anal margin depending on the primary location. If there has been an entire field change of VIN involving large areas of the vulva there may be more than one primary tumour present. More distant spread occurs by embolisation to the inguinal lymph nodes. This is usually to the nodes on the same side as the lesion, but contralateral nodal spread does occur, especially with large and centrally-located tumours. Later, the pelvic nodes become involved. Distant haematogenous spread to the lungs, liver or bone is rare. The verrucous carcinoma is a particularly slow-growing tumour which rarely spreads to lymph nodes. In contrast, the malignant melanoma is characterised by rapid nodal and distant spread, and has a particularly poor prognosis.

Clinical features

The most common primary site is the labia majora. An indurated ulcer with an irregular margin is characteristic. The woman may complain of pruritus, pain, bleeding, discharge or ulceration. In very elderly women the presentation is sometimes at an advanced stage with a large infected exophytic mass. When lymphatic spread has occurred, a groin mass may be present. Malignant melanoma appears as a raised pigmented lesion. A carcinoma of Bartholin's gland begins as a lump below the surface. The verrucous carcinoma appears as a large warty lesion.

Diagnosis and staging

The diagnosis is confirmed by biopsy. This is performed under general anaesthetic if the patient is fit enough. The size, mobility and degree of fixation of the tumour to surrounding structures must be assessed, with regard to planning of treatment (see Box 71). Multiple biopsies may be required to determine the true extent of the tumour, especially when there is encroachment on to the urethra, anus and vagina. The groin nodes are carefully palpated. If there is evidence of enlargement or fixation, a fine needle aspiration for cytological examination can be performed.

Treatment

Surgery is the cornerstone of treatment for vulval carcinoma. The extent of surgery is dictated by the size, depth

---

Box 70 Pathology of vulval cancer

• **Common**	Squamous cell carcinoma
• **Rare**	Verrucous carcinoma
	Basal cell carcinoma
	Melanoma
	Carcinoma of Bartholin's gland
	Sarcoma
	Urethral carcinoma

Box 71 Vulval carcinoma: staging

Stage I	Tumour confined to vulva and <2 cm diameter. No nodes palpable
Stage II	Tumour confined to vulva but >2 cm diameter. No nodes palpable
Stage III	Tumour extends to lower urethra, vagina, or anus, or to unilateral inguinal nodes
Stage IVa	Tumour involves upper urethra, bladder, rectum, pelvic side wall, or bilateral inguinal nodes
Stage IVb	Distant spread

of invasion, location and histological type of the primary tumour. The aim is to excise all the primary tumour with at least a 1 cm margin of normal skin, and excise the regional lymph nodes when there is a significant risk of tumour involvement. Small tumours of less than 2 cm diameter may be treated by wide local excision, but larger ones will usually require radical vulvectomy in order to obtain adequate local clearance. When the depth of invasion is less than 1 mm the chance of lymph node metastases is small, so groin node dissection is unnecessary. When the depth of invasion exceeds 1 mm, the risks of nodal involvement increase, so surgery should include inguinal and femoral lymphadenectomy. Ipsilateral lymphadenectomy is performed for laterally-placed small tumours, whilst bilateral lymphadenectomy is performed for centrally-placed and large tumours. Radical vulvectomy is an extensive surgical procedure, involving excision of the entire vulval skin including the labia minora, labia majora and clitoris, together with the subcutaneous tissues and a wide margin of normal skin. The groin nodes are usually removed via separate incisions. It is an effective but morbid operation.

Radiotherapy is mainly reserved for nodal disease and local recurrence. If more than three groin nodes are involved, or if the pelvic lymph nodes are involved a course of pelvic radiotherapy is usually given. This gives better results and is less morbid than pelvic lymphadenectomy. Radiotherapy can also be given preoperatively in combination with chemotherapy to reduce the size of large tumours which are encroaching onto the anus or urethra. The aim is to reduce the extent of the subsequent surgery and thus preserve the integrity of the bowel or urinary tract.

Complications of treatment

Wound breakdown and infection are major problems following radical vulvectomy. In this situation, wound healing occurs by secondary intention, over many weeks. The risk of venous thromboembolism is especially high in elderly women, and early mobilisation is therefore desirable. Considerable psychological difficulties may be experienced following such extensive vulval surgery. Careful individual counselling is essential in helping individuals come to terms with the alteration in both appearance and function of the genitalia. Radiotherapy is limited in its application to the vulva, because the skin folds make it difficult to deliver an adequate dose to the primary tumour without causing considerable morbidity to the surrounding skin in terms of discomfort and desquamation.

Prognosis

Survival is related to the stage of disease and in particular the involvement of lymph nodes (see Box 72). If the pelvic nodes are involved the 5-year survival drops to 20%.

Box 72 Vulval carcinoma: prognosis

Stage	5-year survival
I	70%
II	50%
III	32%
IV	13%

Improving the outlook in vulval cancer

- Increased awareness of pruritus as a common presenting symptom
- Urgent biopsy of any suspicious lesion
- Close follow-up of at-risk groups such as those with lichen sclerosus and VIN
- Referral to cancer centres for specialist multidisciplinary team management
- Excision of all tumour with at least 1 cm margin of normal tissue
- Less radical surgery for early disease.

17.4 Vaginal neoplasia

Learning objectives

You should understand:

- the significance of vaginal intraepithelial neoplasia
- the importance of examination under anaesthetic in vaginal cancer

Benign vaginal tumours

These include:

- epidermoid cysts
- condyloma acuminata (warts)
- mesonephric duct remnants
- endometriotic cysts.

Epidermoid cysts

Epidermoid cysts are usually seen as painless swellings at the posterior vaginal fourchette. They are caused by secretions from dermal tissue which has been inadvertently buried during previous episiotomy repair.

Vaginal warts

Vaginal warts result from HPV infection. They are usually an asymptomatic finding in association with vulval warts.

Mesonephric duct cysts

Mesonephric duct cysts are remnants of the Mesonephric duct and are seen as small swellings on the lateral aspect of the vagina. They are rarely noticed by the patient and are only excised if troublesome.

Endometriotic deposits

Tender endometriotic deposits can occur in the rectovaginal septum or in the vaginal vault after hysterectomy.

Vaginal intraepithelial neoplasia (VAIN)

Like VIN, this condition has malignant potential and therefore requires either surveillance or treatment. It is asymptomatic, and usually seen in the upper vagina in association with cervical intraepithelial neoplasia (CIN) at the time of colposcopy. Sometimes VAIN is seen at the vaginal vault following a previous hysterectomy for CIN. It is then particularly difficult to visualise because it becomes buried beneath the vaginal suture line. Treatment is by laser ablation or excision, with the latter being preferred where there is suspicion of invasive change.

Vaginal cancer

Primary vaginal cancer is rare, accounting for just 2% of all gynaecological malignancies. Secondary spread from a primary tumour of the endometrium or cervix is more common. Vulval or rectal carcinoma may rarely spread to involve the vagina.

Pathology of vaginal cancer

- Squamous cell carcinoma
- Clear cell carcinoma
- Embryonal rhabdomyosarcoma (sarcoma botryoides)
- Malignant melanoma.

Squamous cell carcinoma of the vagina
The majority of primary tumours are squamous cell carcinomas. Spread occurs by local invasion and lymphatic permeation, and by embolisation to the inguinal and pelvic nodes.

Clear cell carcinoma of the vagina
Clear cell carcinoma is a rare form of vaginal cancer, seen particularly in young women whose mothers were given stilboestrol during pregnancy to prevent miscarriage.

Embryonal rhabdomyosarcoma
Embryonal rhabdomyosarcoma is a very rare type of vaginal sarcoma seen in young girls. It presents with vaginal bleeding and a grape-like mass. Treatment is with combination chemotherapy. Surgery and radiotherapy are reserved for advanced disease. The 5-year survival is 80%.

Vaginal cancer: clinical features

Most vaginal cancers present in elderly women with post-menopausal bleeding and discharge. The most common site is in the upper posterior third of the vagina. Examination reveals either an ulcer or a polypoid mass.

Diagnosis and staging

Examination and biopsy are performed under general anaesthetic, when tumour size and mobility are more easily assessed (Box 73). Cystoscopy and sigmoidoscopy are used to examine for evidence of bladder or rectal involvement. Computerised tomography is useful to identify nodal spread.

Treatment

Radiotherapy is the preferred method of treatment for vaginal carcinoma. This consists of brachytherapy directed to the primary tumour and external beam pelvic radiotherapy to the regional lymph nodes. An intravaginal template is often used for brachytherapy, through which iridium wires are afterloaded and implanted directly into the tumour.

Box 73 Vaginal cancer: staging

- Stage I   Tumour confined to vaginal wall
- Stage II   Tumour involves subvaginal tissues, but not pelvic side wall
- Stage III   Tumour extends to pelvic side wall
- Stage IV   Tumour involves bladder or rectum, or has extended outside the pelvis

Box 74	Vaginal carcinoma: survival

Stage	5-year survival
I	70%
II	45%
III	30%
IV	10%

Survival

This depends on stage (see Box 74).

17.5 Cervical neoplasia

Learning objectives

You should understand:

- how the natural history of cervical neoplasia makes it suitable for screening
- how to explain the benefits of cervical screening to a woman
- which women are at greatest risk of cervical cancer
- the importance of accurate staging in cervical cancer
- how the outlook in cervical cancer can be improved

Cancer of the cervix is usually preceded by a pre-invasive stage called cervical intraepithelial neoplasia (CIN). CIN takes up to 20 years to progress to invasive cancer. This presents an opportunity for detection of the disease at an early stage in the natural history, before it becomes invasive, and when a simple and curative treatment is possible. This is the theory on which cervical screening is based. In order to understand how neoplasia develops it is first necessary to see what happens in the normal cervix under the effects of oestrogen.

The normal cervix

The vagina and ectocervix are lined by squamous epithelium. The endocervix is lined by columnar epithelium, containing mucus-secreting crypts. These two epithelia meet at the squamocolumnar junction. Before puberty and after the menopause, the squamocolumnar junction is situated inside the cervical canal (Fig. 27A), and is not visible on vaginal examination. At puberty, the lips of the cervix enlarge and evert, which results in the squamocolumnar junction being carried out onto the vaginal portion of the cervix (Fig. 27B). The columnar epithelium is then visible on the ectocervix as a red, vascular area, often erroneously referred to as an erosion. After the menopause, as a result of falling oestrogen levels, the squamocolumnar junction retreats to within the confines of the endocervical canal.

When the columnar epithelium on the ectocervix becomes exposed to the vaginal environment, it is gradually replaced by squamous epithelium. This process is called squamous metaplasia. The underlying crypts continue to secrete mucus through gland openings in the metaplastic squamous epithelium. These gland openings have a tendency to become blocked, which results in a mucus retention cyst. These cysts are often visible as smooth swellings on the ectocervix, called Nabothian follicles.

The area on the cervix which undergoes metaplasia from columnar to squamous epithelium is called the transformation zone. This is the area where cervical smears should be taken from, as it is here that both CIN and cervical cancers originate.

Cervical intraepithelial neoplasia

Disruption of the normal metaplastic process results in squamous neoplasia. In the early stages, this is confined to within the surface epithelium, and it is called cervical intraepithelial neoplasia. CIN consists of disordered maturation of the cells of the epithelium, characterised by increased numbers of mitoses, and an increased nuclear to cytoplasmic ratio. The change to invasion occurs when the neoplastic cells extend below the basement membrane.

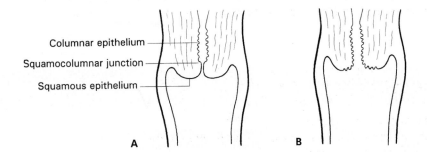

Columnar epithelium
Squamocolumnar junction
Squamous epithelium

A   B

Fig. 27 (A) Before puberty and after menopause, the squamocolumnar junction is situated inside the cervical canal. **(B)** At puberty, the squamocolumnar junction is carried out onto the vaginal portion of the cervix.

Natural history of CIN

The grades of CIN are stages in a continuous process from the smallest CIN I lesion through to invasive cancer (see Box 75). The exact rate and incidence of this progression is not known, but there is evidence to suggest that approximately 30% of CIN III lesions will eventually progress to cancer. Many other cases of CIN will either not progress or undergo regression if left untreated. The time taken for invasion to develop appears to be variable. The peak incidence for CIN is between 30 and 40 years of age, whilst for carcinoma of the cervix it is 50 years. This would suggest the timescale is of the order of 15 years on average (see Box 76).

Aetiology of cervical neoplasia

Both CIN and cervical cancer are closely related to sexual activity. Known risk factors include an early age at first intercourse, multiple sexual partners, and smoking. Cervical cancer is rare amongst virgins. There is increasing evidence that the human papillomavirus (HPV) plays a central role in the aetiology, with DNA from HPV types 16 and 18 having been identified in both cervical cancer tissues and in CIN.

Risk factors for cancer of the cervix

These are:

- early age at first intercourse
- multiple sexual partners
- sexually transmitted disease
- smoking
- low socioeconomic status.

Cervical screening

Following the introduction of a National Cervical Screening Programme all sexually active women between the ages of 20 and 64 years are invited to attend for a cervical smear on a 3-yearly basis. The smear aims to detect CIN, and thus allow treatment before a cancer develops. Although treatment of CIN reduces the incidence of cervical cancer amongst women who are screened, a major problem is that those women most at risk of cancer tend not to come for their smears. This may explain why there has been only a small reduction in the overall incidence of cervical cancer in this country despite the widespread availability of screening. It could be argued that screening has prevented a rise in cancer rates, as there has been a large increase in the reported incidence of CIN.

How to take a cervical smear

The cervix is exposed and inspected using a Cusco's vaginal speculum. The smear is taken from the squamocolumnar junction by scraping it with a wooden spatula, rotating it through 360 degrees, making sure that the whole area is sampled. The squamocolumnar junction is

---

Box 75 CIN: grades

- CIN I — Neoplastic changes are confined to the lowest layers of the epithelium
- CIN II — Neoplastic changes extend to middle third of epithelium
- CIN III — Neoplastic changes extend throughout entire thickness of epithelium

---

Box 76 CIN: natural history

Normal events
Squamous epithelium → columnar epithelium → squamous metaplasia

Abnormal events (progression over 15 years)
Squamous metaplasia → CIN I → CIN II → CIN III → early invasive → invasive cancer

---

Box 77 Unsatisfactory cervical smears

Cause	Remedy
Inadequate cells present for diagnosis	Repeat, using firmer pressure
Cells obscured by blood	Repeat, in between periods
Cells poorly fixed	Repeat, and fix slide immediately
Slide incorrectly labelled	Repeat, and label slide correctly using a pencil

usually situated on the ectocervix, and can be recognised by where the colour changes from red in the centre of the cervix to pink at the periphery. The cells obtained are spread thinly onto the surface of a microscope slide and fixed using alcohol. They are then examined under a microscope for evidence of dyskaryosis. Dyskaryosis is a cytological term used to describe cells compatible with origin from CIN. All women having a smear must be informed of the result, even if it is normal, as screening causes considerable anxiety. To obtain maximum benefit and to avoid the need for repeat testing it is essential that the smear is taken properly and by a suitably trained person (Box 76). Recent developments in cervical screening are currently being trialed to see if they can provide improvements. HPV testing of women with smears showing borderline nuclear change or mild dyskaryosis may enable identification of those at highest risk of developing cervical cancer. Liquid based cytology may reduce the number of false negative test results as well as the number of inadequate specimens.

The abnormal smear

5% of smears are reported as abnormal. The different abnormalities are graded in a similar manner to CIN. Dyskaryotic cells are characterised by a larger nucleus and increased nuclear to cytoplasmic ratio. It is important to emphasise that dyskaryosis is a cytological diagnosis, made on the appearance of individual cells. By contrast, CIN is a pathological diagnosis that can only be made by histological examination of a biopsy. Cytology is a reliable but not infallible indicator of cervical pathology, and as such should never be used as the sole diagnostic test of either CIN or invasive cancer, as both false negative and false positive smear results can occur (Box 78).

Management of the abnormal smear

All women with dyskaryotic smears require investigation by colposcopy as soon as possible (Box 79). If local resources do not permit such a policy, referral of women with mildly dyskaryotic smears can be deferred whilst the smear is repeated every 6 months. If the smear reverts back to normal on two successive occasions the woman can re-enter the routine screening programme, but if mild dyskaryosis persists then referral for colposcopy is indicated.

Colposcopy

The colposcope allows examination of the cervix and vagina with binocular magnification and a strong light source. This gives information regarding the nature, size and location of any abnormality. The patient sits in a couch in the lithotomy position, with legs supported in stirrups. A bimanual examination is done in order to feel the cervix, and detect any pelvic masses. The cervix is

Box 78 Abnormal smears: interpretation

Report	Explanation
Inflammatory change	Probable vaginal infection or intra-uterine device present
Koilocytosis/HPV changes	Empty-looking cells seen in association with HPV infection
Borderline nuclear change	Minor nuclear abnormalities, not amounting to dyskaryosis
Mild dyskaryosis	Compatible with a CIN I lesion. (Risk of CIN II/III = 30–50%)
Moderate dyskaryosis	Compatible with a CIN II lesion. (Risk of CIN II/III = 50–70%)
Severe dyskaryosis	Compatible with a CIN III lesion. (Risk of CIN II/III = 80–90%)
Malignant cells	Compatible with invasive carcinoma

Box 79 Abnormal smears: management

Cytology	Management
Unsatisfactory	Repeat smear
Negative	Routine recall in 3 years
Borderline nuclear change	Repeat in 6 months, treat any infection. Refer for colposcopy if it persists
Mild dyskaryosis	Refer for colposcopy
Moderate dyskaryosis	Refer for colposcopy
Severe dyskaryosis	Refer for urgent colposcopy

then exposed using a Cusco's speculum. A smear is taken if necessary, and the appearance of the cervix is observed under magnification. Particular note is taken of the appearance of any blood vessels. Dilute acetic acid is then applied, which stains abnormal epithelium white. The degree of acetowhite change, the size of the area and the vascular pattern of the underlying capillaries allow any CIN to be graded. Lugol's iodine may also be used as a stain to differentiate between normal and abnormal epithelium. Punch biopsies can be taken for histological confirmation of any colposcopic abnormalities.

Indications for colposcopy
- Abnormal cervical smear
- Suspicious clinical appearance of cervix
- Persistent unexplained abnormal bleeding, such as post-coital or intermenstrual bleeding
- Genital warts.

Treatment of CIN

All cases of CIN II and III should be treated. Treatment of CIN I can be delayed for 6 months following colposcopic assessment, as a significant proportion will undergo spontaneous regression. Treatment of CIN can be by ablation or excision. Excision has the advantage that the entire lesion can be sent for histological examination, whereas ablation destroys the abnormal area and relies on the smaller punch biopsy for histology, which is not always representative. Furthermore, a small percentage of colposcopically diagnosed CIN III lesions will show unsuspected invasive change on histology, which would not be detected if the lesion had been ablated. Excision is most easily performed using a wire loop diathermy. The laser is an alternative tool but is more time-consuming. These treatments are usually performed as out patient procedures under local anaesthetic, and have few complications. Large lesions may require treatment under general anaesthetic. Knife cone biopsy is indicated when the lesion extends out of sight up the endocervical canal, when a central cone of tissue is excised, containing the entire transformation zone. Unlike the loop and laser, knife cone biopsy produces no thermal tissue damage, which allows easier histological interpretation. Vaginal hysterectomy is considered when there are additional indications such as menorrhagia, or when CIN extends onto the vagina.

Treatment modalities for CIN
- Wire loop excision
- Laser excision or ablation
- Cold coagulation
- Diathermy
- Cryotherapy

- Cone biopsy
- Hysterectomy.

Healing takes between 4 and 6 weeks after treatment, during which time there is a variable amount of bleeding and discharge. If bleeding is heavy, suturing may be required. Rare complications include cervical stenosis causing painful or absent menstruation, and cervical incompetence.

Follow-up after treatment for CIN

95% of women are successfully cured of CIN by one single treatment. Follow-up is essential to detect the 5% who are not. A check colposcopy and smear 4–6 months after treatment is followed by annual smears for 5 years. If these tests are all normal, the woman re-enters the 3-yearly screening programme. A persistently abnormal smear after treatment usually indicates inadequate primary treatment rather than recurrent disease.

Carcinoma of the cervix

Cervical cancer is the second most common female cancer worldwide. The main risk factor is infection with the sexually transmitted HPV. It is a disease of developing countries, and of sexually active women. In the UK the overall incidence of cervical cancer is falling, although this trend is not seen in young women. The aetiology is the same as for pre-invasive disease of the cervix. Squamous carcinoma accounts for 90% with adenocarcinoma making up most of the rest. Primary lymphoma and sarcoma of the cervix are very rare.

Cervical carcinoma: natural history

The majority of cervical cancers arise as a result of progression of CIN. In the earliest stages, tiny prongs of malignant cells are seen to be invading below the basement membrane from within an area of CIN III. Unchecked growth results in the tumour becoming visible and palpable on the cervix. Later the upper vagina and paracervical tissues become infiltrated. This can result in ureteric obstruction, a common cause of death from cervical cancer. Tumour may extend anteriorly into the bladder causing a vesicovaginal fistula, or posteriorly into the rectum. Lymphatic spread occurs to the pelvic and then to the para-aortic nodes. Haematogenous spread is rare.

Clinical features

CIN is asymptomatic, and is usually detected by cervical screening. Symptoms of invasive cancer (see Box 80) occur when the tumour erodes into blood vessels or becomes infected.

Box 80 Symptoms of cervical cancer

Early	Late
• Post-coital bleeding	• Pelvic pain
• Intermenstrual bleeding	• Leg pain
• Post-menopausal bleeding	• Urinary leakage
• Vaginal discharge	• Uraemic coma

Most of the tumours are on the ectocervix, when they are visible on speculum examination, appearing as a necrotic ulcer or a raised polypoid lesion. Tumours arising from the endocervix are more difficult to recognise as they arise from within the cervical canal. They tend to grow and expand the cervix into a barrel shape.

Diagnosis and staging

Any women with persistent irregular vaginal bleeding should be investigated by bimanual and speculum examination, and a cervical smear. Any suspicious nodules or ulcers on the cervix should be referred for immediate biopsy. When a carcinoma is suspected or confirmed on a biopsy, staging under anaesthetic is carried out (Box 81). This is to allow the extent of disease to be estimated with a view to planning the most appropriate treatment. Abdominal, pelvic and rectal examination is performed, and a representative biopsy taken from the lesion on the cervix. A cystoscopy is performed to exclude bladder involvement. If the tumour appears confined to the cervix, this is stage I disease. Treatment is then equally successful using either surgery or radiotherapy. Careful assessment as to whether or not the tumour has invaded the parametrium is most important, as if it has, radiotherapy is preferred to surgery. Computerised tomography (CT) or magnetic resonance imaging (MRI) is used to identify both parametrial and pelvic lymph node involvement. An intravenous urogram may be performed to assess any ureteric obstruction by tumour.

Treatment

Superficial invasive cervical carcinoma (stage Ia)

The term 'microinvasive carcinoma of the cervix', although still extensively used, was replaced by the term 'superficial invasive cervical carcinoma' in 1995. Superficial invasive carcinoma is defined by a depth of tumour invasion not exceeding 5 mm and a width not exceeding 7 mm. The diagnosis is made by measurement on histological examination of the specimen after it has been excised. There are usually no symptoms, and the disease is picked up on screening. Colposcopy may reveal atypical blood vessels, surface irregularities, or extensive acetowhite change. If the depth of invasion is less than 3 mm (stage Iai), the risk of pelvic node metastases is extremely low. Cone biopsy is therefore sufficient treatment. If invasion exceeds 3 mm depth, more extensive treatment is required because of the higher risk of parametrial and nodal spread. This is usually by radical hysterectomy and bilateral pelvic lymphadenectomy. The prognosis is excellent, but close follow-up is required.

Invasive cervical cancer

For stage Ib disease treatment is either by surgery or radiotherapy (Box 82). The survival is the same for each modality, but surgery is preferable in young women with small stage I tumours because ovarian function can be preserved.

Surgery consists of radical hysterectomy and bilateral pelvic lymphadenectomy. The uterus, upper third of the vagina and parametria are excised en bloc after mobilisation and lateral reflection of the ureters. The pelvic lymph nodes are excised from where they sit alongside the major vessels of the pelvic side wall. If the lymph nodes are found to contain tumour, post-operative radiotherapy may be given to reduce the risk of pelvic recurrence.

Radiotherapy is preferred to surgery in older women and in those with larger tumours who are at higher risk

---

Box 81 Cervical carcinoma: staging

Stage	Features	
0	Pre-invasive disease (CIN)	
Ia	Superficial invasive cervical carcinoma (microinvasion)	Iai: up to 3 mm depth, <7 mm wide
		Iaii: depth 3–5 mm, <7 mm wide
Ib	Carcinoma confined to cervix	Ibi <4 cm in size
		Ibii >4 cm in size
IIa	Carcinoma extends onto upper vagina	
IIb	Carcinoma extends into parametrium, but does not reach pelvic side wall	
IIIa	Carcinoma extends onto lower vagina	
IIIb	Carcinoma extends to the pelvic side wall or causes ureteric obstruction	
IVa	Carcinoma involves bladder or rectum	
IVb	Distant blood-borne spread	

Box 82 Invasive cervical cancer treatment

Advantages of surgery
- Preservation of ovarian function
- Prognostic information from histology
- Easier to detect recurrent disease

Complications of surgery
- Infection
- Bladder or ureteric injury
- Post-operative voiding problems
- Lymphocyst
- Thromboembolism

Advantages of radiotherapy
- Better tolerated by older women
- Major surgery avoided
- Useful in advanced disease

Complications of radiotherapy
- Vaginal stenosis
- Haematuria
- Dysuria
- Diarrhoea

of having pelvic lymph node metastases. External radiation is given in fractionated doses to the whole pelvis over 5 weeks. Brachytherapy is then given to the cervix and parametria, usually via catheters placed under general anaesthetic in the cervical canal and lateral vaginal fornices, into which radioactive sources are later placed. Such delayed placement of the radioactive source into the patient is called afterloading. It reduces radiation leakage and contamination.

Advanced and recurrent disease

Advanced disease is treated mainly by radiotherapy. However, recent studies suggest that women with advanced or bulky disease who are fit enough should be considered for chemotherapy using cisplatin, given concurrently with radiotherapy. The commonest site for disease recurrence is in the pelvis. This is isolated and centrally placed, anterior pelvic exenteration may cure the patient. This involves total cystectomy and urinary diversion by means of an ileal conduit. By contrast, pelvic side wall recurrence is usually not curable. This presents with pain, leg swelling and ureteric obstruction. Ureteric stenting or nephrostomy is occasionally of benefit whilst radiotherapy is given, but survival is limited. Death results from uraemia or cachexia.

Survival

Tumour volume and stage at presentation are the most important prognostic factors. See Box 83.

Box 83 Cervical carcinoma: 5-year survival by stage

Stage	5-year survival
I	80%
II	50%
III	30%
IV	5%

Improving the outlook in cervical cancer

- Management by specialist multidisciplinary teams working in cancer centres
- Increase cervical screening coverage amongst sexually active women over 20 years of age
- Improve follow-up after treatment for CIN
- Ensure cervix is fully visualised when smear is taken
- Reduce the percentage of unsatisfactory smears by improving smear-taking techniques
- Investigate intermenstrual and post-coital bleeding even if smear result is normal
- Develop improved methods of screening the cervix
- Develop HPV vaccine.

17.6 Uterine neoplasia

Learning objectives

You should understand:

- the mechanisms by which fibroids may cause symptoms
- the significance of post-menopausal bleeding
- the different way in which trophoblastic disease may present

Benign uterine tumours include fibroids and endometrial polyps.

Fibroids

Fibroids are the most common uterine tumours. They are benign smooth muscle tumours called leiomyomas, which arise from the myometrium. They vary in size from small seedlings to large masses, and are frequently multiple. They are sensitive to ovarian hormones, tending to grow in pregnancy and regress after the

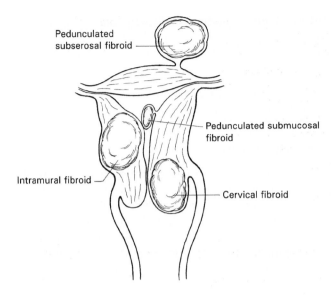

Fig. 28 Uterine fibroids.

menopause. In old age they may become calcified. Most fibroids are intramural in position, but they may also be subserous or submucous (see Fig. 28).

Symptoms

Most fibroids do not cause any symptoms, in which case they do not require treatment. When they do it is usually as a result of their size or location (Box 84). Acute accidents, degeneration and malignant change are all rare.

Fibroids which enlarge or distort the uterine cavity may cause menorrhagia and anaemia. Very heavy bleeding occasionally occurs with pedunculated submucous fibroids. As with any large pelvic tumour the woman may experience pelvic pain, or feel a mass. Frequency of micturition results from pressure on the bladder. Malignant change to a leiomyosarcoma is extremely rare but should be suspected if there is rapid enlargement. Severe pain usually indicates an acute accident such as torsion of a pedunculated fibroid resulting in strangulation. Degeneration of uterine fibroids occurs in pregnancy, as a result of rapid growth under the effects of oestrogen, and outstripping the blood supply. Painful infarction occurs, then a localised tender mass becomes palpable. The process is called red degeneration. A large

---

Box 84 Fibroids: symptoms

Common	Rare
• Menorrhagia	• Infertility
• Abdominal swelling	• Miscarriage
• Frequency of micturition	
• Pain	

---

fibroid situated in the cervix may obstruct labour, but this is a rare occurrence. Finally, submucosal fibroids which distort the endometrial cavity are a potential cause of infertility and miscarriage, due to interference with the process of implantation.

Treatment

Any large pelvic mass of uncertain nature requires removal to exclude malignancy and relieve pressure symptoms, providing the woman is fit to undergo surgery. Smaller uterine fibroids only require treatment if symptomatic. Heavy or prolonged bleeding unresponsive to hormonal therapy is the most troublesome symptom.

Surgical removal by myomectomy or total hysterectomy is the treatment of choice in this situation. Hysterectomy is generally preferred for patients over the age of 40 years.

Myomectomy is used when the patient wishes to preserve her uterus or fertility. This can be achieved abdominally, laparoscopically or vaginally, depending on the size and position of the fibroids and the particular skills of the surgeon. Myomectomy involves enucleation of fibroids from the uterus. It can be a more difficult operation than hysterectomy if there are many fibroids present, and blood loss can be heavy. Furthermore, the fibroids may recur. Prior to myomectomy, pre-operative treatment with LHRH agonists is sometimes used to bring about shrinkage of fibroids and a reduction in vascularity, so allowing easier removal. Submucosal fibroids can be treated by transcervical resection, allowing the uterus to be conserved. A recently developed alternative treatment for symptomatic uterine fibroids is trans-arterial embolisation. Success rates of between 80 and 100% have been claimed, in terms of improvement in menorrhagia, pain and pressure symptoms.

Endometrial polyps

Endometrial polyps are benign adenomas consisting of endometrium with underlying stroma. They are often pedunculated and are seen as small red fleshy tumours protruding through the cervix. They may be found in association with heavy or intermenstrual bleeding, but most are asymptomatic. All polyps should be removed and sent for histological examination to exclude malignancy.

Endometrial hyperplasia

Simple hyperplasia (cystic glandular hyperplasia)

Simple hyperplasia describes the histological appearance of the endometrium which occurs secondary to unopposed oestrogen stimulation. It is associated with heavy irregular vaginal bleeding, and is treated with cyclical progestogen therapy.

Atypical hyperplasia

The aetiology of atypical hyperplasia is the same as for simple hyperplasia, but atypical hyperplasia has the capacity to progress to endometrial carcinoma. The risk is of the order of 20% over 10 years. In young women the atypia may be reversed with progestogen therapy, but follow-up with regular endometrial sampling is essential. The remainder are treated by hysterectomy.

Malignant tumours of the uterus

These are listed in Box 85.

Endometrial carcinoma

Endometrial carcinoma is a disease of post-menopausal women. The median age of presentation is 60 years, and it is rarely seen below the age of 40 years. It usually presents with post-menopausal bleeding. It has a better prognosis than both cervical and ovarian cancer. However, 25% of women with endometrial cancer still die within 5 years of diagnosis.

Aetiology

Most of the risk factors for endometrial carcinoma relate to excessive oestrogen stimulation of the endometrium. Examples include obesity, whereby excessive endogenous oestrogen production occurs, due to an increased conversion of androstenedione to oestrone in peripheral fat, and with the rare oestrogen-secreting granulosa-cell tumour of the ovary. Giving exogenous unopposed oestrogen therapy increases the risk of endometrial carcinoma but this practice has now virtually ceased. Long-term therapy with tamoxifen has been associated with an increased incidence of endometrial carcinoma, probably due to the weak oestrogenic properties of this drug.

> **Box 85** Malignant tumours of the uterus
>
> | **Common** | **Rare** |
> | --- | --- |
> | • Endometrial carcinoma | • Leiomyosarcoma |
> | | • Endometrial stromal sarcoma |
> | | • Mixed mesodermal tumour |
> | | • Gestational trophoblastic disease |

Risk factors for endometrial carcinoma

- Obesity
- Nulliparity
- Late menopause
- Unopposed oestrogen stimulation
- Diabetes mellitus.

Natural history

The tumour starts in the endometrium, but soon grows to occupy the endometrial cavity and may spread to involve the cervix or fallopian tubes. It invades the myometrium and may penetrate through to the peritoneal surface of the uterus and so invade other pelvic organs. Lymphatic spread occurs to the pelvic, para-aortic, and rarely the inguinal lymph nodes. Haematogenous spread to the lungs is a late feature.

Clinical features

Symptoms of primary disease

Post-menopausal bleeding is the most common presentation. The urgent investigation of this symptom by transvaginal ultrasound and endometrial biopsy provides an opportunity for early diagnosis. Many hospitals have dedicated rapid assessment out-patient clinics for post-menopausal bleeding. Pre-menopausal women with endometrial cancer are less commonly seen. They may experience intermenstrual bleeding, or occasionally just heavier menstrual periods making diagnosis more difficult. Occasionally the tumour obstructs the endocervical canal, causing the uterus to distend with blood and secretions. When this becomes infected it is called a pyometra. This presents with an offensive, bloodstained vaginal discharge.

Symptoms of secondary disease

Secondary disease symptoms are rarely the presenting symptoms, and usually signify disease recurrence sometimes following treatment. See Box 86.

Diagnosis and staging

The tumour is usually confined to the uterus at presentation. Examination occasionally reveals uterine enlarge-

> **Box 86** Endometrial carcinoma: secondary disease
>
> | **Symptom** | **Cause** |
> | --- | --- |
> | • Vaginal bleeding | Vaginal metastasis |
> | • Shortness of breath | Pulmonary metastases |
> | • Abdominal pain | Enlarged para-aortic lymph nodes |

ment. Pelvic ultrasound may show increased endometrial thickness. Friable malignant-looking tissue is obtained from the uterine cavity at dilatation and curettage or hysteroscopy, and the diagnosis is confirmed by histological examination of this material. The disease is sometimes discovered by the finding of malignant endometrial cells on a cervical smear. The staging is shown in Box 87.

Treatment

In stage I disease, treatment is by hysterectomy and bilateral salpingo-oophorectomy. At operation the pelvic and para-aortic lymph nodes, liver and omentum are carefully inspected for evidence of metastatic tumour. Biopsies are taken of any suspicious areas and peritoneal washings are sent for cytology. Bilateral pelvic lymphadenectomy may be undertaken in patients with a high risk of node involvement. Postoperative external beam pelvic radiotherapy may be given when the tumour is poorly differentiated or is penetrating the myometrium, because of the increased risk of lymph node metastases. Postoperative irradiation of the vaginal vault using caesium reduces the incidence of vault recurrence.

Treatment of advanced and recurrent disease

In stage II disease when the tumour involves the cervix, post-operative pelvic radiotherapy is indicated. Advanced disease with tumour extending outside the uterus is often only discovered at the time of surgery. Hysterectomy should still be performed wherever possible, to control symptoms of bleeding and discharge. A thorough assessment is made of the degree and location of all metastatic disease to allow tailoring of postoperative radiotherapy.

In recurrent disease radiotherapy is useful for palliation of symptoms such as pain caused by pelvic side wall invasion, or bleeding from a vaginal metastasis. Urinary or bowel diversion may be used for palliative treatment of fistulae. Curative treatment at this stage is rarely possible as systemic disease is usually present, making the prognosis limited. Hormonal therapy with medroxyprogesterone acetate or tamoxifen can be use-

ful in this situation with response rates of up to 60%. Chemotherapy with adriamycin or cisplatin may also be useful, but many patients are elderly and unable to withstand cytotoxic treatments.

Survival

This is mainly determined by stage (Box 88), but also by the particular histological type of tumour. The poorly differentiated serous papillary and adenosquamous varieties have a particularly bad prognosis.

Improving the outlook for endometrial cancer

- Avoidance or reduction of risk factors such as unopposed oestrogen therapy and obesity
- Development of effective screening techniques
- Urgent investigation of all cases of persistent irregular vaginal bleeding
- Targetting poor prognosis patients with more aggressive treatment.

Uterine sarcomas

- Leiomyosarcoma
- Endometrial stromal sarcoma
- Mixed mesodermal tumour.

These are rare and usually highly malignant uterine tumours. They present as a rapidly growing pelvic mass or with uterine bleeding. The definitive diagnosis is usually made on histological examination after hysterectomy although the uterine curettings may suggest a

---

Box 88 Endometrial carcinoma: 5-year survival by stage

Stage	5-year survival
I	75%
II	50%
III	30%
IV	10%

Box 87 Endometrial carcinoma: staging

- Stage Ia   Tumour confined to endometrium
- Stage Ib   Tumour invades myometrium, less than 50% penetration
- Stage Ic   Tumour invades myometrium, more than 50% penetration
- Stage II   Tumour involves the cervix
- Stage III   Spread to involve lymph nodes, uterine serosa, adnexae or vagina
- Stage IV   Tumour involves bladder or rectum, or spread out of pelvis

sarcoma. Grading of these tumours and a guide to their behaviour is obtained by counting the number of mitotic cells per ten high powered fields. Tumours are defined as low grade if there are less than ten mitoses per ten high powered fields, and high grade if there are more than ten.

The leiomyosarcoma arises from the uterine smooth muscle. The macroscopic appearance is similar to a fibroid. The endometrial stromal sarcoma has a tendency to infiltrate veins and is occasionally found growing up the vena cava. The mixed mesodermal tumour contains both carcinomatous and sarcomatous elements. Characteristically a large encephaloid tumour is found filling the uterine cavity.

All sarcomas have a tendency to early and distant haematogenous spread, which accounts for their poor prognosis. Treatment is by hysterectomy and bilateral salpingo-oophorectomy, together with excision of any extra-uterine tumour masses. Sarcomas are not particularly sensitive to either radiotherapy or chemotherapy, but both these treatment modalities are sometimes used in advanced or recurrent disease.

Trophoblastic disease

Trophoblastic diseases comprise a spectrum of tumours which arise from the trophoblast (Box 89). They comprise the benign hydatidiform mole and partial mole, the invasive mole, and the highly malignant choriocarcinoma. All secrete the hormone human chorionic gonadotrophin (HCG), which is used in the monitoring of treatment and in follow-up.

All forms of trophoblastic disease are potentially curable with the correct treatment.

Aetiology

The hydatidiform mole arises from fertilisation of an ovum from which the maternal genetic material is lost. The sperm then duplicates, making 46 chromosomes, which are thus all paternally derived. No embryonic tissue is present, and the chromosomal pattern is usually 46XX. Partial moles differ in that the maternal genetic component is retained, giving a triploid chromosomal pattern with partial moles, a fetus may be present, but survival beyond 8 weeks is rare. An invasive mole

occurs as a result of local invasion of the myometrium by a hydatidiform or partial mole. Choriocarcinoma is a malignant tumour of trophoblast. It may occur following hydatidiform mole, normal pregnancy, miscarriage or ectopic pregnancy.

Incidence

There is considerable ethnic variation in the incidence of trophoblastic disease. The highest incidence is seen in South-East Asia. In the UK, the incidence of hydatidiform mole is 1 in 2000 pregnancies, and for choriocarcinoma it is 1 in 20 000.

Clinical features

Hydatidiform mole
Vaginal bleeding in the first trimester is the most common symptom. Vesicles may be passed or the entire mole may spontaneously abort. Less common presentations are with hyperemesis gravidarum, pre-eclampsia or thyrotoxicosis. The uterine size is often larger than dates would suggest, but fetal heart sounds are absent. The ovaries may be enlarged due to the presence of thecalutein cysts. Ultrasound examination of the uterus shows a characteristic snowstorm appearance (Fig. 29). The tumour consists of hydropic chorionic villi and hyperplastic trophoblast tissue, and has the macroscopic appearance of a bunch of grapes.

Invasive mole and choriocarcinoma
Those cases which develop following a molar pregnancy may be predicted before the development of symptoms by the finding of elevated HCG levels (see below). Alternatively, persistent or heavy vaginal bleeding may occur some months after otherwise unremarkable childbirth or miscarriage due to the invasion of the myometrium by malignant trophoblast. The diagnosis is then made by histological examination of tissue

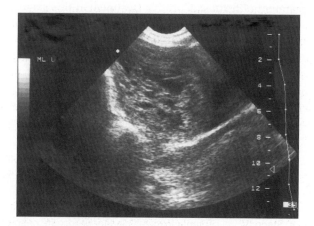

Fig. 29 Hydatidiform mole: ultrasound examination.

Box 89 Trophoblastic disease: classification

Benign	Malignant (gestational trophoblastic disease)
• Hydatidiform mole	• Invasive mole
• Partial mole	• Choriocarcinoma

obtained from curettage of the uterus. One third of cases of choriocarcinoma present with symptoms of metastatic disease. Common sites are the lungs, liver and brain. These deposits are often extremely vascular. Biopsy requires caution because of the risk of haemorrhage, and may be unnecessary if the HCG level is grossly elevated.

Treatment

Treatment of hydatidiform mole

Serum is sent for HCG measurement. Blood should be taken for cross-matching as bleeding can be significant and require transfusion. The uterus is emptied by suction evacuation under general anaesthetic, whilst intravenous syntocinon is given to minimise blood loss. The vesicles are sent for histological examination. All patients with molar pregnancy require careful follow-up because 8% go on to develop invasive mole or choriocarcinoma. Such patients are identified by persistent elevation of both serum and urinary HCG levels following evacuation of the uterus. All patients with hydatidiform mole and partial mole are registered at one of three specialist UK centres which coordinate the collection and measurement of regular urinary and serum samples. Urinary HCG levels are measured every 2 weeks until they have returned to normal, and then continued on a less frequent basis for a further 6 months to 2 years depending on the rate of fall. Advice is given to use reliable contraception until follow-up is complete, because pregnancy will cause a rise in HCG levels and mask any rise due to development of malignancy. HCG levels are checked 6 weeks after any subsequent pregnancy because of the persisting small increased risk of choriocarcinoma.

Treatment of invasive mole and choriocarcinoma

Chemotherapy is the prime modality of treatment for choriocarcinoma and invasive mole. The response is monitored by serial measurements of HCG levels. Those patients who develop invasive disease after a hydatidiform mole are usually identified on the basis of rising HCG levels following evacuation of the uterus. This enables treatment to be started before life-threatening complications develop. There is a wide spectrum of behaviour of trophoblastic disease, and patients are assigned to low, medium or high risk groups based on prognostic factors. For low risk patients, treatment is with methotrexate followed by folinic acid rescue. Medium and high risk patients receive more intensive combination chemotherapy regimens.

Survival

With appropriate treatment in specialist centres, long-term survival in choriocarcinoma is excellent, with 98% of patients being cured.

17.7 Tumours of the fallopian tube

Learning objective

You should understand:

- that fallopian tube cancer is managed in the same way as ovarian cancer

Primary fallopian tumours are extremely rare. Diagnosis is often at a late stage because of lack of early symptoms and the difficulty in detection. Presentation is with a pelvic mass accompanied by a blood-stained vaginal discharge, by which time the tumour has usually invaded other pelvic organs. Most are adenocarcinomas, and the treatment is with cytoreductive surgery and chemotherapy. The fallopian tube is more commonly a site of secondary invasion from a primary ovarian or endometrial carcinoma.

17.8 Ovarian neoplasia

Learning objectives

You should understand:

- the wide pathological variety of ovarian neoplasias

- that most ovarian tumours in women under the age of 40 are benign

- how to investigate a woman with a pelvic mass

- why the prognosis in ovarian cancer is poor

- the role of chemotherapy and surgery in ovarian cancer

- the role of serum CA125 measurement in the management of ovarian cancer

There is a wide diversity in the pathology of tumours of the ovary, reflecting the different tissue types found there. Tumours may be cystic or solid, unilateral or bilateral, benign, low grade malignant or frankly malignant (Box 90). Malignant tumours are not uncommon and may occur

Box 90 Ovarian tumours: classification by tissue of origin

Pathological type	Tissue of origin
● Epithelial tumours	Surface epithelium of the ovary
● Sex cord tumours	Sex cord cells of ovarian cortex
● Germ cell tumours	Primordial germ cells
● Metastatic tumours	Gastrointestinal or breast

in all age groups. Functional ovarian cysts are included here although they are not strictly speaking neoplastic.

Functional ovarian cysts

Functional ovarian cysts account for the majority of cases of ovarian enlargement in young women, and include:

- follicular cysts
- corpus luteum cysts
- theca-lutein cysts
- polycystic ovarian disease
- endometriotic cysts.

Follicular cysts

Follicular cysts are thin-walled cysts, filled with fluid. They rarely grow larger than 5 cm in diameter. They are derived from the Graafian follicle and arise as a result of disordered follicular growth. They may be associated with menstrual irregularity, be asymptomatic, or present as a result of an acute accidental complication, such as torsion. Uncomplicated cysts of less than 5 cm diameter often resolve spontaneously, and only require treatment if they persist or cause symptoms. Persistent cysts over 5 cm diameter are usually treated by laparoscopic drainage or cystectomy.

Corpus luteum cysts

Corpus luteum cysts arise as a result of bleeding into an otherwise normal corpus luteum. Pain arises from distension of the ovary or from peritoneal irritation if there is free blood. Menstruation is sometimes delayed, so the symptoms may mimic an ectopic pregnancy. Acute appendicitis may also be suspected. Laparoscopic drainage is usually all that is required.

Theca-lutein cysts

Theca-lutein cysts are usually bilateral and can reach a large size. They are caused by overstimulation of the ovaries by high levels of HCG. They are seen in association with gestational trophoblastic disease or when gonadotrophins are given during infertility treatment. The cysts resolve when the cause is removed.

Polycystic ovarian disease

In a typical case there are numerous small subcapsular cystic follicles, a thickened ovarian capsule and generalised ovarian enlargement. Associated clinical symptoms may be infrequent periods, hirsutism, infertility or obesity.

Endometriotic cysts

Endometriotic cysts arise as a result of ovarian endometriosis, and are characterised by pain, swelling and fixation of the ovaries. They are often referred to as chocolate cysts because of the appearance of the altered blood.

Epithelial ovarian tumours

Epithelial ovarian tumours make up the majority of ovarian neoplasms. They are derived from the epithelial surface of the ovary, and are classified by specific histological type. Histological types of epithelial ovarian tumours include:

- serous
- mucinous
- endometrioid
- Brenner tumour
- clear cell.

Each of these tumours can exist in benign, borderline, or malignant form.

Benign epithelial tumours of the ovary

Serous and mucinous cystadenomas constitute the majority of benign epithelial tumours. The serous cystadenoma consists of a thin-walled cyst filled with fluid (Fig. 30). Most are below 20 cm in diameter. Mucinous tumours are often loculated. They occasionally grow to a large size and can fill the entire abdomen. Rupture of a mucinous cyst can lead to cells seeding on to peritoneal surfaces, where they grow and secrete mucin, resulting in a condition called pseudomyxoma peritonei. In severe cases the abdominal cavity becomes distended with gelatinous mucin.

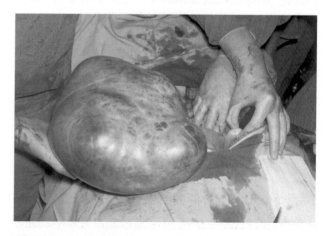

Fig. 30 Large benign ovarian cyst, with normal contralateral ovary.

Clinical features

In the absence of an acute accident such as torsion or haemorrhage these tumours cause remarkably few symptoms, and are often only discovered as a result of a bimanual pelvic examination or an ultrasound scan. Larger cysts may cause abdominal distension or exert pressure on the bladder. An acute presentation with severe localised pain occurs when a cyst undergoes torsion, rupture or haemorrhage. Cysts larger than 5 cm are usually palpable on vaginal examination as a smooth mobile mass separate from the uterus. Larger cysts may be palpable abdominally. Torsion causing strangulation presents with fever, vomiting, peritonism and leucocytosis.

Treatment

These tumours should be surgically excised histological diagnosis. The risk of malignancy is highest if there are solid areas present in the tumour, if the capsule has been breached or if ascites is present. If malignant features are found at operation the whole ovary should be excised and sent for histological examination. When there are no obvious malignant features, all that is required is enucleation of the cyst, taking care to avoid rupture, with conservation of the ovary wherever possible. The contralateral ovary should also be carefully inspected. In post-menopausal women bilateral salpingo-oophorectomy with hysterectomy is usually preferred. In pregnancy, surgery is ideally performed in the second trimester when the risk of miscarriage is lowest.

Ovarian epithelial tumours of borderline malignancy

Up to 20% of epithelial ovarian tumours are classified histologically as borderline. This refers to a tumour possessing some but not all the morphological features of malignancy. The cells exhibit malignant features, but do not invade the stroma. The majority of these tumours are serous or mucinous cystadenomas. They are often found bilaterally, and extra-ovarian spread may be present at the time of initial diagnosis. The treatment is surgical removal. Younger patients are treated with unilateral oophorectomy in order to preserve fertility. Total abdominal hysterectomy and bilateral salpingo-oophorectomy is reserved for cases where the tumours are bilateral or when childbearing is complete.

Malignant epithelial ovarian tumours

90% of all ovarian cancers are epithelial in origin. It is the most common cause of death from cancer of the genital tract in women, with a peak incidence at 60–70 years of age. The majority of cases present with advanced disease because the early stages have only vague or even absent symptoms. This largely accounts for the poor survival in ovarian cancer. The development of an effective screening programme to allow earlier detection and improved treatment for advanced disease would considerably improve the outlook in ovarian cancer.

Aetiology

The cause of ovarian cancer is unknown. Nulliparity, early menarche and late menopause are associated with an increased risk of the disease, whereas oral contraceptive use offers protection. This suggests that ovulation may be an important risk factor in the aetiology of ovarian cancer. A small percentage of ovarian cancer is familial and has a genetic origin. The risk is associated with the possession of certain mutations on the BRCA1 gene. Women who have had two or more first degree relatives with the disease should therefore be offered genetic counselling.

Natural history

Ovarian cancer spreads initially by local infiltration (Box 91). This involves the surface of the ovary and then any other pelvic organs. Malignant cells are transported throughout the peritoneal cavity by transcoelomic spread. This results in multiple small superficial tumour seedlings on the omentum and peritoneal surfaces of the liver and bowel. Large areas of the bowel may become coated with tumour. This inhibits peristalsis and results in subacute obstruction at multiple sites. Tumour spread across the diaphragm causes pleural effusions. In some cases the primary tumour remains small with the main feature being widespread miliary peritoneal implants. Large bowel obstruction in the pelvis may mimic a colonic carcinoma. Lymphatic spread also occurs, to the pelvic and para-aortic nodes, and thence to the supraclavicular nodes. Blood spread to the liver and lungs is less common. Death usually occurs from cachexia secondary to chronic bowel dysfunction.

Box 91 Ovarian cancer: spread

Method of spread	Site
● Local infiltration	Pelvic organs
● Transcoelomic spread	Any peritoneal surfaces
● Lymphatic spread	Pelvic and para-aortic lymph nodes
● Blood spread	Lungs, liver

Clinical features

The disease has an insidious onset and produces few early symptoms. A high index of suspicion is therefore required in any woman with vague abdominal symptoms and pelvic discomfort. When symptoms do arise they are often more suggestive of gastrointestinal disease. The majority of patients present with advanced disease with ascitic abdominal distension, pain or a mass. Extrinsic compression and invasion of the large bowel by tumour can be difficult to distinguish from primary bowel cancer.

Symptoms of ovarian cancer

- Anorexia
- Weight loss
- Indigestion
- Abdominal bloating
- Pelvic discomfort
- Vaginal bleeding.

Clinical examination may be unremarkable in the early stages, but pelvic examination should always be performed, looking for signs of ovarian enlargement. In advanced disease a pelvic mass is nearly always present. On rectal examination irregular, firm tumour deposits may be felt in the pouch of Douglas. Omental metastases may be palpable as a diffuse upper abdominal mass. In end stage disease the patient is thin and cachectic, with an abdomen distended by tumour and ascites. There may be bilateral pleural effusions, and an enlarged mass of supraclavicular nodes.

Diagnosis and staging

Pelvic ultrasound and laparoscopy are both used to investigate symptoms suggestive of ovarian cancer in the absence of clinical signs of disease. The majority of women with symptoms will not be found to have any serious disease. Ultrasound imaging is useful, but will not detect all cases, particularly those of small volume disease. Making an early diagnosis can thus be difficult, and the patient may be referred for gastrointestinal endoscopy with the incorrect label of irritable bowel syndrome or diverticular disease. If ascites is the only clinical feature, paracentesis to obtain a sample of ascitic fluid to look for malignant cells may be helpful. The finding of an elevated serum level of the tumour marker CA125 is suggestive but not diagnostic of epithelial ovarian cancer.

Most patients with a suspicious pelvic mass will ultimately require laparotomy, both for diagnosis and staging of disease (Box 92).

The staging of ovarian cancer is done at laparotomy, and is particularly important in order to direct appropriate treatment. A thorough search of the entire peritoneal cavity is made for metastatic disease. This includes cytological examination of peritoneal washings, multiple peritoneal biopsies, palpation of the pelvic and para-aortic lymph nodes, and omentectomy. In cases when advanced disease is unexpectedly discovered at laparotomy, the diagnosis should be confirmed with a biopsy prior to major surgery, because other conditions such as endometriosis and actinomycosis can closely resemble ovarian cancer.

Treatment of ovarian cancer

Stage I disease

The treatment for stage I ovarian cancer is surgical removal of the involved ovary. In stage IA disease unilateral oophorectomy is sufficient in young women, but consideration should be given to removing the other ovary and uterus when childbearing is complete. Postmenopausal women are usually offered removal of both ovaries and the uterus. In stage IB and C disease, adjuvant chemotherapy may be given to decrease the risk of recurrence.

Advanced disease

Advanced disease is treated by cytoreductive surgery (Box 93) followed by chemotherapy. Radiotherapy and hormones may also be used.

Surgery allows diagnosis, staging and treatment. Cytoreductive surgery aims to excise all visible tumour masses. This may necessitate very extensive procedures

---

Box 92 Ovarian cancer: staging

Stage IA	Tumour confined to one ovary
Stage IB	Tumour involving both ovaries
Stage IC	Tumour on one or both ovaries, with ascites or positive peritoneal washings
Stage II	Tumour spread beyond the ovaries but confined to the pelvis
Stage III	Spread outside the pelvis but confined to the abdominal cavity. Retroperitoneal spread to pelvic or para-aortic lymph nodes
Stage IV	Distant spread

- Diagnosis
- Staging
- Cytoreduction of tumour masses
- Drainage of ascites
- Relief of bowel or urinary obstruction
- Second look laparotomy/laparoscopy

Box 94 Ovarian cancer: 5-year survival by stage

Stage	5-year survival
I	70%
II	40%
III	20%
IV	5%

such as resection of bowel or urinary tract. Cytoreductive surgery can confer substantial symptomatic improvement and offers the best chance of response to chemotherapy, but the impact on survival is probably small. In very advanced and recurrent disease surgery has a limited but useful role in the palliative treatment of urinary and faecal fistulae. Most cases of bowel obstruction can be managed without the need for surgery.

Chemotherapy is the most effective treatment for advanced disease. It improves survival by an average of 18 months. Current evidence suggests that paclitaxel/carboplatin in combination is the most effective, with single agent carboplatin being reserved for women who may not be able to tolerate the combination. Chemotherapy is most effective when only minimal residual disease remains following cytoreductive surgery. Progress and response to chemotherapy are monitored by clinical examination, imaging of tumour deposits, and serial measurement of serum CA125 levels. Patients who relapse or do not respond to chemotherapy have a poor outlook. They may respond to second line agents or derive limited benefit from hormonal therapy with progestogens or tamoxifen.

Chemotherapeutic agents include: platinum compounds, e.g. cisplatin, carboplatin; Taxanes, e.g. paclitaxel; alkylating agents, e.g. chlorambucil, cyclophosphamide, ifosphamide; doxorubicin.

Radiotherapy has a limited role in the treatment of ovarian cancer because of the difficulty in delivering an effective dose of radiation to the entire abdomino-pelvic cavity without causing significant bowel damage. Small peritoneal tumour seedlings can be treated by instillation of radioactive isotopes in solution into the peritoneal cavity, but there is no proven survival benefit. Painful bony metastases can occasionally be palliated by a short course of localised external beam radiotherapy.

Prognosis

The overall 5-year survival for all stages is 30% (Box 94). Poor prognostic factors include residual disease greater than 2 cm after primary surgery, age over 70 years, and poorly differentiated tumours.

Improving the outlook for ovarian cancer

- Bimanual pelvic examination at the time of cervical smear
- Development of an effective screening test
- Identification and testing for BRCA1 gene mutations in familial ovarian cancer
- Prophylactic oophorectomy in high risk patients
- Accurate staging so that patients receive appropriate treatment
- Development of better treatments for advanced disease.

Whole population screening has not as yet been shown to reduce the mortality from ovarian cancer but is being subjected to trials. Since the true natural history of the disease is unknown, the impact of earlier diagnosis and treatment on survival is hard to ascertain. Unlike cervical carcinoma, there is no pre-cancerous stage when simple and preventative treatment can be given. Furthermore, none of the tests which have been developed are sufficiently reliable when used in isolation, so a combination of investigations is required. These include bimanual pelvic examination, ultrasound imaging, measurement of flow patterns in ovarian vessels with transvaginal colour Doppler, and measurement of serum tumour markers, such as CA125. Bimanual pelvic examination is the least accurate of these. Ultrasound and Doppler are more sensitive, but are expensive as screening tests, and abnormal findings require further investigation by laparoscopy or laparotomy. Elevated levels of the tumour marker CA125 may precede clinically detectable cancer, but more sensitive and specific markers are needed because only 50% of women with stage I disease have elevated levels, and some women with elevated levels have benign conditions such as endometriosis.

Sex cord stromal tumours of the ovary

- Granulosa cell tumour
- Fibroma
- Androblastoma.

These tumours are derived from the stromal cortex of the ovary. They comprise 6% of all ovarian neoplasms, and are usually seen in post-menopausal women. The granulosa cell tumour is white or yellow, and usually around 10–12 cm in diameter. It secretes oestrogen, which can result in both endometrial hyperplasia or carcinoma. The benign ovarian fibroma occasionally presents with ascites and a pleural effusion, when it is called Meigs' syndrome. The androblastoma contains Sertoli or Leydig cells. It is a small tumour which may secrete large amounts of androgens, resulting in virilisation.

Treatment

The majority of sex cord tumours are of low grade malignancy and are confined to the ovary at presentation. Hysterectomy, bilateral salpingo-oophorectomy and omentectomy is usually sufficient treatment. The 5-year survival is 80%. Late recurrences are characteristic of these tumours and are usually managed by further excision.

Germ cell tumours of the ovary

Benign
- Benign cystic teratoma.

Malignant
- Malignant teratoma
- Dysgerminoma
- Yolk sac tumours
- Choriocarcinoma.

Germ cell tumours arise from cells having the potential to develop into embryonic or extra-embryonic tissues. They occur in young women, accounting for 70% of all ovarian neoplasms under the age of 20 years.

Benign cystic teratoma

The benign cystic teratoma, or dermoid cyst as it is commonly called, is by far the most common germ cell tumour. It may contain tissues derived from endoderm, ectoderm and mesoderm, which may include cartilage, teeth, muscle, thyroid and neural tissue. Calcification may be seen on a pelvic X-ray, and on ultrasound scan both solid and cystic areas are commonly seen. Treatment is by ovarian cystectomy. 20% of dermoids are bilateral, so the other ovary should be carefully inspected.

Malignant germ cell tumours

The dysgerminoma accounts for 50% of malignant germ cell tumours. 90% occur in women under 30 years old. They are solid, rubbery tumours, which are bilateral in 10–20% of cases. Malignant teratomas account for 20% of malignant germ cell tumours. Yolk sac tumours are rare, highly malignant, and secrete alpha-fetoprotein. The ovarian choriocarcinoma is a non-gestational tumour, but is histologically indistinguishable from gestational choriocarcinoma. It secretes HCG.

Chemotherapy is the main treatment modality for malignant germ cell tumours, and this has greatly improved the prognosis. Surgery is limited to unilateral oophorectomy, and also to allow thorough staging. Radical surgery does not improve the prognosis and should therefore be avoided. All these tumours are uncommon, and should be referred to specialised centres for treatment and follow-up. Measurement of serum tumour markers is useful, as rises are often the first sign of disease recurrence.

Secondary tumours of the ovary

Metastatic carcinoma in the ovaries most commonly arises from a primary in the breast or bowel. These may be seen as bilateral solid ovarian masses, called Krukenberg tumours. Endometrial carcinoma may also spread to the ovary.

17.9 Palliative care in advanced gynaecological malignancy

Learning objective

You should understand:

- the role of palliative care in gynaecological cancer

Palliative care is indicated in advanced malignancy when a cure is no longer possible. A variety of interventions may be appropriate, ranging from further radical treatment or palliative surgery (for example, to relieve bowel obstruction) to radiotherapy or medical treatment. The aims are to relieve distressing symptoms, improve the quality of life, and allow the patient to remain at home wherever possible and have a dignified death. The common causes of death from gynaecological cancer are uraemia secondary to ureteric obstruction, and cachexia resulting from chronic subacute bowel obstruction.

Common problems in advanced gynaecological malignancy
- Pain
- Anorexia
- Bowel obstruction
- Ureteric obstruction

- Vaginal bleeding or discharge
- Urinary or faecal fistulae
- Recurrent pleural effusions or ascites.

Pain

Particular attention should be given to adequate pain control. Treatment requires an understanding of the cause. For example, the pain from a bony metastasis may be successfully relieved by radiotherapy. Alleviating anxiety by listening, supporting and providing accurate and sensitive information can alter the perception of pain. Pain relief should be started using mild analgesics such as paracetamol taken on a regular basis, with progression to moderate analgesics such as co-proxamol when these are no longer effective. In severe chronic pain, opioids are indicated. The patient should be reassured that morphine is not being given to hasten death. It can be given by slow release oral preparation or by subcutaneous infusion. Opiates cause both constipation and nausea, so stool softeners and laxatives should be prescribed from the outset. Steroids, antidepressants and non-steroidal analgesics are also useful and can reduce opioid requirements.

Anorexia

This may respond to treatment with steroids, or a high protein, low residue diet.

Bowel obstruction

This is commonly seen in advanced ovarian cancer when median survival is around 14 weeks. It is usually managed conservatively because there is rarely one discrete point of obstruction and the morbidity of surgery is high. A combination of an anti-emetic such as haloperidol with an anticholinergic drug such as hyoscine can be given by subcutaneous infusion via a syringe driver. Octreotide is given to stimulate gut absorption and inhibit peristalsis.

Ureteric obstruction

Uraemia can be relieved by the insertion of ureteric stents. The decision to insert stents in the presence of incurable disease requires careful consideration because uraemia can provide the patient with a relatively gentle passage into unconsciousness and death.

Fistulae

A diverting colostomy can relieve the soiling and odour from a rectovaginal fistula. Urinary diversion using an ileal conduit may be used as treatment for a vesicovaginal fistula.

Ascites

Drainage of ascites by paracentesis, and tapping pleural effusions may relieve abdominal discomfort and shortness of breath respectively. All women with advanced gynaecological cancer should have access to specialist palliative care on a 24 hour basis, and should be helped to remain in the place they prefer, be it home, hospital or hospice, and should be allowed to choose where they wish to die.

Self-assessment: questions

Multiple choice questions

1. Which of the following statements are true: regarding gynaecological cancer in this country?
   a. The incidence of cancer of the cervix is falling
   b. The mortality from ovarian cancer is rising
   c. The number of women dying each year from ovarian cancer exceeds that from both cervical and endometrial cancer combined
   d. The overall 5-year survival rate in endometrial cancer is 66%
   e. Gynaecological cancer develops in 1.5% of women

2. Which of the following statements are true?
   a. Barrier methods of contraception confer protection from carcinoma of the cervix
   b. Pregnancy increases the risk of ovarian cancer
   c. Obesity is a risk factor for carcinoma of the endometrium
   d. Use of the oral contraceptive pill reduces the risk of both ovarian and endometrial cancer
   e. There is an effective screening programme for ovarian cancer

3. A 70-year-old woman presents with a 1 cm diameter infected ulcer on the left labium majus, and an enlarged palpable inguinal lymph node. Biopsy of the ulcer shows this to be a squamous cell carcinoma of the vulva. Which of the following are true?
   a. Lichen sclerosus may be present in the surrounding vulval skin
   b. Radical vulvectomy is required
   c. The inguinal lymph node enlargement is almost certainly due to a metastasis
   d. If excision of the primary tumour shows the depth of invasion to be 5 mm there is no need for inguino-femoral lymphadenectomy
   e. Pelvic lymphadenectomy is required if the groin nodes are extensively involved with tumour

4. Which of the following are true regarding cervical screening?
   a. The majority of women who die from cervical cancer have never had a smear
   b. Screening is not designed to detect adenocarcinoma
   c. The smear is always abnormal in carcinoma of the cervix
   d. The presence of an intra-uterine device can change the appearance of the cells on a smear
   e. A systematic computerised call and recall system is fundamental to a screening programme

5. A 55-year-old woman presents with a 4 cm diameter cervical carcinoma, with extension into the right parametrium. It does not extend to the pelvic side wall, and an intravenous urogram shows no ureteric obstruction. Which of the following are true?
   a. She has stage III disease
   b. She should be treated by radiotherapy
   c. She has a better than 40% 5-year survival
   d. The chances of recurrence are highest within 3 years of treatment
   e. Hormone replacement therapy is contraindicated

6. Which of the following are poor prognostic indicators in patients with endometrial carcinoma?
   a. Poorly differentiated tumour
   b. Obesity
   c. > 50% myometrial penetration by the tumour
   d. Serous papillary endometrial carcinoma
   e. Past history of using unopposed oestrogen therapy

7. Concerning choriocarcinoma:
   a. It is 1500 times more common after a molar pregnancy than after a term delivery
   b. Consists of malignant fetal tissue
   c. Presenting symptoms include haemoptysis and stroke
   d. HCG levels usually exceed 20 000 IU/L
   e. Hysterectomy is rarely necessary

8. Side-effects of chemotherapy include:
   a. Myelosuppression
   b. Lymphoedema
   c. Intestinal obstruction
   d. Nausea
   e. Alopecia

Short notes

1. A study into the frequency of cervical screening has estimated that the incidence of invasive carcinoma of the cervix could be reduced by 84% by screening all women aged 20–64 years every 5 years, by 91% by screening every 3 years and by 93% by screening annually. If you were responsible for organising the provision of health care, which screening programme would you choose and why?

2. What are the complications of radical vulvectomy and bilateral groin node excision?

3. Name the risk factors associated with the development of endometrial carcinoma.

4. What proportion of women presenting with post-menopausal bleeding will have endometrial cancer? What are the other possible diagnoses? What investigations can be performed to investigate post-menopausal bleeding?

5. A 55-year-old woman presents with shortness of breath 6 months following surgery for a leiomyosarcoma of the uterus. A chest X-ray shows multiple nodular opacities. What is the likely explanation, and what is the management? What is the prognosis?

6. Follicular cysts are often associated with menstrual disturbance. Why? Why is the incidence of functional ovarian cysts reduced in women taking the combined oral contraceptive pill? Is the risk of ovarian cancer altered with use of the oral contraceptive pill?

7. How is the staging of ovarian cancer performed? Why is accurate staging important in this disease?

8. With regard to ovarian cancer, what is meant by intervention debulking surgery?

9. A 29-year-old lady has a sister and mother who have both died from ovarian cancer. She wants to know what her risk is of developing ovarian cancer, and whether there is anything she can do to reduce it. What advice would you give her?

Self-assessment: answers

Multiple choice answers

1. a. **True.**
    b. **True.**
    c. **True.**
    d. **True.**
    e. **False.** Gynaecological cancer develops in 5% of women.

2. a. **True.** Cancer of the cervix behaves like a sexually transmitted disease, and the human papillomavirus (HPV) appears to play a key role. All barrier methods of contraception lower the risk by reducing exposure of the cervix to viruses, semen and other possible agents. In addition many spermicides have antiviral properties. Other known risk factors include an early age of first sexual intercourse, a high number of sexual partners, and smoking.
    b. **False.** Pregnancy confers protection against ovarian cancer. The mechanism is thought to be by inhibition of ovulation.
    c. **True.** Obesity is a known risk factor for endometrial carcinoma due to the associated raised levels of circulating oestrogens.
    d. **True.** The oral contraceptive pill confers protection against both endometrial and ovarian cancer.
    e. **False.** There is currently no screening test for ovarian cancer that has been shown to reduce the death rate from this disease.

3. a. **True.** Changes of lichen sclerosus are frequently seen in the skin adjacent to vulval carcinoma, but it is uncertain whether the carcinoma arises directly from it. 3% of cases of lichen sclerosus are associated with the subsequent development of invasive carcinoma.
    b. **False.** The primary tumour may be treated by wide local excision if adequate tumour clearance can be achieved.
    c. **False.** Enlarged palpable lymph nodes may be due to involvement with metastatic tumour, but infection in the primary tumour may cause regional nodal enlargement in the absence of metastases. Fine needle aspiration looking for malignant cells is useful to differentiate between these two conditions.
    d. **False.** Lesions of 5 mm depth have a significant risk of lymph node metastases and inguinofemoral lymphadenectomy is required.

Lymphadenectomy can normally be avoided when the cancer invades to a depth of less than 1 mm.
    e. **False.** When there is extensive tumour involvement of the inguinal nodes there is a high chance of pelvic node involvement. However, pelvic radiotherapy is more effective than surgery.

4. a. **True.** The major problem with screening is that women most at risk use the service least.
    b. **True.** Adenocarcinoma accounts for 10–15% of invasive cervical cancers.
    c. **False.** The cervix should always be visually inspected and digitally examined when a smear is taken because a necrotic tumour can give a negative result. If the clinical appearance of the cervix is suspicious, colposcopy should be performed regardless of the smear result.
    d. **True.**
    e. **True.** It is recommended that all screening programmes operate a computerised call and recall system to invite women to attend for smears.

5. a. **False.** She has stage IIb disease.
    b. **True.** Advanced carcinoma of the cervix is treated by radiotherapy.
    c. **True.** The survival in stage II disease is 50%.
    d. **True.** Most recurrences occur within 3 years of treatment.
    e. **False.** HRT is not contraindicated and may help to alleviate radiation-induced dyspareunia.

6. a. **True.** Poorly differentiated tumours tend to behave more aggressively.
    b. **False.** Obesity and unopposed oestrogen therapy are only risk factors for the development of endometrial carcinoma.
    c. **True.** Myometrial penetration by the tumour is associated with a higher incidence of pelvic lymph node metastases.
    d. **True.** The serous papillary endometrial carcinoma is a particularly aggressive variety, characterised by rapid and widespread dissemination.
    e. **False.** Those cancers which develop in association with unopposed oestrogen therapy tend to be well differentiated and are of relatively good prognosis.

7. a. **True.** 50% of all choriocarcinomas occur following a molar pregnancy, and it is 1500 times more likely after a mole than after a term delivery.
   b. **False.** The tumour arises from the trophoblast and consists of cytotrophoblast and syncytiotrophoblast. There are no fetal elements.
   c. **True.** Haemoptysis and stroke may be the presenting symptoms of choriocarcinoma due to haemorrhage from metastases in the lung or brain.
   d. **True.** HCG levels are characteristically very high.
   e. **True.** Surgery is rarely needed as it is usually possible to control vaginal bleeding with chemotherapy.

8. a. **True.**
   b. **False.** Lymphoedema occurs following pelvic lymphadenectomy or radiotherapy.
   c. **False.** Bowel obstruction can be caused by radiation stenosis but not by chemotherapy.
   d. **True.**
   e. **True.**

Short notes answers

1. Cervical screening should be seen as a risk reduction programme, rather than as a prevention programme. Screening and treatment of CIN confers protection from the development of cervical cancer. The increased protection conferred by annual screening has to be balanced against the greater cost. A 2% reduction in the incidence of invasive disease would be gained from a three-fold increase in expenditure, and it could be argued that this does not represent best use of limited resources. In addition there would be increased inconvenience and anxiety caused to women because of the necessity of annual examinations. Most health authorities have therefore compromised on a 3-yearly screening interval. There is a good case to be made for spending any additional resources on improved targeting of non-attenders, who represent a high risk group, rather than introducing more frequent screening.

2. Early complications include wound infection, wound breakdown, thromboembolic disease and urinary infection.
   Late complications include secondary haemorrhage from the femoral vessels, chronic lymphoedema of the legs, narrowing of the vaginal introitus and psychological problems.

3. The following are all risk factors for endometrial carcinoma: obesity, nulliparity, late menopause, unopposed exogenous oestrogen therapy, tamoxifen therapy, granulosa cell tumour of the ovary, previous pelvic radiotherapy.

4. Approximately 10% of women who present with post-menopausal bleeding will be found to have endometrial cancer.
   Other causes of post-menopausal bleeding include genital tract atrophy resulting from oestrogen deficiency, and bleeding caused by hormone replacement therapy. However, even when signs of oestrogen deficiency can be seen post-menopausal bleeding requires further investigation. In addition to endometrial carcinoma other tumours such as cancer of the cervix, ovary, fallopian tube and vagina may also present in this way. Post-menopausal bleeding should be investigated by history, pelvic and abdominal examination, ultrasound measurement of endometrial thickness, and endometrial biopsy if this exceeds 5 mm. This is usually carried out in one-step rapid access post-menopausal bleeding clinics. The aim is to identify the small percentage of women who require endometrial biopsy. This can often be achieved without general anaesthetic, either by using a small plastic tube which is inserted through the cervix, or by hysterectomy.

5. Widespread pulmonary metastases from haematogenous tumour spread is the likely diagnosis. This should be confirmed by transbronchial biopsy before treatment is commenced, and the extent of disease should be assessed by thoracic, abdominal and pelvic computed tomography (CT) scan. Systemic therapy with hormones such as medroxyprogesterone acetate or with chemotherapy will produce a 30% response rate, but the prognosis remains very poor. Survival beyond 6 months is unlikely.

6. The menstrual disturbances commonly seen in association with follicular cysts occur because of disordered ovarian function. Normally the Graafian follicle reaches 1.5 cm diameter just prior to ovulation. If ovulation does not take place, further enlargement results in a cystic follicle. There are rarely symptoms due to the cyst unless an acute accident occurs, but in the absence of ovulation there is no corpus luteum and no progesterone production. Menstruation thus becomes irregular.
   Ovulation is suppressed by the combined oral contraceptive pill. Follicular development is thus inhibited, and follicular cysts are thus less common.
   The risk of ovarian cancer is decreased with oral contraceptive use. The exact reason is unknown but it may be by prevention of the repetitive trauma to

the surface epithelium of the ovary which normally occurs as a result of ovulation.

7. Staging is done by laparotomy via a mid-line abdominal incision. It consists of: assessment of the site and extent of the primary tumour; cytological examination of peritoneal washings; examination of all peritoneal surfaces, including the diaphragmatic surface of the liver; multiple peritoneal biopsies; excision of the omentum; palpation of the pelvic and para-aortic lymph nodes.

   Meticulous staging is important because ovarian cancer seeds via transcoelomic spread to all peritoneal surfaces early in the course of the disease. If staging is not performed adequately, there is a risk that women with stage III disease, by virtue of microscopic tumour deposits in the omentum or other extra-pelvic sites will be wrongly ascribed to stage I disease. Such incorrect staging may result in inadequate treatment and incorrect prognostic information.

8. Intervention debulking surgery is defined as a planned laparotomy performed during primary chemotherapy in patients adjudged to be responding to that chemotherapy. It may confer a survival advantage in those patients with bulky residual disease, as it is believed that surgical reduction of tumour volume is crucial to chemoresponse. However, the survival of patients who undergo failed cytoreductive surgery may be worse than that of those who just receive chemotherapy alone. Trials are in progress.

9. Ovarian cancer affects 1% of women by the age of 70 years. However, this risk is increased if an individual has a positive family history. With two affected first-degree relatives, the lifetime risk in this lady may be as high as 40%, and referral for genetic counselling should be offered.

   Annual screening using transvaginal ultrasound, with colour Doppler and serum CA125 estimations may provide earlier detection of disease, but has not as yet been shown to confer any survival advantage in randomised trials. The risk of ovarian cancer could be reduced by suppression of ovulation with the combined oral contraceptive pill.

   5–10% of ovarian cancers occur due to a familial inheritance of a single autosomal dominant gene. Where two family members are affected there is a 30% chance that the condition is caused by mutations in the BRCA1 or BRCA2 genes. Unfortunately most families have their own specific mutation. Genetic testing is therefore complicated, and requires genetic material from an affected relative to be available. Carriers of the gene mutation are at high risk of developing both ovarian and breast cancer. The options in this situation rest between regular screening and prophylactic bilateral oophorectomy. The relative merits and disadvantages of both options will require careful discussion.

18 Genital prolapse and urinary disorders

Overview

The main cause of genital prolapse is neuro-muscular damage to the pelvic floor following childbirth. Surgery is the most usual form of treatment for prolapse.

Urinary incontinence has a variety of different causes. Urodynamic studies are often required for accurate diagnosis. Detrusor instability is a common cause of urinary incontinence in the elderly. Treatment is usually with anticholinergic drugs and bladder retraining. Genuine stress incontinence is usually caused by vaginal delivery. Pelvic floor exercises may help many patients, but surgery should be offered if conservative measures fail.

Urinary infections are a significant cause of morbidity in women.

Introduction

Genital prolapse is a common gynaecological disorder, resulting from a failure of the pelvic supporting structures, and may involve both the uterus and vagina. It characteristically affects post-menopausal multiparous women.

18.1 Anatomy of the pelvic floor

Learning objective

You should understand:

- how the uterus and vagina are supported

The uterus is supported by the strong transverse cervical ligaments of Mackenrodt, also called the cardinal ligaments. These consist of thickenings of connective tissue around the uterine vessels in the base of the broad ligament. They extend laterally from the cervix to the side wall of the pelvis. Together with the uterosacral ligaments they impart stability and support to the cervix and uterus (Fig. 31A, B). The round ligaments which run in the top of the broad ligament from the uterine cornua to the deep inguinal ring offer only minimal support.

The vagina and bladder neck are supported by the levator ani muscles, which form a muscular hammock slung from the side walls of the bony pelvis. The urethra, vagina and rectum all pass through this hammock, whose muscular fibres act as sphincters to help maintain continence. Relaxation of these muscles allows micturition, defecation and parturition. They are innervated by the pudendal nerve, the root value of which is S 2,3,4.

18.2 Aetiology of genital prolapse

Learning objective

You should understand:

- the pathophysiology of prolapse

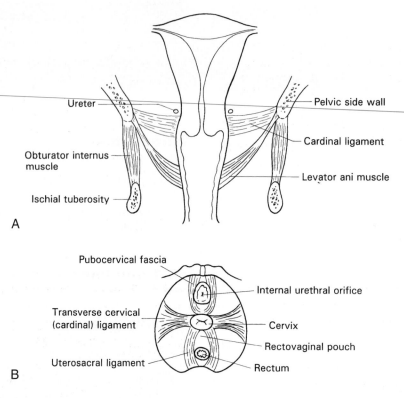

Fig. 31 (A, B) Two views of the female pelvis showing vaginal and uterine supports.

Damage to the pelvic floor from difficult childbirth and prolonged second stage of labour both predispose towards genital prolapse. Studies have shown that even normal childbirth may cause irreversible damage to the nerve supply of the pelvic floor. The combined effects of ageing and post-menopausal oestrogen deficiency cause further insult to the pelvic ligaments and fascia. Increased intra-abdominal pressure from any cause such as constipation, chronic cough, heavy lifting or an abdominal mass will exacerbate prolapse.

18.3 Vaginal prolapse

Learning objective

You should know:

- the anatomical classification of vaginal prolapse

Figure 32A is a sagittal section through the female pelvis showing normal anatomy.

Vaginal prolapse represents a herniation of urethra, bladder, pouch of Douglas or rectum through the supporting fascia (Fig. 32B). The resulting pressure causes indentation of the vaginal wall, which may give rise to a lump at the introitus. The prolapse may consist of:

- urethrocele – lower anterior vaginal wall
- cystocele – upper anterior vaginal wall
- rectocele – posterior vaginal wall
- enterocele – pouch of Douglas.

An enterocele usually contains small bowel or omentum in a peritoneal sac, which prolapses down between the uterosacral ligaments.

18.4 Uterine prolapse

Learning objectives

You should:

- be able to classify uterine prolapse
- understand how prolapse is assessed

Three degrees of uterine prolapse are described:

- first – when there is slight descent of uterus
- second – when the cervix projects beyond the vulva
- third – when the entire uterus prolapses outside the vagina. This is called procidentia.

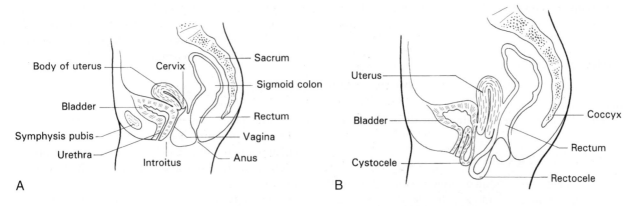

Fig. 32 **(A)** Sagittal section through the female pelvis showing normal anatomy. **(B)** Sagittal section showing types of prolapse.

The severity of symptoms often bears little relationship to the degree of prolapse. Prolonged standing often exacerbates symptoms, whereas they are eased by lying flat.

Common symptoms

Common symptoms of uterine prolapse include:

- dragging sensation in the pelvis
- feeling a lump 'down below'
- leakage of urine on coughing or straining.

Rare symptoms

Rare symptoms include:

- backache
- coital difficulties
- a lump bulging into the vagina on defecation
- bleeding or rubbing on underclothes.

Full general examination should be carried out with particular reference to fitness for anaesthesia. The presence of any abdominal mass should be sought. Pelvic examination should be performed with the patient lying comfortably in the left lateral position, using a Sims speculum and a sponge-holding forceps. The anterior and posterior vaginal walls are assessed in turn for the presence and degree of any prolapse. This may only be visible if the woman is asked to bear down. Urinary leakage may be demonstrated on coughing. Uterine descent is sometimes obvious but is usually more difficult to assess in the conscious woman. Applying traction to the cervix with an instrument is not recommended as this can cause considerable discomfort. The vaginal skin and cervix may exhibit keratinisation or decubitus ulceration if prolapse has been long-standing.

18.5 Treatment of prolapse

Learning objectives

You should:

- understand how conservative measures in the treatment of prolapse work
- be aware of the different surgical options

All women with prolapse should be reassured that they do not have a life-threatening condition and that symptoms do not always worsen with age. The severity of symptoms is in part determined by the degree of physical activity and lifestyle. Patients with mild symptoms and first-degree prolapse are often improved by conservative measures such as avoidance of heavy lifting, treatment of constipation, and pelvic floor exercises (Box 95). Surgical repair of the pelvic floor is the most effective treatment for severe prolapse or where conservative measures have failed. It is most likely to benefit

---

Box 95 Prolapse: treatments

Preventative	Conservative
• avoidance of prolonged labours	• elimination of chronic cough
• careful repair of perineal tears	• reduction in smoking and heavy lifting
• attention to postnatal exercises	• weight loss
• avoidance of constipation	• physiotherapy to the pelvic floor muscles
• hormone replacement therapy	• vaginal ring pessary

those patients who make the necessary lifestyle changes to avoid future excessive demands on their pelvic floor.

Surgery

If the patient is sexually active the surgeon must ensure that the repair does not result in excessive vaginal narrowing. The various operations are described below.

Repair of a cystocele

Repair of a cystocele is called anterior colporrhaphy. It entails support and elevation of the bladder neck via a vertical incision in the anterior vaginal wall. This is achieved by buttressing sutures which aim to approximate the pubocervical fascia beneath the bladder base. Any redundant anterior vaginal wall skin is then excised. Post-operative bladder drainage using a urethral catheter is advisable for 48 hours. If genuine stress incontinence of urine is present, colposuspension is generally preferred.

Repair of a rectocele

Repair of a rectocele is called posterior colporrhaphy. It entails repair of the perineal body and levator muscles via an incision in the posterior vaginal wall. Redundant vaginal skin is again excised. Care is needed to avoid excessive narrowing of the introitus causing subsequent coital difficulties.

Vaginal hysterectomy

Vaginal hysterectomy is the best operation for prolapse of the uterus. Incidental benefits are elimination of menstruation, and the risk of both cervical and endometrial cancer. When performed for prolapse, vaginal hysterectomy is frequently combined with anterior and posterior colporrhaphy. An incision is made around the cervix enabling the vagina and bladder to be reflected away from the uterus. The peritoneum of the pouch of Douglas is incised posteriorly, and three pedicles on each side of the uterus are ligated and divided. These are the uterosacral and cardinal ligaments, the uterine vessels, and the tubo-ovarian and round ligaments. The uterus is thus fully detached and can then be removed. The peritoneum and vagina are closed with absorbable sutures, and the uterosacral ligaments are approximated together and used to support the vaginal vault.

Repair of enterocele

This is also frequently performed at the time of vaginal hysterectomy. The herniating peritoneal sac is identified, separated and opened. The contents are returned to the abdominal cavity and the sac excised. The peritoneum is closed with a pursestring suture and the defect between the uterosacral ligaments repaired to prevent any future recurrence.

Manchester repair

The Manchester repair operation is occasionally performed for prolapse. It entails amputation of the cervix, which is often elongated from long-standing prolapse, together with shortening of the cardinal ligaments. Anterior and posterior repair are added as necessary. Care must be taken to ensure that the cervix is not stenosed in order to allow menstruation to continue in pre-menopausal women and those on hormone replacement therapy.

An in-dwelling urethral catheter and a vaginal pack are left in situ for the first 24–48 hours post-operatively following vaginal surgery for prolapse.

Prolapse may recur many years after surgery, especially if continuing excessive pressures are placed on the pelvic floor. Typically an enterocele appears after a hysterectomy, or the vaginal vault descends. A further vaginal repair can be undertaken, which will carry a slightly increased risk of trauma to the bladder and rectum because of obliteration of tissue planes by scar tissue. Vaginal sacrospinous colpopexy, and abdominal colpopexy using Mersilene mesh to hitch the vaginal vault to the sacral promontory are less commonly used procedures which are reserved for intractable prolapse when conventional surgery has failed.

18.6 Normal bladder function

Learning objective

You should understand:

- the physiology of normal bladder function

Micturition

The desire to pass urine arises from autonomic afferent impulses from stretch receptors within the bladder wall travelling via S 2,3,4, and from sympathetic visceral afferent fibre nerves via T10 to L2. Micturition is inhibited subconsciously by descending central impulses, but with further bladder filling, a conscious desire to void arises. This can be voluntarily suppressed by cortical impulses and voluntary suppressed by cortical impulses and voluntary contraction of the pelvic floor. Micturition is then initiated at a convenient time and place. This is brought about by:

- contraction of the detrusor muscle
- relaxation of both the urethral sphincter and pelvic floor muscles
- contraction of abdominal wall muscles and diaphragm.

When intravesical pressure exceeds intra-urethral pressure, voiding begins. The normal urinary flow rate exceeds 15 ml per second.

Continence

This depends on 3 factors:

- bladder neck support
- external urethral sphincter
- smooth muscle in urethral wall.

These factors help to keep the bladder neck closed and the proximal urethra within the abdominal cavity (see Fig. 33). This results in a pinchcock effect, whereby increases in abdominal pressure are transmitted to the proximal urethra, so maintaining competence of the urethral sphincter mechanism.

18.7 Urinary incontinence

Learning objective

You need to understand:

- the limitations of the history in the differential diagnosis of urinary incontinence

Urinary incontinence is the involuntary loss of urine. It is estimated to occur in approximately 10% of women, but is probably widely under-reported. The causes are listed in Box 96.

> **Box 96** Causes of urinary incontinence
>
> - Genuine stress incontinence
> - Urge incontinence
> - Overflow incontinence
> - Urinary fistulae

The history is an important but unreliable guide to diagnosis. Further investigations are often necessary to direct appropriate treatment.

18.8 Genuine stress incontinence

Learning objective

You need to understand:

- how descent of the bladder neck disrupts the normal mechanism of urinary continence

Genuine stress incontinence is defined as the involuntary loss of urine which occurs when intravesical pressure exceeds the maximum urethral closure pressure in the absence of detrusor activity. It is the commonest cause of female urinary incontinence, accounting for 50% of all cases. The main cause is bladder neck weakness, which allows the bladder base to funnel and descend outside the abdominal cavity. This results in a loss of the normal pinchcock effect (see Fig. 34). Genuine stress incontinence often coexists with uterovaginal prolapse, because they share the same predisposing factors of age, multiparity and oestrogen deficiency.

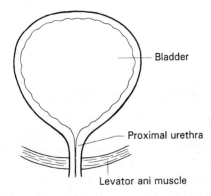

Fig. 33 The position of the proximal urethra within the abdominal cavity.

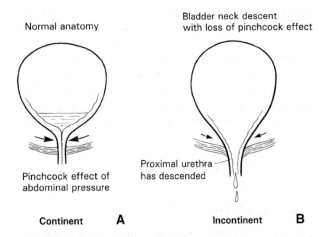

Fig. 34 Genuine stress incontinence. (**A**) normal anatomy; (**B**) loss of pinchcock effect.

Clinical features

Patients may describe any amount of urinary leakage, from a few drops to soaking their underwear. This is typically provoked by coughing, sneezing or other physical activity. It can be demonstrated on coughing with the patient in the left lateral position when the urethral orifice can be visualised. If negative, the patient can be asked to cough whilst standing or bouncing with a full bladder. This may cause embarrassment so a sympathetic approach is essential.

18.9 Treatment of genuine stress incontinence

Learning objective

You should understand:

- why there are several choices of operation for the treatment of genuine stress incontinence

Physiotherapy

Young women with minor degrees of urinary leakage often benefit from physiotherapy to strengthen the pelvic floor muscles, especially after recent childbirth.

Surgery

Surgery should be offered to those women with proven genuine stress incontinence which persists despite physiotherapy. Urodynamic investigation is essential before operating especially in those patients also complaining of urinary urgency or hesitancy. A poor urinary flow rate identifies those cases at increased risk of post-operative voiding problems. Numerous abdominal and vaginal operations are described, but none of them have a long-term cure rate exceeding 90%. The first operation performed has a higher chance of success than any subsequent one. Post-operative bladder drainage for the first 48 hours is advisable to prevent over-distension. A suprapubic catheter has the dual advantage of allowing an earlier return to spontaneous voiding and easy measurement of residual bladder volumes.

Colposuspension

This is widely regarded as the most successful procedure, with a cure rate for genuine stress incontinence of between 75 and 90%, depending on the experience of the surgeon and patient selection. Sutures are used to approximate the paravaginal tissues of each lateral vaginal fornix to the ipsilateral ileopectineal ligament. This results in elevation of the bladder neck and any associated cystocele. It requires a degree of anterior vaginal wall mobility. It is usually performed through a transverse suprapubic incision, but may be done endoscopically. There is a small but definite incidence of post-operative complications from colposuspension. These comprise voiding difficulties, detrusor instability, dyspareunia and enterocele.

Tension free vaginal tape (TVT) operation

This newly developed procedure may become the operation of choice for genuine stress incontinence, and it is currently being compared with the colposuspension in a multi-centre trial.

Stamey procedure

A separate nylon suture is placed on each side of the bladder neck between the rectus sheath and the paraurethral tissue with the aid of specially designed needles. It avoids the need for a large incision, but cystoscopy is necessary to exclude bladder puncture and assess the degree of bladder neck elevation obtained. It is well suited to elderly patients because of the low morbidity.

Suburethral sling

Rectus fascia or silastic material is slung beneath the proximal urethra and hitched to the rectus sheath. Requiring both abdominal and vaginal incisions, it is a complex procedure and rarely performed as a first choice.

Anterior colporrhaphy

This procedure is used where there is marked coexisting anterior vaginal wall laxity, and is usually combined with vaginal hysterectomy. It is not as successful as colposuspension in relieving genuine stress incontinence.

Peri-urethral injections of collagen

Injections of collagen aim to increase urethral closure pressure and thus help to maintain continence. It is a minimally invasive operation carried out via a cystoscope.

18.10 Urinary urgency

Learning objective

You should understand:

- the different mechanisms which can give rise to urinary urgency

Urinary urgency is a symptom with varied aetiology. When accompanied by frequency and nocturia the most likely diagnosis is detrusor instability. Organic causes must be excluded. Causes are listed in Box 97.

Investigation

A well-directed history may suggest a likely cause. Abdominal and pelvic examination will detect any mass such as a fibroid uterus pressing on the bladder. Urinary tract infection should be excluded by a midstream specimen of urine sent for microscopy, culture and sensitivity. Microscopic haematuria requires investigation by renal ultrasound.

18.11 Detrusor instability

Learning objectives

You should:

- be able to recognise detrusor instability from examination of a cystometry filling profile
- understand why it is important to diagnose detrusor instability from the other causes of urinary incontinence

Detrusor instability is the second most common cause of female urinary incontinence. It is usually idiopathic, and is characterised by involuntary contractions of the detrusor muscle, which give rise to symptoms of urinary frequency, nocturia and urgency. The diagnosis cannot be reliably made from the history alone. It often coexists with genuine stress incontinence, and may even be stress induced, for instance in response to coughing. For this reason urodynamic studies are required for diagnosis. These are described below.

Treatment of detrusor instability

Bladder retraining and drug therapy are the mainstay of treatment. Surgery is rarely helpful.

Box 97 Causes of urinary urgency

• Urethral	urethral syndrome, urethritis, diverticulum
• Bladder	inflammation, infection, tumour, stone, instability, radiation
• Gynaecological	prolapse, pelvic mass or pregnancy
• Psychosomatic	stress induced, anxiety states
• Neurological	multiple sclerosis
• Endocrine	diabetes mellitus

Simple measures

Simple measures should initially be tried such as reducing fluid intake and avoiding caffeine or alcohol.

Drugs

Most cases will need further treatment using a combination of drug therapy and bladder retraining. Drugs such as tolterodine, oxybutinin or amitriptyline may help symptoms but their usefulness may be limited by anticholinergic side-effects.

Bladder retraining

This involves voiding by the clock rather than by desire, using progressively longer time intervals, with the aim of retraining the bladder to hold larger volumes again.

Surgery

If all conservative measures fail, cystodistension may help but relief is often temporary. Major surgery in the form of augmentation ileocystoplasty is reserved for patients with intractable symptoms.

18.12 Urodynamic studies

Learning objective

You should understand:

- the role of urodynamic studies in the investigation of urinary incontinence

Urine flow test

The patient voids with a full bladder into a receiving vessel, which measures both volume passed and flow rate. This test is indicated to investigate hesitancy and poor stream, and is useful prior to bladder neck surgery.

Filling cystometry

Detrusor pressure is measured whilst the bladder is being filled via a catheter. This is calculated by subtracting abdominal pressure from intravesical pressure. Abdominal pressure is measured via a rectal catheter fitted with a pressure transducer, whilst intravesical pressure is measured via a second small urethral catheter. The normal bladder is compliant and exhibits only a small rise in detrusor pressure during filling (Fig. 35A). Instability is characterised by marked detrusor contractions, which may be strong enough to cause incontinence (Fig. 35B).

Graph showing normal cystometry filling profile

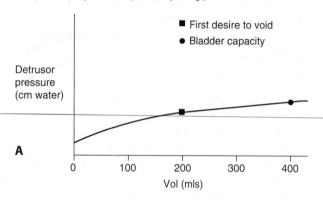

Graph showing abnormal cystometry filling profile

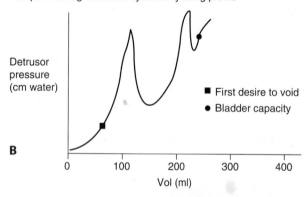

Fig. 35 Filling cystometry. (**A**) Normal bladder shows small rise in detrusor pressure during filling. (**B**) Marked detrusor contractions indicate instability.

Voiding cystometry

This measures the power of the detrusor muscle during voiding. When detrusor function is poor, voiding is sometimes achieved by contraction of the abdominal muscles.

Urethral pressure profile

This test is of limited value in clinical practice. A resting urethral pressure profile is measured by withdrawing the catheter containing the transducer along the length of the urethra.

18.13 Urinary infection

Learning objective

You should know:

- how to manage female urinary tract infection

Urinary infection is extremely common in women, largely due to both an anatomical and bacteriological susceptibility. The female urethra is only 5 cm long, and the distal third is normally colonised by bacteria.

Other predisposing factors include pregnancy, sexual intercourse, and catheterisation. Clinical features are shown in Table 22.

Treatment is with antibiotics and increased fluid intake after a midstream specimen of urine has been sent for microscopy, culture and sensitivity. 70% of urinary infections are caused by coliform bacteria, and the antibiotic of first choice is trimethoprim. Other common urinary pathogens include klebsiella, pseudomonas and proteus. Treatment of pyelonephritis requires more aggressive action using parenteral antibiotics to prevent septicaemia. Repeated urinary infections require investigation by renal ultrasound, intravenous pyelogram and cystoscopy to exclude reflux and intravesical pathology. Recurrent proteus infections are associated with renal staghorn calculi. Fastidious organisms such as *Mycoplasma hominis* and *Ureaplasma urealyticum* occasionally cause urinary symptoms but are difficult to isolate.

Urinary infection may follow sexual intercourse, and some women are prone to recurrent bouts as a result of this. Symptomatic relief may be obtained by emptying the bladder both before and directly after intercourse, as this may prevent bacteria gaining access to the upper urethra.

18.14 Urinary retention

Learning objective

You should understand:

- the ways in which female urinary retention can arise

Retention and voiding difficulties are rare in women so may go unrecognised. Painless overdistension of the bladder can occur following epidural anaesthesia in the absence of regular catheterisation during labour, and result in long-term voiding problems. Chronic voiding difficulty due to bladder denervation may occur following

Table 22	Urinary infection: clinical features	
Urethritis	**Cystitis**	**Pyelonephritis**
Frequency	Frequency	Joint pain
Urgency	Urgency	Vomiting
Dysuria	Dysuria	Rigors

radical hysterectomy for cervical cancer. This is usually treated by intermittent clean self-catheterisation.

Acute urinary retention is painful and may be caused by:

- vulval herpes
- bladder neck surgery
- pelvic mass
- urethral stenosis or foreign body
- retroverted gravid uterus.

Treatment is directed at the cause. A urinary catheter is needed to empty the bladder and allow the detrusor muscle to recover from overdistension.

18.15 Urinary fistulae

Learning objectives

You should understand:

- how urinary fistulae can arise
- why obstetric fistulae are most common in countries with poor provision of obstetric care

Urinary fistulae are rare but should always be considered in the investigation of urinary incontinence. The commonly encountered fistulae are:

- vesicovaginal
- vesicocolic
- ureterovaginal.

Vesicovaginal fistulae may result from advanced pelvic malignancy, surgical trauma or prolonged obstructed labour. Vesicocolic fistulae may result from diverticular disease, and present with pneumaturia and recurrent urinary infection. This diagnosis was once made by a patient, who grew a tomato plant from the ingested seeds which he passed in his urine.

Self-assessment: questions

Multiple choice questions

1. Which of the following may exacerbate uterovaginal prolapse?
   a. Menopause
   b. Childbirth
   c. Chronic bronchitis
   d. Anterior repair
   e. Diuretic therapy

2. Management of genuine stress incontinence includes:
   a. Anticholinergic drugs
   b. Pelvic floor exercises
   c. Bladder training exercises
   d. Colposuspension
   e. Intermittent self-catheterisation

3. Which of the following are correctly matched?
   a. Cystocele   Bulge in anterior vaginal wall
   b. Enterocele   Prolapse of bladder
   c. Anterior colporrhaphy   Treatment for cystocele
   d. Manchester repair   Treatment for procidentia
   e. Rectocele   Prolapse of rectum through anal canal

4. Which of the following may cause symptoms suggestive of bladder instability?
   a. Urinary infection
   b. Bladder tumour
   c. Bladder calculi
   d. Multiple sclerosis
   e. Colposuspension

5. Regarding urinary incontinence:
   a. The cause can be reliably diagnosed from the history
   b. Symptoms may be improved by limiting fluid intake
   c. It may be caused by a vesicovaginal fistula
   d. It is often due to weakness of the urethral sphincter mechanism
   e. Urge incontinence can be treated with cholinergic drugs

Short notes

1. What is a urethral caruncle?
2. (i) What abnormality is seen in Figure 36?
   (ii) What are the possible complications?
   (iii) What are the treatment options?
   (iv) What preoperative measures would be appropriate?

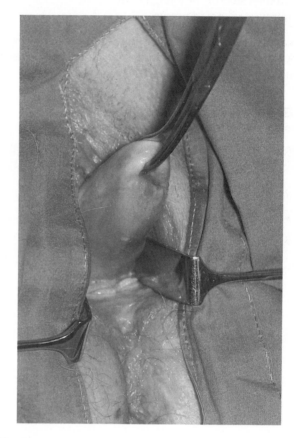

Fig. 36

Case histories

Case history 1

A 37-year-old woman is referred by her GP complaining of backache and a dragging feeling in her vagina. On examination she is found to have first-degree uterine descent and a cystocele.

1. What other history would you elicit?
2. What factors are important in deciding the most appropriate treatment?

Case history 2

A 75-year-old lady complains of continuous urinary leakage 10 days following a vaginal hysterectomy and anterior repair. She takes tricyclic antidepressant medication.

1. What are the possible causes?
2. Outline the management.

Self-assessment: answers

Multiple choice answers

1. a. **True.** Post-menopausal atrophy of the pelvic floor supports is associated with prolapse.
    b. **True.** Pelvic nerve damage following childbirth is also an aetiological factor.
    c. **True.** Chronic coughing increases the abdominal pressure which is transmitted to the pelvic floor.
    d. **False.**
    e. **False.** Diuretic therapy may exacerbate urinary incontinence but does not cause prolapse.

2. a. **False.** Anticholinergic drugs are used in the treatment of bladder instability.
    b. **True.**
    c. **False.** Bladder training exercises are used in the treatment of bladder instability.
    d. **True.**
    e. **False.** Intermittent self-catheterisation is used for chronic voiding difficulties.

3. a. **True.**
    b. **False.** An enterocele is a prolapse of the pouch of Douglas.
    c. **True.**
    d. **False.** Procidentia consists of complete uterine prolapse and is treated by vaginal hysterectomy and pelvic floor repair. Manchester repair is reserved for lesser degrees of prolapse. Only the cervix is removed, whilst the transverse cervical ligaments are tightened and the vaginal walls repaired.
    e. **False.** A rectocele is a prolapse of the rectum and posterior vaginal wall forwards into the vagina. Prolapse of the rectum through the anal canal is called rectal prolapse.

4. a. **True.** A diagnosis of idiopathic bladder instability should only be made when causative factors such as urinary infection, bladder tumours and calculi have been excluded.
    b. **True.**
    c. **True.**
    d. **True.** Neurological disease such as multiple sclerosis may rarely present with symptoms of bladder instability.
    e. **True.** 10% of women undergoing colposuspension for genuine stress incontinence will develop bladder instability.

5. a. **False.** It is not always possible to differentiate between the causes of urinary incontinence from the history alone, and further investigation with urodynamic studies is often required.
    b. **True.** Limiting fluid intake is a simple measure that may be of help in both genuine stress and urge incontinence as symptoms may only be present when the bladder is full.
    c. **True.**
    d. **True.**
    e. **False.** Urge incontinence can be treated with anticholinergic drugs.

Short notes answers

1. A urethral caruncle is a benign granuloma which develops at the external urethral meatus in post-menopausal women, due to prolapse of the posterior urethral mucosa. It has a characteristic appearance, and may cause symptoms of dysuria and haematuria. It should be distinguished from the much rarer urethral carcinoma.

2. This is complete procidentia, in which the entire uterus prolapses outside. The squamous epithelium of the vagina and cervix become keratinised. Ulceration, bleeding and infection may occur due to rubbing. Very rarely, the downward displacement of the bladder can produce kinking of the ureters causing renal failure. The most effective treatment is vaginal hysterectomy with anterior and posterior colporrhaphy. Preoperative measures include assessment of fitness for surgery, and treatment of any vaginal infection or ulceration with antibiotics, vaginal antiseptics and oestrogen cream. A vaginal ring pessary can be useful if the patient refuses or is unfit for surgery. This flexible polythene ring sits in the vaginal rather like a contraceptive cap and once it is in place the patient should be unaware of its presence. Another alternative is a vaginal shelf pessary. Pessaries need to be checked every 4 months as they may cause vaginal wall ulceration. Oestrogen vaginal cream is useful to treat coexisting vaginal wall atrophy.

Case history answers

Case history 1

1. Specific questions should be asked about further plans for pregnancy, the presence of urinary symptoms and menstrual problems. Backache is

only rarely caused by prolapse and a history of musculoskeletal problems should be sought.

2. Treatment with pelvic floor exercises should be tried initially but if unsuccessful anterior colporrhaphy with vaginal hysterectomy should be considered. Co-existing menstrual problems would favour vaginal hysterectomy as first-line treatment. If genuine stress incontinence is diagnosed, bladder neck surgery such as colposuspension can be combined with hysterectomy. Vaginal delivery will severely stress a vaginal repair so surgery is usually delayed until after the family has been completed.

Case history 2

Urinary retention with overflow is the most likely diagnosis. Any form of bladder neck surgery aims to increase bladder outflow resistance, and some women, especially those with poor preoperative detrusor activity are at risk of postoperative voiding problems.

For this reason, preoperative flow rate measurement is useful to predict those patients at risk of this complication. The detrusor muscle has a parasympathetic motor innervation and the anticholinergic activity of tricyclic antidepressant drugs tends to inhibit bladder emptying. An enlarged bladder may be palpable, and catheterisation or ultrasound would be diagnostic. Intermittent clean self-catheterisation, suprapubic catheterisation, or cholinergic agents such as carbachol may be used in treatment. If the bladder has been chronically overdistended it may take some time for detrusor activity to return.

A less likely possibility would be a vesicovaginal fistula from inadvertent intraoperative bladder trauma. A cystogram will demonstrate a fistula, and an IVP is required to exclude ureteric trauma. A small fistula may heal spontaneously with continuous bladder drainage and antibiotics, but the remainder will require surgical repair.

Overview

The menopause is a physiological event, which occurs as a result of ovarian failure. It is characterised by the cessation of monthly periods, and varying symptoms of oestrogen deficiency.

Due to an increase in life expectancy, a woman today can expect to spend 30% of her life in the menopause. Although hormone replacement therapy can alleviate many of the symptoms of oestrogen deficiency, the decision to take it should be an individual one for each woman. Hormone replacement therapy may protect against both osteoporosis and cardiovascular disease, but carries a small increase in the risk of breast cancer.

Introduction

The menopause is defined as the cessation of menstrual periods for a minimum of 6 months, in the absence of a cause such as pregnancy. The diagnosis can only therefore be made in retrospect. The average age of the menopause is 51 years. The time leading up to it is called the climacteric.

There is a growing awareness of the consequences of long-term oestrogen deficiency after the menopause the most important of which are an increase in the risk of both osteoporosis and cardiovascular disease. Hormone replacement therapy (HRT) is widely used not only to treat the immediate symptoms of oestrogen deficiency, but also to provide protection against osteoporosis and cardiovascular disease. The increased life expectancy of women after the menopause has emphasised the potential benefits of HRT.

19.1 Aetiology of menopause

Learning objective

You should understand:

- why monthly periods cease at the menopause

The menopause occurs due to ovarian failure. This occurs as a natural event because of an ageing process in the ovary which involves a gradual depletion in the number of ova, from a peak of approximately 7 million at 20 weeks' gestation. In the climateric, ovarian function steadily declines, and ovulation becomes erratic. This accounts for the high incidence of menstrual irregularities seen during this time. By the menopause, only a few ova remain, and these are resistant to follicle-stimulating hormone (FSH) stimulation.

The menopause may be iatrogenically induced if the ovaries are surgically removed or destroyed by radiation.

19.2 Symptoms of menopause

Learning objective

You should be able:

- to take a directed history to ascertain whether or not a woman is menopausal

During the climacteric the usual monthly cycle may become either longer or shorter, before periods cease altogether. Over 80% of women experience hot flushes during the menopause but the frequency of these declines to 20% after 4 years. Flushes are related to falling oestrogen levels. Typically the skin temperature rises and is accompanied by visible reddening of the neck and chest.

The low oestrogen levels commonly result in symptoms of vaginal dryness and dyspareunia, due to thinning and loss of elasticity of the skin. The distal urethra may also be affected, resulting in the urethral syndrome, characterised by urinary frequency, dysuria and urgency.

Psychological symptoms are also commonly seen. These are more likely to result from concerns regarding loss of fertility and femininity rather than as a direct consequence of oestrogen lack.

In the long term, oestrogen deficiency results in atrophy of the genital tract. The vulva, vagina and uterus all become smaller and less vascular, and the breasts diminish in size. There is accelerated loss of calcium from the skeleton, which can lead to osteoporosis. The incidence of cardiovascular disease also increases. All these physiological effects can be prevented or slowed by hormone replacement therapy.

Symptoms of menopause

Vasomotor symptoms

- Hot flushes
- Nocturnal sweats
- Insomnia
- Palpitations.

Symptoms of end organ atrophy

- Vaginal dryness
- Dyspareunia
- Recurrent urinary infection
- Breast shrinkage.

Psychological symptoms

- Anxiety
- Poor concentration
- Lack of confidence
- Depression.

19.3 Diagnosis of menopause

Learning objective

You should understand:

- the hormonal profile of a menopausal woman, and how this differs from a pre-menopausal woman

A history of absent menstruation combined with hot flushes, night sweats and vaginal dryness is characteristic. The biochemical findings are a low serum oestrogen and raised gonadotrophin levels, but measurement is rarely necessary and indeed is often unhelpful because of the marked cyclical variations in FSH levels. In practice, symptoms often precede the biochemical changes, so if the diagnosis is in doubt, a therapeutic trial of HRT is more useful.

19.4 Treatment of menopause

Learning objectives

You should understand:

- the aims of treatment with HRT
- why women with a uterus must be given a progestogen if they are taking HRT

The main aims of treatment with HRT are the relief of oestrogen deficiency symptoms and a reduction in the risk of both osteoporotic fractures and cardiovascular disease. The main concerns with HRT are a small increased risk of breast cancer associated with long-term use, and an increased risk of endometrial cancer if unopposed oestrogen is given. Despite popular opinion, not all women choose to take HRT at the menopause. The possible reasons for this include a lack of awareness, a dislike of long-term medication, a positive family history of breast cancer and the inconvenience of continued menstruation. In practice, each woman should be given the opportunity to make an informed choice regarding whether or not to take HRT, and if so for how long.

Types of therapy

Hormonal

- Oestrogen
- Progestogen
- Testosterone
- Tibolone.

Oestrogens
Natural oestrogens are preferred to synthetic ones, as the latter have less favourable metabolic effects. See Box 98.

Oestrogen must always be given in combination with a progestogen in women with a uterus. This is to prevent the risk of developing endometrial hyperplasia and carcinoma, which results from prolonged unopposed oestrogen therapy.

Natural
- Oestradiol
- Oestrone
- Oestriol
- Conjugated equine oestrogen

Synthetic
- Ethinylestradiol
- Mestranol

Progestogens

The progestogens used in HRT formulations are of two main types:

- 17-hydroxyprogesterone derivatives, e.g. medroxyprogesterone acetate
- 19-nortestosterone derivatives, e.g. norethisterone.

There are many different regimens for giving these hormones. The most popular is combined sequential therapy, whereby oestrogen is given continuously and a progestogen is given for 12 days per month. On this regimen most women will have slight cyclical withdrawal bleeds. A minority will not have any bleeding at all, but occasionally bleeding can be heavy and troublesome. The continued presence of a monthly bleed can be a major drawback to the acceptability of HRT to some women, who welcome the cessation of menstruation that the menopause brings. Prevention of uterine bleeding is the aim of continuous combined oestrogen and progestogen therapy. This is achieved by inducing endometrial atrophy. Continuous combined therapy (CCT) should be given only to women who report 12 months of amenhorroea and who are thought to be menopausal. The main disadvantage of CCT is erratic bleeding during the first few months of treatment.

Hysterectomised women can safely take oestrogen only preparations.

Testosterone

Testosterone is only occasionally used in HRT regimens, to increase libido.

Tibolone

Tibolone is a synthetic steroid having weak oestrogenic, progestogenic and androgenic properties, and is used as HRT in post-menopausal women. It induces endometrial hypoplasia so has the advantage that it does not cause bleeding. It does act on the vagina where it improves symptoms of dryness and painful intercourse. It also improves libido. Tibolone may prove to be the HRT of choice for those women with a personal history of breast cancer, in view of its progestogenic effect on the breast.

Non-hormonal

Non-hormonal treatments are especially useful when oestrogen therapy is contraindicated. Vaginal lubricants and moisturisers can help to relieve dyspareunia. Clonidine can be useful for the alleviation of hot flushes.

19.5 Routes of administration of HRT

- oral
- transdermal
- subcutaneous
- vaginal.

Oral

Oral administration results in rapid transfer of absorbed oestrogen to the liver via the portal venous system, where much of it is metabolised before it reaches the systemic circulation.

By contrast, the other routes of oestrogen administration avoid this first-pass liver metabolism, so lower doses can be used.

Transdermal

Oestrogen can be given by the transdermal route, either via small adhesive patches or as a gel applied directly onto the skin. These require changing once or twice a week. Progestogen can also be given via skin patches.

Implants

Oestradiol implants are small pellets which are inserted subcutaneously under local anaesthetic. They release a continuous small amount of oestrogen over many months. They are replaced when menopausal symptoms recur. Implants are most commonly used after hysterectomy when there is no need to give any progestogen.

Vaginal

The vagina, urethra, bladder and pelvic floor tissues all have oestrogen receptors. Vaginal creams and pessaries deliver a high local concentration of oestrogen and are thus useful for treatment of genital tract symptoms. Systemic absorption does occur, so a progestogen should be added if vaginal oestrogens are given for more than a few weeks to women with a uterus.

19.6 Side-effects of HRT

Learning objective

You should understand:

- the reasons for poor compliance with HRT

Most side-effects are transient and disappear within a few months. However, they are responsible for a significant proportion of women discontinuing treatment. The common side-effects include irregular uterine bleeding, breast tenderness, and progestogen-related symptoms such as abdominal bloating and oedema. Persistent irregular bleeding requires investigation. Rare side-effects include skin irritation from patches, and exacerbation of migraine or epilepsy. With such a wide choice of preparations and routes of administration, it should be possible to find a formulation to suit most women who wish to use HRT.

19.7 Benefits of HRT

Learning objective

You should be able:
- to advise on the health benefits of HRT

Short-term

In the short term, HRT effectively relieves symptoms of oestrogen deficiency such as hot flushes, vaginal dryness and dyspareunia. The generalised atrophic changes which occur in connective tissues after the menopause such as skin thinning, hair loss, brittle nails and aching joints may also improve. Some women report a feeling of improved energy, confidence and quality of life whilst taking HRT.

Long-term

The two major long-term benefits of HRT are a lowered risk of osteoporosis and cardiovascular disease.

Osteoporosis

Loss of boney-calcium after the menopause is the major factor predisposing to osteoporosis. The resulting lowered bone mass increases the susceptibility to fracture. Such fractures are a significant cause of morbidity and mortality amongst elderly women. Those at greatest risk are light in weight, smoke, or have an early menopause. Areas most affected are the trabecular bone of the hip, spine and wrist. Identification of women at increased risk of osteoporosis allows them to be targeted for long-term HRT, so preventing excessive loss of calcium from bone. Dual energy X-ray absorptiometry (DEXA) can be used to measure bone density at different sites and thus provide an assessment of fracture risk.

Hormone replacement therapy is the most effective way of preserving bone mass in post-menopausal women. If oestrogen is contraindicated or poorly tolerated there are a number of alternatives. The most useful are the biphosphonates such as etidronate and alendronate. These act primarily on the skeleton to inhibit bone resorption, and do not alleviate symptoms of oestrogen deficiency. Selective oestrogen receptor modulators (SERMs) such as raloxifene act preferentially on bone, but not on breast or endometrium. They are being developed for both prevention and treatment of osteoporosis, and may prove particularly beneficial when conventional HRT is contraindicated. Dietary calcium supplementation, exercise and avoidance of smoking all play useful preventative roles in osteoporosis. Calcitonin inhibits the resorption of bone by osteoclasts, so may have a preventative role to play, but it is expensive and requires further evaluation. See Box 100.

Cardiovascular disease

Cardiovascular disease is the leading cause of death in women. This means that even small alterations in the degree of risk can have a major impact on health. Susceptibility is influenced by many factors such as family history, smoking, exercise, obesity and hypertension. Women have a lower incidence of cardiovascular disease than men, and this appears to be due to a beneficial effect which oestrogen exerts on the blood lipid profile. This consists of a lowering of cholesterol and low-density lipoprotein levels, and an increase in high-density

---

Box 100 Prevention of osteoporosis

- Dietary calcium
- Exercise
- Avoidance of smoking
- HRT
- Biphosphates
- SERMs
- Calcitonin

lipoproteins. After the menopause when oestrogen levels decline, the difference in the incidence of cardiovascular disease between the sexes gradually disappears. Observational studies suggest that oestrogen replacement therapy reduces the risk of both coronary heart disease and stroke. There is controversy over the role of progestogens with regard to the risk of cardiovascular disease. Progestogens have opposing effects to oestrogen on lipid metabolism, so in theory their addition to HRT regimens could diminish the cardio-protective effect.

19.8 Risks of HRT

> **Learning objective**
>
> You should be able:
>
> • to advise on the health risks of HRT

These are:

• Breast cancer
• Endometrial cancer
• Venous thromboembolism.

Breast cancer

Evidence that oestrogens play a role in the aetiology of breast cancer is supported by the observations that a late menopause and the use of oral contraceptives in late reproductive life both confer an increased risk of the disease. Conversely, an early menopause is protective. The fact that HRT may confer an increase in the risk of breast cancer is of great concern to women and their doctors, and is often sited as a reason for stopping treatment. The duration of treatment appears important, with the risk only becoming apparent after 10 or more years of HRT use. Women who use HRT should therefore be advised to participate in the national screening programme.

Endometrial cancer

Endometrial cancer is associated with unbalanced oestrogen stimulation of the endometrium. This will occur if oestrogen-only replacement therapy is given to women with a uterus. This risk is eliminated by the addition of a progestogen such as norethisterone, in a dose of 1 mg daily for a minimum of 10 days per month.

Venous thromboembolism

There appears to be a small increased risk of venous thromboembolism, particularly in the early years of HRT use. That risk is estimated to be around 1 in 5000 users per year.

19.9 Commencement and monitoring of HRT

> **Learning objective**
>
> You should understand:
>
> • the importance of education in facilitating a decision about starting HRT

Prior to making a decision about HRT, each woman must be given the opportunity for a full discussion regarding the benefits and risks for treatment. A thorough and accurate understanding will help to dispel any anxieties or wrong information which may have been gained from other sources, and will help to maximise compliance with treatment.

A gynaecological and medical history is necessary to identify any potential contraindications to treatment, such as breast or endometrial cancer. Blood pressure, weight and height should be measured, and a screening pelvic and breast examination offered. Urinalysis is performed and a cervical smear should be taken if due. HRT can then be commenced, with a preparation and route of administration that the woman feels happy with.

A 3-month check is arranged to enquire about side-effects, and thereafter yearly checks to allow breast and blood pressure assessment; 3-yearly mammographic screening should be offered to women aged between 50–64 years.

19.10 Premature menopause

> **Learning objective**
>
> You should understand:
>
> • the health implications of a premature menopause

Premature menopause is defined as ovarian failure which occurs before the age of 40 years. It occurs in 1% of women.

Aetiology

Many cases are idiopathic, but it may follow surgical removal of the ovaries, pelvic radiotherapy or chemotherapy (Box 101). In some cases ovarian function returns spontaneously, when the term resistant ovary syndrome is used.

Box 101 Premature menopause: aetiology

Common	Rare
• Idiopathic	• Autoimmune disease
• Surgery	• Infection
• Irradiation	• Ovarian dysgenesis
• Chemotherapy	

Clinical features

The symptoms of ovarian failure are the same regardless of the age at which it occurs, so the diagnosis should be suspected in any woman complaining of hot flushes, vaginal dryness or dyspareunia. Psychological problems relating to a loss of fertility and femininity are also common. The diagnosis can be confirmed by a hormone profile, which shows a reduced serum oestrogen level together with elevated gonadotrophins.

Treatment

Hormone replacement therapy is indicated because of the increased risk of both osteoporosis and cardiovascular disease associated with premature ovarian failure, and also to alleviate menopausal symptoms.

Pregnancy following premature ovarian failure

Further pregnancies may be desired if ovarian failure occurs prior to the completion of a family. Under these circumstances it is necessary to perform an ovarian biopsy to look for the presence of primordial follicles. If follicles are present, attempts to stimulate ovulation using gonadotrophins may be successful. If there are no follicles present, pregnancy is only possible using donor eggs. Exogenous hormonal administration is then needed both to prepare the endometrium and to provide support during the early stages of a pregnancy.

Self-assessment: questions

Multiple choice questions

1. Which of the following are true of an early menopause?
   a. There is an increased risk of breast cancer
   b. There is an increased risk of osteomalacia
   c. Many cases are due to a lack of primordial follicles in the ovary
   d. It usually presents with secondary amenorrhoea
   e. It should nearly always be treated
   f. Karyotyping may be considered

2. Regarding osteoporosis:
   a. It affects around 1 million people in the UK
   b. Hip fracture causes more deaths than cancer of the cervix, uterus and ovaries combined
   c. Bone densitometry can be used to screen individuals at risk
   d. There is reduced loss of bone after the menopause
   e. May be associated with hypogonadism

3. Which of the following are associated with an increased risk of osteoporosis?
   a. Late menopause
   b. History of anorexia
   c. Malabsorption syndrome
   d. Steroid therapy
   e. Hyperparathyroidism

4. Regarding the menopause:
   a. The vaginal pH is reduced
   b. There are reduced numbers of lactobacilli
   c. Over 50% of women will experience hot flushes
   d. The endometrium becomes unresponsive to oestrogen and progesterone
   e. Repeated urinary infections may occur secondary to urethral atrophy

5. Which of the following are true?
   a. There is no systemic absorption with vaginal oestrogen therapy
   b. Transdermal oestrogens have no measurable effect on clotting factors
   c. Compliance with HRT is known to be poor
   d. Anovulatory cycles are common in the climacteric
   e. HRT can alleviate symptoms of oestrogen deficiency prior to the cessation of menstruation

6. Which of the following statements are true?
   a. HRT provides contraception
   b. The risk of breast cancer is significantly increased by taking HRT for 5 years
   c. Short courses of HRT decrease the risk of osteoporosis
   d. Gonadotrophin levels are elevated after the menopause
   e. The ovary becomes resistant to FSH stimulation after the menopause

7. Which of the following are true?
   a. Prevention of bone loss is the most effective means of avoiding osteoporotic fractures
   b. Increased physical activity is a risk factor for osteoporosis
   c. Treatment of osteoporosis with biphosphonates reduces the incidence of vertebral fractures
   d. Osteoporotic fractures are most common in the hip, radius and spine
   e. HRT is more expensive than biphosphonates

Short notes

1. Why do the ovaries fail at an earlier age in hysterectomised women? How is the menopause diagnosed in a hysterectomised woman? What are the other possible causes of hot flushes?

2. Is it safe for a woman who has had a previous deep vein thrombosis to take HRT?

3. What is the role of testosterone in HRT regimens?

4. What are the contraindications to HRT? What are the common side-effects? How long should treatment be continued for?

5. If oestrogen is contraindicated, what other measures can a postmenopausal woman take to reduce her risk of osteoporosis?

Case histories

Case history 1

A 40-year-old woman complains of tiredness, depression and pain on sexual intercourse. She has had no periods over the last 4 months.

What is the differential diagnosis and what investigations should be performed?

Case history 2

A 45-year-old woman who is using the progestogen-only pill for contraception states that her periods, which were previously regular, have stopped. She has not missed any pills, and her pregnancy test is negative. She has not had any hot flushes. She asks you if she has gone through the menopause.

How could you tell, and what advice would you give her regarding contraception?

Self-assessment: answers

Multiple choice answers

1. a. **False.** The risk of breast cancer is reduced in women having an early menopause.
   b. **False.** There is an increased risk of osteoporosis.
   c. **True.** Ovarian biopsy usually shows a lack of primordial follicles. This could be due to a deficiency in the original number of oocytes or excessive atresia.
   d. **True.** Ovarian failure usually presents with secondary amenorrhoea together with symptoms of oestrogen deficiency.
   e. **True.** It should be treated to alleviate symptoms and reduce the risk of osteoporosis in almost all cases. Contraindications are rare, such as the presence of an oestrogen-dependent tumour.
   f. **True.** Women with chromosomal abnormalities such as Turner's syndrome may present with secondary amenorrhoea, so karyotyping should be considered if the woman is of short stature.

2. a. **False.** Osteoporosis affects 3 million people in the UK.
   b. **True.** Osteoporotic fractures constitute a major public health problem: there are more than 50 000 femoral neck fractures each year in the UK, with a mortality of 20% within the first year.
   c. **True.** Assessment of bone density using dual energy X-ray absorptiometry (DEXA) at specific sites such as the hip can provide a prediction of the risk of fracture.
   d. **False.** There is increased loss of bone after the menopause.
   e. **True.** Untreated hypogonadism predisposes to osteoporosis because of low oestrogen levels.

3. a. **False.** It is an early menopause that predisposes to osteoporosis.
   b. **True.** Anorexia is associated with amenorrhoea and low oestrogen levels due to hypogonadotrophic hypogonadism.
   c. **True.**
   d. **True.**
   e. **True.**

4. a. **False.** The vaginal pH is increased after the menopause. This renders the vagina more susceptible to infection.
   b. **True.** There is a reduction in the glycogen content of the vaginal epithelial cells, which reduces the numbers of lactobacilli. These bacteria normally metabolise glycogen to lactic acid, thus maintaining vaginal acidity.
   c. **True.** 80% of women experience hot flushes at the time of the menopause, but the incidence reduces after a few years.
   d. **False.** The endometrium remains responsive to both oestrogen and progesterone. The periods stop because of a failure in ovarian production of these hormones.
   e. **True.** Oestrogen deficiency results in atrophy of both the vaginal epithelium and the distal urethra, which increases the susceptibility to infection. Both the vaginal epithelium and the distal urethra contain oestrogen receptors, so local oestrogen therapy can be beneficial in treating urogenital atrophy. This increases the resistance to both vaginal and urinary infections.

5. a. **False.** There may be appreciable systemic absorption with vaginal oestrogen therapy, so progestogens should also be given to non-hysterectomised women if treatment is continued for more than a few weeks.
   b. **True.** Transdermal absorption of oestrogen occurs directly into the systemic circulation, and avoids first-pass metabolism in the liver. Oestradiol levels are therefore higher, but there are no effects on clotting factors. This route of administration is therefore preferred in women with a history of thromboembolic disease.
   c. **True.** Studies suggest that long-term compliance with HRT is only of the order of 20%.
   d. **True.** The high incidence of anovulatory cycles during the climacteric accounts for the high incidence of menstrual irregularity.
   e. **True.** Symptoms of oestrogen deficiency frequently occur prior to the cessation of menstruation, and these often respond to treatment with HRT.

6. a. **False.** HRT does not provide contraception, as it does not inhibit ovulation.
   b. **False.** The risk of breast cancer is only increased by use of HRT for 10 years or more.
   c. **False.** Short courses of HRT do not confer protection against osteoporosis – treatment must be for at least 5–10 years.
   d. **True.**
   e. **True.**

7. a. **True.**
   b. **False.** Physical activity is protective against osteoporosis.
   c. **True.**
   d. **True.**
   e. **False.** The biphosphonates are more expensive than the majority of HRT preparations.

Short notes answers

1. The age of the menopause is advanced by up to 4 years by hysterectomy. This is probably due to interference with the ovarian blood supply. Branches of the uterine arteries ascend in the broad ligament to supply the ovaries, and these may be ligated at the time of hysterectomy.

   After hysterectomy, the absence of amenorrhoea as a symptom makes the diagnosis of the menopause more difficult. A recent onset of hot flushes, night sweats and vaginal dryness are suggestive of an early menopause. In the first instance, a therapeutic trial of oestrogen is indicated. If this relieves the symptoms, no further investigation is required. Serum FSH, luteinising hormone (LH) and oestradiol levels can be checked where there is any doubt

   Thyrotoxicosis, phaeochromocytoma and carcinoid syndrome are all rare causes of flushes which should be considered if there is no response to oestrogen replacement therapy.

2. Until 1996, there was no evidence that HRT increased the risk of deep venous thrombosis or pulmonary embolism. Recent studies, however, have shown a 2–4-fold increase in the risk of thromboembolism in association with current HRT use. For women with no previous history, this additional risk of thromboembolic disease is around 1 in 5000 users per year, and for pulmonary embolism, around 5 per 100 000. In other words, the absolute risks are low.

   In women with a past history of deep vein thrombosis, the orally administered oestrogens do cause a small increase in the hepatic production of certain coagulation factors. Transdermal oestrogens avoid first-pass metabolism in the liver and have no effect on clotting factors, so are probably a better choice in such women.

3. Testosterone increases libido in the female. It is produced in small amounts by the ovary, but levels decline after the menopause. Testosterone implants are occasionally used in HRT regimens when lack of libido or energy is a particular problem.

4. Contraindications to HRT are undiagnosed abnormal uterine bleeding, oestrogen-dependent tumours such as breast and endometrial cancer, active thromboembolism and chronic liver disease. Hypertension and ischaemic heart disease are not contraindications. Unlike the synthetic oestrogens used in the contraceptive pill, the natural oestrogens used in HRT do not appear to have any significant effect on blood pressure, and actually reduce the risk of myocardial infarction and stroke.

   Relative contraindications include uterine fibroids, which may enlarge slightly, endometriosis, migraine, diabetes and benign breast disease. Most women with these conditions can still take HRT but particular care needs to be taken with monitoring, for example of diabetic and blood pressure control.

   Withdrawal bleeding is an inconvenient side-effect of HRT, and is the most commonly cited reason for poor compliance with treatment. Irregular bleeding and poor cycle control may be reduced by using continuous combined oestrogen and progestogen therapy, as this induces endometrial atrophy.

   The duration of HRT depends on the wishes of the individual woman. The benefits of long-term use, namely a reduction in the incidence of fractures, heart attacks and stroke, must be weighed up against the increased risk of breast cancer associated with long-term use, and any inconvenience caused by bleeding.

5. Regular exercise, daily calcium supplementation and avoidance of cigarette smoking all help to reduce osteoporosis. Treatment with the biphosphonate disodium etidronate for 2 years has been shown to reduce the rate of vertebral fractures by 50%. Selective oestrogen receptor modulators, such as raloxifene, may confer protection against both breast cancer and osteoporosis. Further studies are awaited as to the role of SERMS.

Case history answers

Case history 1

A premature menopause is the most likely diagnosis, but pregnancy, thyroid dysfunction and hyperprolactinaemia should be considered. Clinical examination and a pregnancy test will exclude a pregnancy. Hyperprolactinaemia from a pituitary adenoma may cause secondary amenorrhoea and headache. Hypothyroidism may cause symptoms of tiredness and amenorrhoea. Measurement of serum prolactin, FSH, LH, oestrogen and thyroid function is indicated. FSH and LH levels above 50 U/L and oestradiol below 50 pmol/L would confirm a diagnosis of premature menopause.

Case history 2

Contraceptive advice in the climacteric can prove tricky. Most women taking the progestogen-only pill (POP) have normal periods, but some will experience amenorrhoea. The POP does not suppress the rise in FSH at the menopause, so measurement of FSH levels can be used to determine the cause of the amenorrhoea. If FSH levels are normal, the woman is not menopausal, and is still potentially fertile. The amenorrhoea is then due to the POP, and she should be advised of the continual need for contraception. If the FSH level is in the menopausal range (> 30 IU/L) it should be repeated in 3 months' time, and if still elevated, is suggestive of the menopause. The POP can be stopped, but non-hormonal contraception should still be used for the next 12 months.

Index

'Q' indicates a topic alluded to or mentioned in a question. In some cases the topic may not be mentioned in the question but only in the corresponding answer.